W. Eicher G. Kockott (Eds.)

Sexology

H.-J. Vogt V. Herms R. Wille (Coeds.)

With 72 Figures and 133 Tables

Springer-Verlag Berlin Heidelberg New York
London Paris Tokyo

Editors

Professor Dr. med. Wolf Eicher

Frauenklinik am Diakonissenkrankenhaus Mannheim,
Akademisches Lehrkrankenhaus der Universität Heidelberg,
Speyerer Straße 91, 6800 Mannheim 1

Professor Dr. med. Götz Kokott

Psychiatrische Klinik und Poliklinik der Technischen Universität,
Möhlstraße 26, 8000 München 80

Co-Editors

PD Dr. Hermann-J. Vogt

Dermatologische Klinik und Poliklinik der Technischen Universität, München,
Biedersteiner Straße 29, 8000 München 40

PD Dr. Volker Herms

Gynäkologische und Geburtshilfliche Abteilung Kreiskrankenhaus,
Krankenhausstraße 46, 8765 Erlenbach/Main

Professor Dr. med. Dr. jur. Reinhard Wille

Sexualmedizinische Forschungs- und Beratungsstelle im
Klinikum der Christian-Albrecht-Universität Kiel,
Hospitalstraße 17–19, 2300 Kiel

ISBN-13:978-3-642-73796-1 e-ISBN-13:978-3-642-73794-7
DOI: 10.1007/978-3-642-73794-7

Library of Congress Cataloging in Publication Data.
Sexology / W. Eicher, G. Kockott, eds. p. cm. Includes index.
1. Sexual disorders. 2. Psychosexual disorders. 3. Sex. 4. Birth control. I. Eicher, Wolf. II. Kockott, G. (Götz). [DNLM: 1. Acquired Immunodeficiency Syndrome. 2. Family Planning. 3. Sex. 4. Sex Behavior. 5. Sex Disorders. HQ 21 S5138] RC875.S48 1988 613.9–dc19 DNLM/DLC
for Library of Congress 88-16087 CIP
ISBN-13:978-3-642-73796-1 (U.S.)

Softcover reprint of the hardcover 1st edition 1988

Typesetting: : Brühlsche Universitätsdruckerei, Giessen

2121/3020-543210

Preface

Sexology is concerned with a basic human need. Sexuality is the fundamental energy and a driving force of human existence. From the very beginning, human beings have provided evidence of this, both pictorially and in writing. Artists and philosophers were the first to illustrate and explain sexuality, and the representatives of religion sought to control and regulate it by rituals and codes of behavior.

With the advent of the natural sciences, the question of reproduction and medicine came to the fore. The desire to have children and the problem of sterility are still issues of major importance today. Then, at the end of the nineteenth century, psychoanalysis, primarily through Sigmund Freud, revolutionized our concept of sexuality. Havelock Ellis's multi-volume studies into the psychology of sexuality were published in America.

In Germany, the scientific study of sexuality blossomed for the first time in the early 1920s. However, sexology had to fight like few sciences before it for recognition as a fully-fledged scientific discipline. It had to hold its own not only against the prejudices of laymen, but also against bias on the part of the academic and scientific establishment. The battle referred to in these lines by Arthur Kronfeld (1919) is not over even yet.

In 1921, Magnus Hirschfeldt organized the first international conference on sexual reform on a sexological basis in Berlin, which dealt with the subjects "Sexual Endocrinology," "Sexuality and the Law," "Birth Control," and "Sexual Education." This conference was followed by four more international congresses, in Copenhagen, London, Vienna, and Brünn. In hardly any other field has there been a greater clash of opposing views than in sexology. Hirschfeldt's colleague Albert Moll condemned the congress as pure propaganda and, 5 years later, organized the first "purely scientific" international congress for sexual research, likewise in Berlin, followed by another in London.

Sexology in Germany underwent savage destruction at the hands of the National Socialists but continued to develop in the rest of the world. At the end of the 1930s, Alfred Kinsey and his coworkers brought us a wealth of statistical data on sexual behavior. After the Second World War Hans Giese helped the discipline onto its feet again in Germany, while somewhat less than 20 years after Kinsey, William Masters and Virginia Johnson published the results of their research into the physiology of the sexual response and the therapy of sexual dysfunctions.

A further revolution was the advent of a generally available, reliable method of contraception – "the pill," developed by Pinkus. At the end of the nineteenth century Freud had described the moment at which the responsible act of procreation is successfully elevated to an act of will and intention, freed from its association with the necessary satisfaction of a natural urge, as one of the greatest triumphs of mankind. It was now possible for a woman particularly, to experience sexuality more freely. She could now determine for herself whether and when she became pregnant. This aided her in her striving for emancipation, a development which, at least in Western societies, is bringing with it far-reaching changes in the relations between the sexes and has a particular influence on the experience of sexuality.

The last few decades have seen an increase in sexual permissiveness in our society which has been fostered, but by no means solely brought about, by the availability of reliable methods of contraception. The threat posed by the epidemic-like spread of AIDS and the relentlessness and deadliness of the disease will turn back the clock and lead to a restoration of old values of lasting partnership and faithfulness, since at the present time it is only possible to prevent AIDS – not to cure it.

The first post-war congress was the International Congress for Medical Sexology held in Paris in 1974. The next congresses, in Montreal, Rome, Mexico, Jerusalem, Washington, and New Delhi, gave full recognition to the breadth of the subject and its interdisciplinarity. Medicine was no longer given special prominence in the title – psychological and sociological questions had equal status. Since its foundation in Rome in 1978, these congresses have been held under the auspices of the World Association for Sexology.

The Eighth World Congress for Sexology took place on June 14–20, 1987, in Heidelberg. At the official opening the Prorector, Prof. Rau, spoke on behalf of the University of Heidelberg, and Prof. Rita Süssmuth, Minister for Youth, Family, Women, and Health, spoke as a representative of the Government of the Federal Republic of Germany. From the wealth of scientific presentations, with over 500 papers, we have concentrated on the central medical themes and have selected the best papers for publication in book form. The subjects covered are topical and stimulating and include items of historical interest (e.g., accounts of Harry Benjamin's 10 first cases of transsexual patients) and transcultural comparisons, (e.g., the report on vasectomy in India). In many fields we have deliberately included controversial views in the hope of spurring the reader on to form his or her own opinions, as for instance, in the case of AIDS.

Some good contributions to the Congress could not be included, either because manuscripts were unavailable or incomplete, or because they could not be assigned to any of the selected central themes. The volume cannot claim to reflect the congress as a whole – only the state of discussion in the most important fields of sexual medicine. Other subjects, such as art, religion, sexuality in the media, sociology, and sexual education have not been touched on here.

The views of the authors to the individual papers do not always coincide with those of the editors, who have endeavoured to show the broad complexity of sexology and, in the process, allow opinions to be aired which are currently at the center of controversy.

Prof. Dr. Wolf Eicher Prof. Dr. Götz Kockott

Contributors

Aiuti, F.
Apfelbaum, B.

Bähren, W.
Banthien, V.
Bertini, M.
Beutel, M.
Blachere, P.
Blanchard, R.
Block, T.
Brand, H. J.
Braun-Falco, O.
Bruinsma, I.
Buddeberg, C.

Clemmensen, L. H.
Cohen-Kettenis, P.
Comhaire, F. H.
Costa, M.
Couture, M.
Crenshaw, T. L.

Deichert, U.
Dickey, R.
Döring, G.
Dupont, A.

Ellison, C. C.
Ernst, G.
Everaerd, W.

Farley, T.
Francoeur, R. T.
Fröschl, M.

Gindin, L. R.
Goldman, J. A.

Hachen, H. J.
Haeberle, E.
Halhuber, M. J.
Henrichs, H. R.
Hutner, G.

Jensen, P.
Jensen, S. B.
Junge, A.

Keep, P. A. van
Koch, M.
Kothari, P.
Kraft, H, G.
Krause, W.
Kremer, J.
Kuiper, A. J.

Labhardt, F.
Labrie, F.
Langer, D.
Lehfeldt, H.
Loewit, K.
Lundström, B.

Manara, I.
Mergury, A.
Mezzaroma, I.
Mohl, B.

Ortlieb, A.

Paeslack, V.
Pardanani, D.
Parekh, N.
Parulkar, B.
Patel, R.
Petah-Tikva, I. L.
Pfäfflin, F.
Pöldinger, W.
Pons, C.
Potts, M.

Ray, I.
Rechenberger, H.-G.
Rechenberger, I.
Rekers, H.
Richardson, J. D.
Richter, D.
Ring, J.
Rousseau, L.
Rowe, P.

Salvati, S.
Schaefer, L. C.
Schätzler, T. G.
Scherzer, N. A.
Schicketanz, R.
Sheth, A.
Silvia Caldiz, L. L.
Simonelli, C.
Slob, A. K.
Solano, L.
Sorensen, P. S.
Springer, A.
Springer-Kremser, M.
Steiner, B. W.

Stichting, R.
Sturm, W.

Täschner, K.-L.
Tordjman, G.

Wetterauer, U.
Wheeler, C. C.
Widhalm, R.
Wiesbeck, G. A.

Winther, G.
Wolfram, G.

Zwanikken, W.

Contents

I. Family Planning

II. Sterility and Sexuality

I. Family Planning

Reproductive Behavior and Family Planning

M. Potts

Family Health International, Research Triangle Park, NC 27709, USA

Introduction

Darwin published *The Origin of the Species* in 1859. Today, anyone who accepts the facts of Darwinian evolution is also, by definition, a sociobiologist – in the sense that we must also accept that our reproductive behavior, like the anatomy of our gait or the neurophysiology of our retina, has been finely tuned by natural selection to perform in a certain way.

We test drugs on baboons, we have a common blood group with rhesus monkeys, and we almost certainly caught the HIV infection from some other primate. We smile in greeting and touch one another for reassurance. What can biology tell us about human reproductive behavior and family planning?

Patterns of Fertility

Biologically, human beings have an exceptionally late age of puberty; they are nonseasonal breeders that separate pregnancies by anovulation associated with lactation, and ovulation, when it occurs, is not marked by any external signs or changes in behavior in the female. Both sexes consistently cover up their genitals and copulate in the quietest part of the 24 h; adults share the same nest at night; and females have a very distinct menopause. In all these ways we are a very remarkable ape!

We are probably the slowest breeding vertebrate that evolution has produced, and it is a paradox that we have come to dominate the globe and threaten the biosphere through our numbers. Whereas when experimental animals are put in crowded conditions, the age of puberty rises, pregnancy intervals lengthen and infant mortality rises, among human beings the opposite is happening.

The onset of the menarche has fallen substantially in the past 100 years and seems to have been even higher in preliterate societies. Among the hunter-gatherers, such as the contemporary Kalahari !Kung, whose life-style made up the great majority of human history, the menarche occurred very late in life. Among some of the clans in the highlands of New Guinea, such as the Gainj, who did not see a white person until 1954, the mean age of the onset of menstruation is 20.9 years (Wood et al. 1985). The later a woman begins to menstruate, the more anovulatory cycles she is likely to enjoy and Gainj women, on average, do not have their first child until they are about 25 years old.

Teenage sexuality and pregnancy is an unnatural product of civilized living, and it demands artificial solutions.

Sexology
Eds.: W. Eicher, G. Kockott

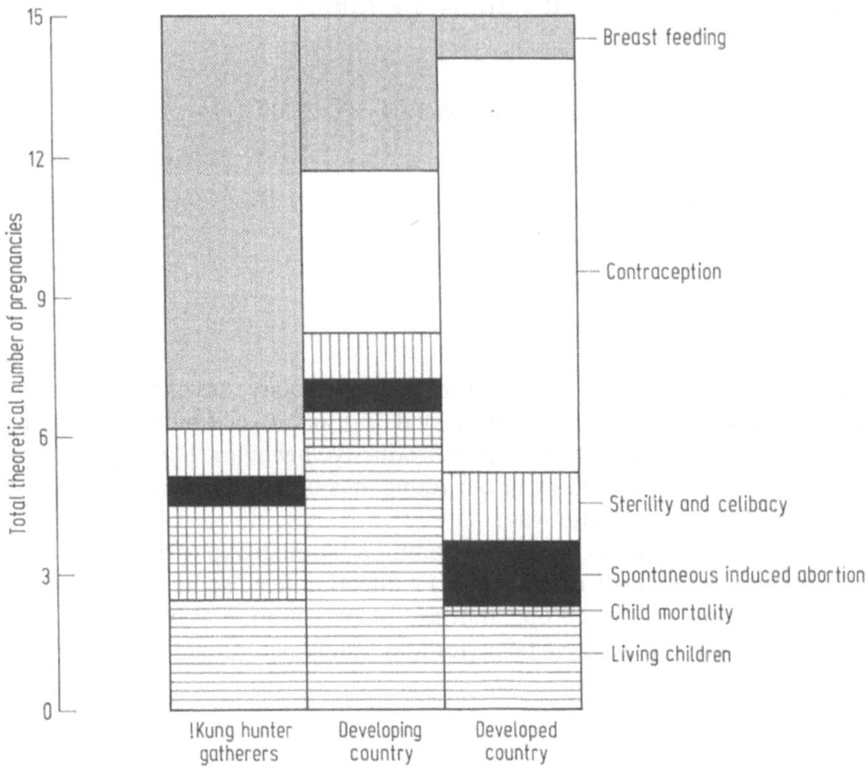

Fig. 1. Natural and artificial restraints on feritility. The figure assumes that, in the absence of breast-feeding or any method of contraception, a woman could have 15 pregnancies

Our hunter-gatherer ancestors (Fig. 1) had a late menarche and four to five live-born children in a fertile lifetime – probably half of whom died before they themselves reached puberty. Historical societies and contemporary agricultural and industrial societies have an earlier menarche and have abandoned or modified patterns of breast-feeding. If, like the Hutterites, you belong to the modern world but reject artificial contraception, then you can expect, on average, to have ten or more liveborn children in a lifetime. The problem is how to restore family size to the *natural* pattern of two children surviving into the next generation.

In contemporary developing countries, fertility is falling because the age of marriage has risen and because the adoption of artificial contraception and abortion more than outweighs the fertility-enhancing effect of shorter intervals of breast-feeding (Fig. 2).

The impact of lactation on pregnancy spacing depends on two factors. One is the duration of lactation and the other is the pattern of breast-feeding. There is a general relationship between the duration of breast-feeding and the duration of postpartum amenorrhea. However, more detailed studies show that some patterns of breast-feeding appear to be more effective in suppressing ovulation than others. Again, to return to our hunter-gatherer ancestors, a !Kung woman breast-feeds her infant, on average, every 14 min (Konner and Worthman 1980). Feed-

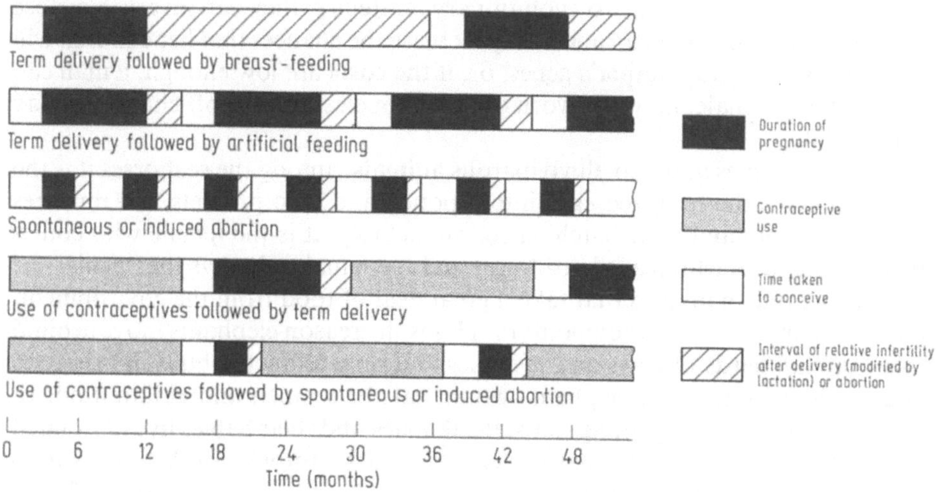

Fig. 2. Patterns of human reproduction

ing on demand, the maintenance of the night feed and avoiding the artificially early introduction of supplementary food all prolong anovulation.

In chimpanzees, the birth interval is 4.5–7.5 years (Konner and Worthman 1980). Among the !Kung it averages 44 months. Chimpanzees do not use contraceptives and the !Kung have never seen a pill or condom.

Bottle feeding is a *conceptive* human behavior, that is it raises fertility. Those nations with the highest achieved fertility (e.g., 8 in Kenya) are using their reproductive systems much more intensively than nature intended.

Reproductive Strategies

Pregnancy and lactation demand a much greater investment from the female than sperm production and copulation do from the male. In genuinely monogamous species, the female, in order to adapt her to the strains of reproduction, is either the same size as the male, as in the marmoset monkey, or even larger than the male, as a blue whale or a beaver. In the struggle for existence, the male, after all, is little more than a pair of testicles on legs.

Among polygamous mammals, where males compete among themselves, as do lions or elephant seals, the males are larger than the females. Biologically we are an indubitably polygamous species. One man, if sufficiently ruthless, can always father more children than one woman can bear in the same interval of time.

As a woman puts such enormous physical and emotional effort into pregnancy, lactation, and parenting to produce a single child, it is always in her interest to be sexually coy and to make a strong, lasting bond with one partner.

A culture may emphasize or negate biological differences, but I do not believe babies are a totally blank slate waiting for cultural messages to be written upon them. We are dimorphic in our reproductive behavior, just as we are in our anatomy.

Biology has given men two evolutionary strategies: they can invest in a close relationship with one woman and vastly increase the chances that her children will survive to pass on their father's genes, or, if the costs are low enough, a man can mate with any female, however worn out and hopeless, on the off chance he may father a child.

These principles apply to all viviparous animals: among the seahorses it is the *male* who takes the fertilized eggs into a pouch and who protects and nurtures the young before and after hatching so, predictably, it is the female who courts the male, the male who plays hard to get and the female who has the "penis."

Among large mammals that take a great deal of food from the environment, males and females become competitors. This is the reason elephants move around in matriarchal herds of cows and juveniles and only allow the bulls in briefly to mate – otherwise the bull elephants would eat the women and children out of house and home. Among orangutans, the females and their babies live in isolated pairs, only meeting with the males every few years. Among gorillas, one silver-back male and several mature females and their offspring live in a troop. The female is the rate-limiting resource in reproductive terms and therefore sets the pace of evolution.

The VIIIth International Conference on Sexology was held in Heidelberg. Eighty years ago one of the first hominid fossils was discovered in Heidelberg and has now been assigned to the genus *Homo erectus*, a designation not based on our ancestors' sexual proclivities but on their posture. Since in reality, the female is the rate-limiting resource in reproductive terms, we really ought to speak about *Femina erectus* and *Femina sapiens*. It is part of our blinkered approach to sex that there have been volumes of speculation about the brain size, the tooth design, the ability to walk upright and the use of tools in our ancestors such as the owner of the Heidelberg jaw, but little speculation about his or her reproductive behavior. What can we guess about Frau *Femina erectus Heidelberg* is that she certainly menstruated; she had probably lost the vulval swellings that characterize ovulation in chimpanzees for the simple reason that she had already learned to walk upright on two legs. But did her breasts develop at puberty as in *Homo sapiens*, or at the first pregnancy as in *Pan troglodytes*? She certainly breast-fed her infants for long intervals, but did she pair-bond with one male for some length of time? Did she gather tubers and share them with males who were beginning to specialize as hunters?

Chimpanzees, with whom we share 99% of our DNA, have an unusual social behavior where a number of related males defend a moderately large territory. Females mate promiscuously as they come into heat. Mothers and sons stay in the same troop throughout life, but at puberty females leave the troop of their birth and enter new troops. Sometimes the females are attacked by the older, more mature females in the troop (Jolly 1985).

We share much of this unusual pattern of social behavior. In most human societies the bride is "given away" by her family and enters her husband's troop, where quite often, like a young chimp, she may come into conflict with her mother-in-law.

However, we do not regularly engage in chimpanzee-like "gang bangs," but establish defined polygamous, monogamous, or serially monogamous sexual relationships. In the process, we have acquired two biologically unique attributes – we share our food and the female conceals ovulation.

Although we are big animals that require a large range to supply our food, we can live in mixed-sex bands because men and women exploit somewhat different food supplies. Among the Kalahari bush people, the women provide most of the family's calories from vegetable sources and the men most of the animal protein. Chimpanzees kill other monkeys and eat meat, when a sort of tolerated scrounging may arise, but we are the only mammals that explicitly share food.

Ecologically, men and women are more like two different, partly noncompetitive species, rather than like two sexes of the same species eating the same type of food. Among the few other species to evolve the same tricks are certain hawks, which pair monogamously and where the male is smaller than the female and therefore more maneuverable in flight and better adapted to prey on small birds than is the stockier female.

In biological terms, marriage is a compromise between the conflicting reproductive agendas of the two sexes united by their complementarity in exploiting food supplies. A woman gives sex for love and a man gives love in order to obtain sex, and both give one another food. Different cultures at different times have promoted the sexual agenda of one sex at the expense of the other.

What we see with homosexuality is each sex implementing its own biological drives without the need for compromise with the opposite sex. The "cruising" homosexual chooses his partners purely on physical grounds, often not knowing their names, seeking a high degree of eroticism, and often having many sexual outlets in a single evening and persisting in this way of life for many years. Lesbian lovers tend to be consistently faithful over many years, to place companionship and human relations above erotic experience, and to seek relatively infrequent sexual outlets (Symonds 1979).

Implications and Speculations

Biology does not tell us what to do, but it helps explain our behavior. As we cover up our genitals and usually copulate at night, one may predict that many human beings will be shy about acquiring contraceptives: for many people, it is easier to use a vending machine than to visit a family planning clinic. As women naturally spend many years pregnant or lactating and, for most of human prehistory, rarely ovulated, we guess that methods which suppress menstruation will not necessarily make unpopular methods of contraception (Loudon et al. 1977).

We would expect the two sexes to have different attitudes towards contraception. In certain circumstances women will go to extreme lengths to postpone or limit childbearing. However painful, however dangerous, however socially condemned, some women will always resort to abortion. Women accept sterilization more rapidly than men. It is, after all, only a fertility menopause without the hot flushes.

In the Moslem culture, Siassi (Fig. 3) has shown that if women are offered oral contraceptives, they have a high discontinuation rate, whereas when the same method was given to men to pass on to their wives, more than 90% of women

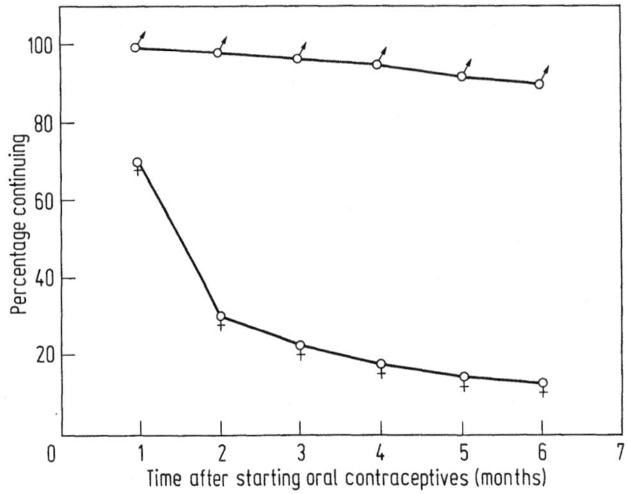

Fig. 3. Continuation rate for oral contraceptives distributed to Iranian women (♀) and to men (♂) to pass on to their wives. (Redrawn from Siassi 1972)

were still using the method after the first 6 months (Siassi 1972). The change in the sociology of decision making is much greater than any alteration in acceptability brought about by differences in pharmacology or formulation.

Men will accept vasectomy if it is offered in a male setting, but the rationale is probably different from a woman's acceptance of the operation. Deys has shown that role-dominant men commonly accept vasectomy before those who share their marital responsibilities, and it may be that there is an element of male control over females in the way the operation is perceived (Deys and Potts 1972). Shanker has pointed out how Orthodox Jewish teaching forbids men to use condoms but permits women to use oral contraceptives and IUDs – a nice religious gloss on a biological drive! Ultimately, male behavior evolved to pass as many genes as possible to the next generation, but in practice many aspects of both male and female behavior focus on proximate patterns of behavior.

A biological model that attempts to explain the adoption of different methods of contraception like a physiological or socioeconomic model leaves a lot of puzzles. Perhaps there are good reasons why this is so. We are a sexy animal programmed by evolution to use our sexuality in an infinite variety of ways in order to exploit many different types of environment. Biological determinism has made us, in large part, unpredictable. Perhaps the multivariant analyses so commonly performed to test hypotheses based on psychological or socioeconomic models of human behavior necessarily have their limitations.

Yet such a conclusion is not an empty one. Indeed, an evolutionary ability to be flexible in sexual behavior is exceptionally important. While it may be difficult to predict who will use an individual method of family planning, we can be certain that any one society needs the widest possible variety of birth control methods. There is no "right" method of contraception. We may conclude that when Japan forbids the pill, as indeed it does, or Egypt sterilization, or the USA fails to make IUDs available, that they are each denying some couples, somewhere, needed birth control choices.

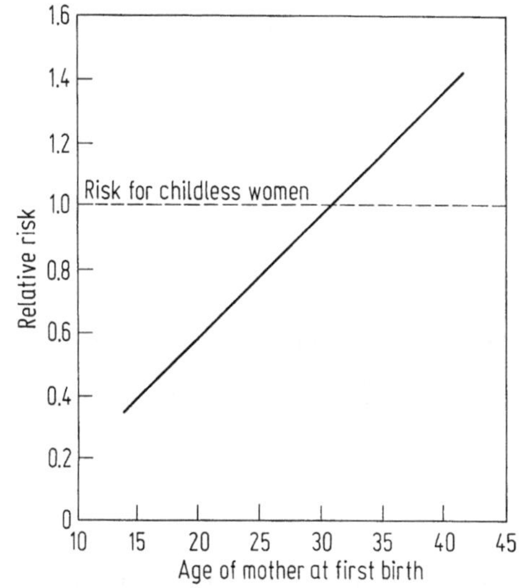

Fig. 4. Relative risk of developing cancer of the breast according to age when first child born. (After MacMahon et al. 1970)

Biology encourages us to look at reproduction over a lifetime rather than at a single menstrual cycle or at one pregnancy and its outcome. An early menarche, few children, and little breast-feeding exposes the modern woman to numerous, repetitive menstrual cycles. This change, or some as yet unidentified part of it, carries in its train certain important pathologies: the more menstrual cycles a woman experiences, the greater her risk of ovarian cancer; uterine cancer also seems to follow a similar pattern. The later a woman bears her first child, the greater the risk of developing breast cancer (MacMahon et al. 1970) around and beyond the menopause (Fig. 4). The modern woman has an approximately one in 5000 lifetime risk of dying in childbirth, but a one in 11 risk of developing breast cancer and a one in 8 risk of dying of that difficult-to-treat malignancy. It seems we pay a very high price for deviating from the reproductive behaviors bequeathed us by evolution.

In a fascinating way, oral contraceptives partially reverse some of the adverse effects of modern living. The pill has been in human use for 30 years and is among the most intensively studied drugs in the pharmacopoeia. Indeed, there is so much information it is difficult to put it together. A number of independent studies show that oral contraceptive use *reduces* the risk of dying of ovarian or endometrial cancers later in life. The longer a woman uses the pill the more marked the effect, and the effect persists after discontinuing its use – perhaps even for a fertile lifetime. By contrast, the harmful effects of the pill on the cardiovascular system begin when a woman first takes and end when she stops using it.

The problem is how to portray the risks and benefits of the pill in a single, grand, Einsteinian equation. One practical way is to ask what is the effect on the expectation of life if a woman uses the pill continuously for 5 years in a specified age group. Basically, the protective effects against cancer more than outweigh the adverse effects on the cardiovascular system. For a woman in the developing world, where the risks of pregnancy are greater, the beneficial effects are correspondingly larger (Fig. 5).

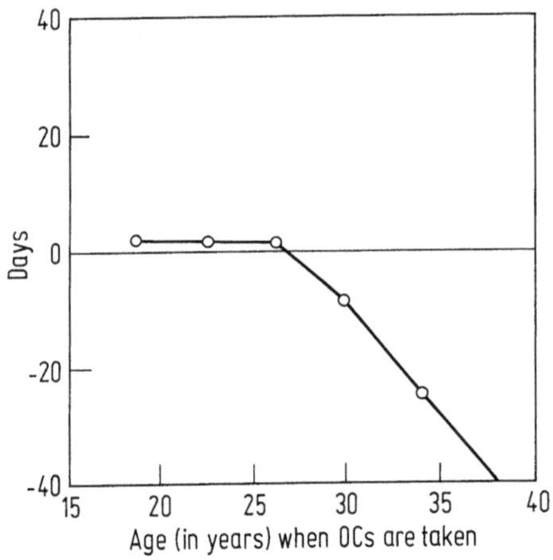

Fig. 5. Change in life expectancy attributable to 5 years of oral contraception in women aged 20 to 40 years, United States, 1978

Overall, both the risks and benefits of the pill are trivial in relation to other risks and benefits of life. Oral contraceptives increase the expectation of life by 12 days. The worst they can do to the expectation of life in older women is shorten life by 40–80 days. Smoking one packet of cigarettes a day decreases the users' expectation of life by an average of 4.6 years. I stand by my aphorism of many years ago that cigarettes should be on prescription and pills in vending machines!

In a way, it is curious that the pill does not have an effect on breast cancer – neither a positive nor a negative one. One of the prime targets to research in the next decade should be how to tease out whether it is possible to formulate a combination of artificial steroids which reduces the risks of breast cancer in the same ways that they do endometrial and ovarian cancers.

It is not that the pill is a philosopher's stone which magically extends human life, but merely that it takes a woman one step nearer to the pattern which evolution intended her reproductive system to experience. Perhaps it should be a dream for the 21st century to so manipulate the dose and formulation of artificial steroids that they not only prevent pregnancy and reduce the risk of ovarian and endometrial cancers, but also, eventually, reduce the risk of breast cancer.

Ethics

If biology tells us a little about contraceptive choices and throws up at least one startling clinical perspective, then it also challenges us ethically.

Wet nursing is surely a greater departure from nature than coitus interruptus – yet St. Augustine condemned the latter while partaking of the former (Noonhan 1967; Potts 1972). To a biologist, a rubber nipple on a glass feeding bottle is more offensive than a rubber condom on an erect penis – one is a latex contraceptive and the other a lactose conceptive – while adults may consent to the use of contraception, infants have no choice as to what is put in their mouths.

In some parts of the world, bottle-fed babies have up to eight times the risk of infant mortality as those that are breast-fed. Every minute, somewhere in the world, one woman dies in childbirth; 99% of these deaths take place in the developing world and half or more involve women that are either over 30 and/or have three or more children – the very groups who would plan their families were contraceptives more fully available. Infant mortality is 50% higher if the birth takes place within 1 year of a previous delivery rather than after a birth interval of 3–4 years (S. Thapa, R. V. Short, and DM Potts 1987, unpublished data). In short, contraceptives save lives.

Ethics relate to the decisions we have to take as our technology carries us further and further from the hunter-gatherer lifestyle in which we evolved. Biology cannot tell us how we ought to behave in the modern world, but it does provide an ethically relevant perspective. We come from a primate line that manifestly copulates for social reasons as well as reasons for fertilization. Women are unique in that (a) they conceal ovulation and (b) accept the male at any time during the monthly cycle, as well as during pregnancy and lactation. Natural family planning, while a valid and useful method of birth control, philosophically is an attempt to turn back the evolutionary clock and make evolution visible once again: it is an attempt to make women into chimpanzees. *Humanae Vitae* argues that every act of intercourse must be open to the possibility of procreation which, to a biologist, must appear as an effort to turn women into rabbits.

Civilization has destroyed natural restraints on fertility. It has burdened women with a pandemic of reproductive cancers. We cannot return to a world where the menarche comes at 20 – would that we could – or where women breastfeed their babies four times an hour. But by looking at where we have come from we can ask sensible questions about where we want to go in relation to social behavior, family life, clinical care, and all important problems of ethics.

References

Deys CV, Potts DM (1972) Condoms and things. Adv Biosci 10:287

Jolly A (1985) The evolution of primate behavior. MacMillan, New York

Konner M, Worthman C (1980) Nursing frequency, gonadal function and birth spacing among !Kung hunter-gatherers. Science 207:788

Loudon NB, Foxwell M, Potts DM, Guild AL, Short RV (1977) Acceptability of an oral contraceptive that reduces the frequency of menstruation: the tri-cycle pill regimen. Br Med J 2:487

MacMahon B, Cole P, Lin TM, Lowe CR, Mirra AP, Ravhihar B, Salber EJ, Valaoras VG, Yuasa S (1970) Age at first birth and risk of breast cancer. WHO Bull 43:209

Noonan JT (1967) Contraception: a history of its treatment by Catholic theologians and canonists. Harvard University Press, Cambridge, Mass

Potts DM (1972) Coitus interruptus. Aust NZ Obstet Gynaecol 241

Siassi I (1972) The psychiatrist's role in family planning. Am J Psychiatry 129:48

Symonds D (1979) The evolution of human sexuality. Oxford University Press, New York

Wood JW, Lai D, Johnson PL, Campbwell KL, Maslar A (1985) Lactation and birth spacing in highland New Guinea. Breastfeeding and fertility. J Bio Soc Sci [Suppl 9]

Trends in Contraception and Contraceptive Research

P. A. van Keep and H. Rekers

Organon International BV, POB 20, 5340 BH Oss, The Netherlands

Introduction

The years around 1960 were, without any doubt, the most important years in the history of contraception. These years brought us the discovery of the pill and the rediscovery of the IUD. These two methods of contraception – both extremely reliable – have changed our world profoundly. Their availability may not have *caused* social changes, but has at least allowed social changes to occur. They have changed the sexual behavior of our generation and will probably have a similar influence on that of the generations to come.

A short history of these two methods of contraception may be useful.

The Pill

It was in 1955 – now 32 years ago – that Gregory Pincus presented at the Congress of the International Planned Parenthood Federation in Tokyo his paper on the effects of oral progestogens on ovarian function in women. According to the chairman of that session, Sir Solly Zuckermann, who was interviewed several years later by the journalist Paul Vaughan, the audience was interested but clearly not aware of the historical value of that moment. Only a posteriori has this moment turned out to be the birth of the pill.

Today about 60 million women worldwide rely on the pill for their contraception, an impressive number, but this has to be seen against the total number of women of fertile age, that is between 15 and 45, in the world: 1000 million and then 60 million looks less impressive. Yet it all looked so simple in those early days of the pill. The pill was effective and induced regular cycles, both clear advantages over existing methods of contraception. The pill was easy to take, hygienic, and did not require the need to touch one's genitals. There was no relation between the taking of the pill and the sex act. The daily ingestion of a small pill was an amulet against the consequences of intercourse. Side effects were minor and transient and concern for health and future fertility hardly played a role. Yet, it is surprising that it took so long for the pill to become accepted to the point where it is now. It took more than 25 years, thousands of studies, numerous campaigns, lectures, and media coverage explaining the relative safety of oral contraception to reach the present degree of acceptance of the pill. It is a horrible thought that all these efforts could be made worthless by the publication of *one* scare story and its subsequent waves of publicity in the lay press. The curves showing the accep-

Sexology
Eds.: W. Eicher, G. Kockott

tance of pill use in the various countries are largely explained by such scare stories and the resulting publicity. Many such events remained limited to one country or a group of countries sharing a language. Other events had a global impact; these events have names that compare to those of battles in a world war.

Humanae Vitae the encyclical in 1967 had a global impact. So did The *Scowen Committee* report in the United Kingdom in 1969, showing that pills with more than 50 μg estrogen were associated with a higher incidence of thromboembolism. The *Nelson* hearings in the United States on oral contraception in 1970 led to a, fortunately, short-lived but massive abandonment of this method of contraception – and even to the abandonment of all contraception – leading to a sudden peak in birth statistics known as the "Nelson babies". The interim report of the *Royal College of General Practitioners* in 1977 expounded the cardiovascular risks of pill use, particularly in women over 35 years of age and in women who smoke. The *Pike Study* in 1983 claimed an increased risk of mammary carcinoma in women who had used the pill before their first full-term pregnancy.

All these events have left scars on the curves of pill use. In retrospect some of these events had little influence, such as Humanae Vitae; others were unjustified, such as the Nelson hearings; and others were only misleading, such as the Pike Study. Some events have been blessings in disguise because, although they temporarily hampered the acceptance of this form of contraception, they have triggered developments which resulted in safer oral contraceptives. Two examples:

The *Scowen report* in 1969 caused the search for OCs with a lower estrogen content; first 50 μg, then 30 μg, and now even 20 μg. This development has drastically lowered the incidence of thromboembolic disease in pill users. The report of the *Royal College of GPs* in the United Kingdom has also had interesting consequences. It triggered the search for pills with less progestogen, sometimes through ingenious dosage schemes, such as the triphasics – which do indeed contain small quantities of hormones and consequently cause only minimal metabolic disturbances – but which are more complicated to take and which may less effectively suppress ovarian activity.

The same report triggered the search for better progestogens, not so much more potent but with an improved hormonal profile; they should have less affinity to androgen receptors in relation to their affinity to the progesterone receptors. As a consequence they should have less effects on metabolism or even, in combination with an estrogen, have beneficial effects on metabolic parameters. This led to the development of the so-called "third-generation oral contraceptives." The *first-generation* progestogens were developed in the late fifties and, with the exception of norethisterone and the structurally related lynestrenol, they disappeared when the *second-generation* progestogen levonorgestrel was introduced. This progestogen could be used in pills in micrograms instead of milligrams. The *third-generation* progestogens, used in the third-generation oral contraceptives, came on the scene in the eigthies. The first one of this generation was Marvelon in 1981 by Organon, based on the progestogen desogestrel, the second one was Cilest introduced in 1986 by Ortho-Cilag, based on norgestimate, and the third one was Femovan introduced in 1987 by Schering and based on gestodene. Although relatively little experience has been gained with the latter two, it seems that they share all three one important quality: minimal impairment of the body's metabolism, in particular the lipid metabolism and, by extrapolation, a virtual absence of cardiovascular risk.

This third-generation range of pills is the result of many years of time- and money-consuming research and only a few industries are still willing to risk their research funds on research for new contraceptives, in particular medicamental approaches. Consequently the development of new forms of contraception will by no means be as dramatic as that we have observed in the past, in particular the years 1957–1967. But also: the third generation of pills are near to perfect. We may predict the development of slightly different dosage schemes and phasic preparations again, but otherwise not much will change in the field of oral contraception in the next decade. The third-generation OCs will be with us for the rest of this century.

Intrauterine Devices

The history of the IUD is infinitely longer than that of the pill. There are stories of camels in ancient times whith a pebble in their uterus to prevent impregnation. Many more such stories exist; they all have in common that they are difficult to check.

Modern IUD history begins with Von Gräfenberg in 1930, who inserted a ring in the uterus of women to obtain a contraceptive effect. His ideas were met with great enthusiasm until, a few years later, they were, as he was almost himself, crushed by opponents who were inspired more by the political arguments of the Third Reich than by scientific arguments. Ohta, the Japanese investigator who developed a comparable device, suffered a similar fate. The IUD seemed to have been efficiently killed. However, after the end of World War II the IUD was still alive. A few enthusiasts used their own devices, but in 1962 – 7 years after the death of Von Gräfenberg in New York City – the IUD was formally rehabilitated, although now as a plastic device. Since then, many developments took place. Several different shapes were developed, and so were long-acting medicated devices – copper, copper-silver, or hormone loaded. Optimum timing for insertion was defined. We learned to define indications and contraindications for the safe and effective use of IUDs and we learned how to identify serious complications and how to prevent or minimize them (Thiery 1987).

Present-day IUDs are effective – also cost-effective – means of contraception. Yet, they are denied to a large portion of the world for a strange reason. Diczfalusy recently wrote "Could Konrad Lorenz rewrite his book *The eight mortal sins of civilized mankind* today, I am convinced that he would change the title from 8 to 9 mortal sins, in order to include: liability suits, American style" (Diczfalusy 1987).

The excessive, even outrageous, claims that IUD manufacturers in the United States have had to fight has discouraged all but one company in the States to continue sales of IUDs. As a consequence, Malcolm Potts stated last year in Singapore, "an American woman, who cannot, for whatever reason use other forms of contraception than the IUD, has only two options, she can either enter into a convent or move across the border." One can only hope that the consequences of this development in the United States will not affect the availability of IUDs in the rest of the world.

What will be the future of IUD technology? New shapes, adaptable to the space that the uterine cavity has to offer? New medicated IUDs with antifertility compounds – spermatotoxic or embryotoxic? IUDs with antiseptic properties?

Intrauterine devices with progestogen are already in use but they have not solved the problem of spotting and menorrhagia. Yet these are major problems of intrauterine contraception. Spotting is disquieting and embarrassing for many women and menorrhagia and metrorrhagia decrease body iron stores, a health hazard, particularly in the developing countries. Will there be frameless, tailless, but medicated IUDs anchored to the uterine wall? Or is the future, as Thiery proposed, for intracervical devices?

Space does not permit to give a similar review of other forms of contraception, quantitatively less important than the pill and the IUD, but nevertheless essential in the "contraceptive mix" that can be offered to today's couple asking for help:
- Sterilization, permanent or temporary
- Natural family planning methods
- Barrier methods, chemical or mechanical
- Postcoital contraception
- Postconception methods

They do have their place now, and will undergo developments in the future. We will come back to that later.

Research in Contraception

Only few companies are still actively engaged in research in this field, three in Europe, one in the United States and none in Japan. The reasons for that are easy to understand. The financial commitment is enormous and the chances of being successful are limited.

Djerassi has wondered, many many years ago, why governments participate financially in the development of new aircraft but refuse to support the development of new contraceptives. Yet, the sums involved are comparable but the impact of a new form of contraception on the future of mankind might be far greater than the impact of a new airplane, even if it is supersonic or able to transport 600 indstead of 300 passengers.

It is the industry – in fact the pharmaceutical industry – which has to decide whether it wants to risk its investments in this area. Sure, there is a need for new approaches to contraception, there are leads; in other words, it is feasible to develop new approaches and it may be economically attractive to do so. However, contraception – or more precisely the use of contraceptives – is certainly determined by the developments in society that will determine which forms of contraception will be acceptable, or needed, in the next decades. How will the fear of AIDS influence contraceptive needs? How will political and religious thoughts about contraception and abortion develop?

We want to elaborate on this last point. Most present-day steroid-based contraception is aimed at the inhibition of ovulation. For most people this is ethically

Table 1. Future fertility planning technologies. (Office of Technology Assessment 1982)

Highly likely before 1990
1. Safer oral contraceptives
2. Improved IUDs
3. Improved barrier contraceptives for women
4. Improved long-acting steroid injections
5. Improved ovulation-detection methods for use with periodic abstinence
6. Steroid implants
7. Steroid vaginal rings
8. LRF-analog contraceptives for women
9. Prostaglandin analogs for self-administered induction of menses

Possible by 1990 but prospects doubtful
1. Monthly steroid-based contraceptive pill
2. Improved monthly steroid injection
3. New types of drug releasing IUDs
4. Mini-dose vaginal rings
5. Antipregnancy vaccine for women
6. Improved barrier contraceptives for men
7. Sperm suppression contraceptives for men
8. Reversible female sterilization
9. Simplified female sterilization techniques
10. Simplified male sterilization techniques
11. LRF analogs for self-administered induction of menses

Unlikely by 1990 but possible by 2000
1. Antifertility vaccine for men
2. Antisperm drugs for men
3. Antisperm maturation drugs for men
4. Lactation-linked oral contraceptives
5. Ovulation prediction methods for use with periodic abstinence
6. New types of antiovulation contraceptive drugs for women
7. Contraceptive drugs for women that disrupt ovum transport
8. Reversible male sterilization
9. Pharmacologic or immunologic sterilization for women
10. Pharmacologic or immunologic sterilization for men
11. Agents other than LRF analog for self-administered induction of menses

acceptable but from the medical point of view it may be better to interfere later in the process of fertilization, for example just before, or at the moment of, nidation. Will this be acceptable for large groups of the population in 10 or 15 years from now? The US Office of Technology Assessment published in 1982 a list of contraceptive technologies for the future. It may be an interesting exercise to review this list with you, now in 1987, only 5 years later (Table 1).

Highly likely before 1990. The easiest part. You only have to study the relevant journals:

1. *Safer oral contraception*. That was not difficult to predict because the first one of the third-generation contraceptives was there in 1981: desogestrel based. The others followed in 1986, norgestimate, and in 1987, gestodene based.
2. *Improved IUDs*. Again an easy one to predict. We have already elaborated on that.

3. *Improved barrier contraceptives for women.* Recent years brought us the sponge, well accepted in some countries, not so in others. The sponge is still based on the well-known spermicide nonoxynol-9. There are, however, more interesting spermicides available for study. The reason why developments here are not faster are, we think, to be found in the limited commercial attractiveness of this form of contraception and the problems in providing the evidence for safety and effectiveness.
4. *Improved long-acting steroid injections.* We know of no major effort in this area. Of course it is possible to develop a delivery system for such an injection but the dispute around the DMPA injection will have had a discouraging effect on anyone who wants to develop such a contraceptive.
5. *Improved ovulation detection methods for use with periodic abstinence.* Several devices were developed but their impact on the contraceptive scene was limited. Such detection systems would narrow the window during which contraception is needed. Mechanical ones are being developed but their acceptance is poor.
6. *Steroid implants.* They are with us, but certainly still open for improvement. Current research is aimed at easier application and at the use of the third-generation progestogens.
7. *Vaginal rings.* Again an easy guess in 1982. Rings are being developed to release both an estrogen and a progestogen. We wonder, however, whether they will be available before 1990.
8. *LRF analog contraceptives for women.* No practical applications in sight.
9. *Prostaglandin analogues for self-administered induction of menses.* The idea has practically disappeared from view.

Let us now look at the developments that were regarded as being possible by 1990 but whose prospects were regarded as being doubtful. As far as we can see none of these will be with us 1990. Only a few leads may find practical applications in or after the year 2000.

The *vaccine against pregnancy.* There are two different approaches, a passive immunization which gives protection during a number of months, and an active immunization which will lead to lifelong sterility.

Male contraception should be mentioned here. There are at present some 120 publications on efforts two use steroids for male contraception, involving some 1100 men (Nieschlag 1987). The leads are there, but it requires optimism to believe that any practical application will be available before the next century. The same goes for Gossypol, the Chinese approach to male contraception. It has been a major deception. Gossypol has probably been the first chemical entity which has been tried extensively in humans *before* it was tested in animals. It proved to be toxic for animals and further research is far from promising.

We cannot comment on a number of surgical techniques, because in this area developments take place along different routes. It seems to us, however, unlikely that developments in this direction will have a significant impact on the worldwide contraceptive landscape in the near future.

The third part of the table produced by the Office of Technology Assessment Survey in 1982 is already now, 5 years later, completely unrealistic.

Table 2. Desirable qualities in a contraceptive for 2001

1.	It must be reversible
2.	It must have no ill effects on health
3.	It must be constantly active; to be switched off rather than on
4.	It must not impinge on intercourse
5.	It must be under female control
6.	It must be applicable on a population basis
7.	It must be suitable for different societies
8.	It must act before rather than after the fact of pregnancy
9.	It must be reliable

Contraception in 2001

We tried, in late 1986, with a group of experts to fantasize about potential approaches to contraception in the distant future, taking the year 2001, after Clark's book 2001 – a space odyssey, as a metaphor for such a technological future. It proved to be difficult to detach ourselves from today's knowledge and we hardly produced any ideas beyond extrapolation of the approaches en vogue today.

One list of requirements of a contraceptive for the next century is worth presenting. It stems from Klopper (1987) from Aberdeen (Table 2).

A few points are worth stressing:

Point 3: it must be constantly active, to be switched off rather than on. In other words, one must *do* something to be fecundable.

Point 6: it must be under female control; this does not mean that the woman should *use* the method, but that she is in control and that is something different.

Point 9: it should act before, rather than after, the fact of pregnancy. For Klopper this meant that the point of attack should be just before, or at, nidation. Others disagreed vehemently and insisted on interference before conception. This reconfirms our earlier point. The type of contraception used in the next century will be determined by the norms and values of society itself at that time. The needs of society will determine the norms and values and hence developments in this field.

At this same meeting Zeilmaker (1986 personal communication), IVF expert in Rotterdam, presented an interesting option: The ovaries of a girl of 17 or so will be stimulated by gonadotrophins during one or two cycles until seven to ten egg cells can be harvested. During harvesting she will be sterilized by closing both her tubes. The egg cells will be frozen. Each time she wants to be pregnant, she presents herself at her "egg bank" with a sperm sample of the man of her choice. The thawed egg cell will be fertilized and implanted. All this can be done during her luncheon breaks. She will never need contraception any more.

One must be brave to live in that new world!

References

Diczfalusy E (1987) Has family planning a future. Contraception 35:1–17
Djerassi C (1970) Birth control after 1984. Science 169:941–945

Djerassi C (1987) In: Van Keep PA, Ellison Davis K, De Wied D (eds) Contraception in the year 2001. Elsevier, Amsterdam

Van Keep PA, Ellison Davis K, De Wied D (eds) (1987) Contraception in the year 2001. Elsevier, Amsterdam

Klopper A (1987) In: Van Keep PA, Ellison Davies K, De Wied D (eds) Contraception in the year 2001. Elsevier, Amsterdam

Nieschlag E (1987) In: Van Keep PA, Ellison Davies K, De Wied D (eds) Contraception in the year 2001. Elsevier, Amsterdam

Pike MC, Henderson BE, Krailo MD et al. (1983) Breast cancer in young women and use of oral contraceptives: possible modifying effect of formulation and age at use. Lancet 2:926–930

The Royal College of General Practitioners (1974) Oral contraceptives and health. Pitman Medical, London

Thiery M (1987) In: Van Keep PA, Ellison Davies K, De Wied D (eds) Contraception in the year 2001. Elsevier, Amsterdam

World Population and Fertility Planning Technologies (1982) Office of Technology Assessment, Washington DC, pp 92–119

New Aspects in Female Contraception

H. Lehfeldt

110, East 82nd St., New York, NY 10128, USA

Contraceptive techniques vary from country to country and change periodically within each one. In Japan, a barrier method, the condom, is virtually the only contraceptive method used, to the almost total exclusion of intrauterine devices (IUDs) and the pill. By contrast, the methods of choice in the People's Republic of China are a stamp-like oral contraceptive and the IUD, with which, according to the latest available statistics, some 55 million Chinese women have been fitted.

In Germany, female barrier methods such as the diaphragm and the cervical cap are rarely used; the plastic cap, which is manufactured in Germany, is unknown to most German physicians. In Britain, a rubber cervical cap has been routinely prescribed in family planning clinics for over 50 years.

In the USA, according to Ory et al. (1982), roughly one-third of couples (slightly more women than men) used sterilization to avoid an unplanned pregnancy, one-third used oral contraception, and one-third used various other methods such as the IUD, the diaphragm, the condom, etc. Almost 2.5 million women of reproductive age used no contraception at all (Table 1).

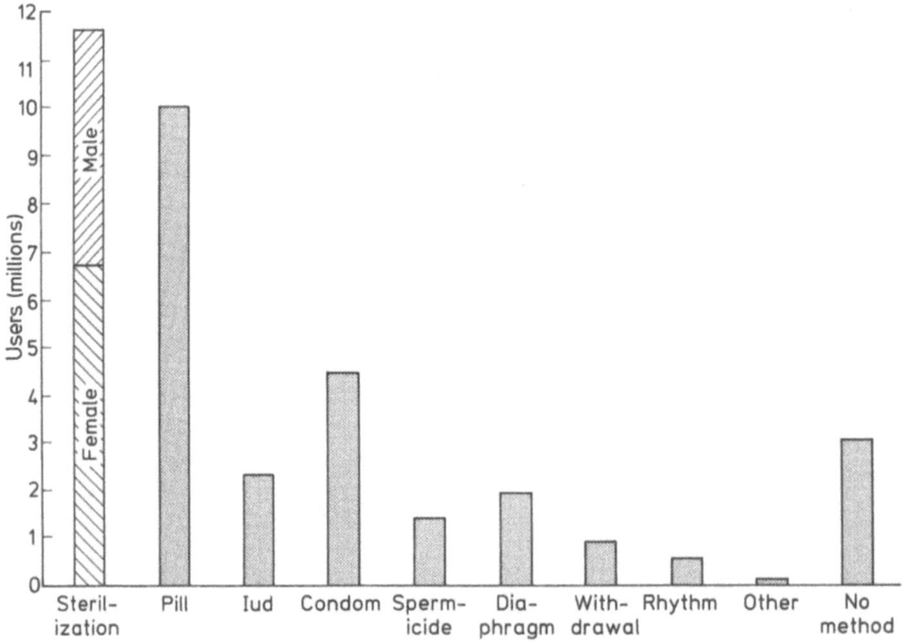

Sexology
Eds.: W. Eicher, G. Kockott

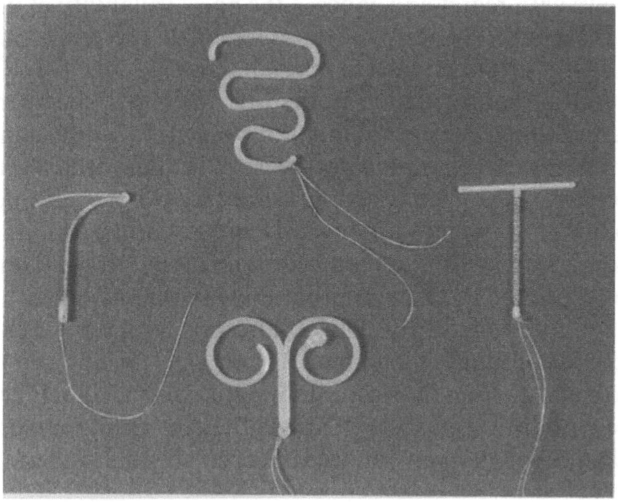

Fig. 1. Lippes loop, Copper-7, Copper-T, Saf-T-coil

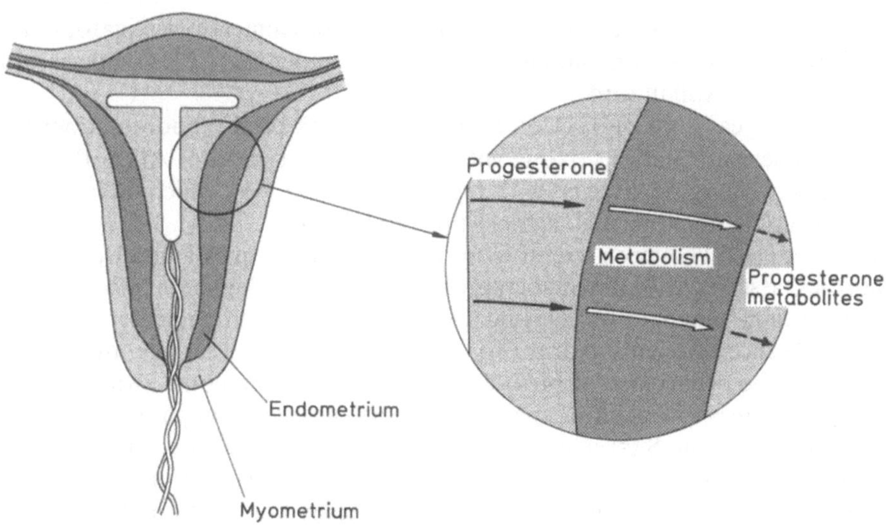

Fig. 2. Progestasert

A bizarre situation has recently developed in the USA: IUDs have become virtually unavailable to physicians because the main manufacturers of the loop, the two copper devices, and the Saf-T-Coil (Fig. 1) have stopped their distribution; the threat of costly liability suits was claimed to be responsible for their decision. The only Food and Drug Administration (FDA)-approved IUD still available is the Progestasert (Fig. 2); it remains effective for only 1 year and it is not considered a method of choice by most gynecologists. At the 12th World Congress on Fertility and Sterility in Singapore in October 1986, the following statement was issued:

The World Congress views with regret and concern the non-availability of inert and copper-bearing IUDs in the USA despite continued FDA approval, and notes that the World Health Organization plans to renew its backing for the IUD as a safe and effective method of contraception in the first week of December, supports criticism of a situation which deprives millions of women of a useful contraceptice choice, and acknowledges the non-medical reasons for the withdrawal of IUDs in the US (i.e., the contingency fee system practiced by US lawyers and the remote but real possibility of very large jury awards making it unprofitable for manufacturers to market a safe method of contraception). The World Congress fully endorses continued use of IUDs in appropriately selected women. It notes that legal problems are not limited to IUDs but also involve, or have the potential to involve, all methods of family planning.

According to Dr. Malcolm Potts (Family Health International, Raleigh, Durham, USA), because of the withdrawal of the IUD from the American market, millions of women in the USA now live in an "underdeveloped" country in terms of family planning options.

The cervical cap had been used in the USA and was a legal contraceptive technique until several years ago when the FDA declared it an experimental and dangerous method. Since then, the use of the cap has been permitted for research purposes only and restricted to one type of rubber cap. Clinical investigators have needed FDA authorization and have had to work under strict FDA supervision. This regulation is still in force.

For many years, the subject of contraception has been taboo on American radio and television stations. Now, with the alarming spread of AIDS this attitude is slowly changing, at least with regard to the condom, which definitely affords protection, albeit partial, against this fatal disease.

Jick et al. (1981), whose scientific findings have been questioned by eminent authorities, asserted that the incidence of birth defects is higher in babies whose mothers became pregnant while using a spermicide containing nonoxynol 9. Despite the absence of scientific proof for any connection between the use of spermicides and the occurrence of birth defects, and American court awarded $ 4.7 million in damages to a plaintiff against the pharmaceutical company Ortho. Following an appeal, the Supreme Court refused to review the case, thus allowing the lower court's decision to stand. This decision may turn spermicides into an "endangered species", as practically all spermicides contain nonoxynol 9 the pharmaceutical companies may stop manufacturing them, to the detriment of our already diminishing contraceptive armamentarium.

In 1985, the American College of Obstetricians and Gynecologists stated that "...no scientific evidence (exists) that spermicides are mutagens... There is no reason to avoid the clinical use of spermicides or to label such products with a consumer-warning label." McCann (1987) warned that "this combination of regulatory caution (by the FDA) with excessive litigation could mean that sexual abstinence will soon be the only way of avoiding unwanted pregnancy."

The failure rates of different contraceptive methods are shown in Table 2 (Williams 1986). Tietze (1979; Table 3) has compared estimated mortality rates associated with pregnancy, childbirth, oral contraception, IUDs, and first-trimester legal abortion; his figures show clearly that the risks to life are lowest

Table 2. Failure rates of different contraceptive methods during first year of use

Methods	Lowest observed failure rate (%)	Failure rate in typical users (%)
Injectable progestin	0.25	0.25
Combined birth control pills	0.5	2
Progestin-only pill	1	2.5
IUD	1.5	5
Condom	2	10
Diaphragm (with spermicide)	2	19
Sponge (with spermicide)	9–11	10–20
Foams, creams, jellies, and vaginal suppositories	3– 5	18
Withdrawal	16	23
Periodic (rhythmic) abstinence	2–20	24
Douche	–	40
Chance (no method of birth control)	90	90

Adapted from Williams (1986).

Table 3. Estimates of mortality rates (per 100000) associated with pregnancy and childbirth, first trimester legal abortion, oral contraceptives, and intrauterine devices

Age group (years)	Pregnancy and childbirth	First trimester legal abortion	Oral contraceptives		Intra-uterine devices
			Nonsmokers	Smokers	
15–19	11.1	1.2	1.2	1.4	0.8
20–24	10.0	1.2	1.2	1.4	0.8
25–29	12.5	1.4	1.2	1.4	1.0
30–34	24.9	1.4	1.8	10.4	1.0
35–39	44.0	1.8	3.9	12.8	1.4
40–44	71.4	1.8	6.6	58.4	1.4

Adapted from Tietze (1977).

for IUD users and for women who resort to first-trimester abortion. The latest report (Atrash et al. 1987) shows a substantial reduction in mortality associated with first-trimester abortion. The rate was 4.1 per 100000 in 1972 and decreased to 0.8 per 100000 in 1982.

The need in developing countries for access to organized family planning was clearly stated by Mahler (1987), director general of WHO:

500000 maternal deaths take place every year – 99% of them in the developing world. In the developed world, there are only 5 to 30 maternal deaths per 100000 life births; in developing countries the figures range from 50 to 800 or more. Women in developing countries run 100 to 200 times the risk of dying in pregnancy and childbirth than do women in an affluent country... The causes of these deaths are tragic indeed. Illegal abortions from unwanted pregnancy cause some 25–50% of these deaths, simply because women do not have access to the family planning services they want and need, or have no access to safe procedures, or

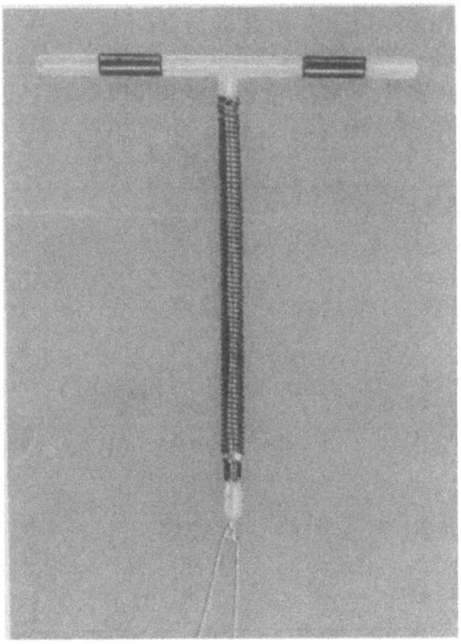

Fig. 3. The new copper IUD: TCu 380A

to humane treatment for the complications of abortion. For the thousands of women who die in pregnancy and childbirth, millions more are permanently disabled... We need to expand family planning and family-life education programs, particularly for young people, and make services for planning families socially, culturally, financially, and geographically accessible.

According to Rosenfield and Maine (1987) "our first concern ought to be that every year hundreds of thousands of women in developing countries die from hemorrhage, untreated sepsis, obstructed labor, or eclamptic convulsions – all for lack of effective medical care..." Recommending a variety of remedies the authors stated: "We hope that foremost will be those that act directly to prevent maternal deaths – i.e. prevention of unwanted pregnancy and early treatment of complications."

Long-term studies of the hormonal contraceptive implant Norplant (Diaz et al. 1987) have shown that the method is highly effective over long periods and does not seem to compromise a woman's future fertility. Norplant has now been approved for general use in the family planning programs of ten countries. The Population Council plans to submit Norplant to the FDA for approval in the USA early in 1988.

The TCu 380A (Fig. 3), which was developed by the Population Council, has been found superior in performance to previous IUDs and has been approved by the FDA. According to newspaper reports, the new device will become available to physicians in the USA in a few months. Unfortunately, its high price – $ 300 – will probably make it unaffordable for nonaffluent women.

References

Atrash HK et al. (1987) Legal abortion mortality in the United States: 1972–1982. Am J Obstet Gynecol 156:605–612

Diaz S et al. (1987) Long-term follow-up of women treated with Norplant implants. Contraception 35:551–567
Jick H et al. (1981) Vaginal spermicides and congenital disorders. JAMA 245:1329–1332
Mahler H (1987) The safe motherhood initiative: a call for action. Lancet I:668–670
McCann MF (1987) Letter to N Engl J Med 316:163
Ory HW et al. (1983) Mortality associated with fertility control. Perspectives 15:57–63
Rosenfield A, Maine D (1987) Letter to Lancet I:691
Tietze C (1977) Fam Plann Perspect 9:74
Tietze C, Lewit S (1979) Life risks associated with reversible methods of fertility regulation. Int J Gynecol Obstet 16:456–459
Williams NB (1986) Contraceptive technology. Irvington, New York

Psychology, Contraception, and Family Planning

I. Ray

Home and Social Science Department, Calcutta University, India
50/1 Hindusthan Park, Calcutta – 700029, India

Introduction

India has adopted family planning as her national policy. A considerable amount of money is being spent on family planning activities and yet there has not been any marked curb in population growth. The people are not sufficiently motivated towards the practice of contraceptives. The reasons behind this are mainly psychological. The author has tried to investigate the reasons.

Study Sample

The study consisted of 200 educated males and females and 100 uneducated females. Uneducated males could not be approached. Both sexes were questioned on 11 independent variables, viz., education, age, age differences between partners, occupation, economic strata, fertility range, duration of marriage, kind of marriage, number of children, and number of living children.

Methodology

The Questionnaire method was applied to educated classes of people and the Interview method was applied to the uneducated women. Twenty-four educated women were also interviewed in order to avoid statistical error. The Stratified Sampling method was used.

Results

After the data were collected they were statistically analyzed. Figures 1 and 2 indicate the distribution of subjects of three broad groups in relation to educational levels and number of issues respectively.

Family planning is accepted by the overwhelming majority of educated males, females, and uneducated females.

It was also observed that there was little difference between the Interview and Questionnaire groups of educated women. The X^2 test showed a highly significant difference between groups. When the question of practising contraceptives

Sexology
Eds.: W. Eicher, G. Kockott

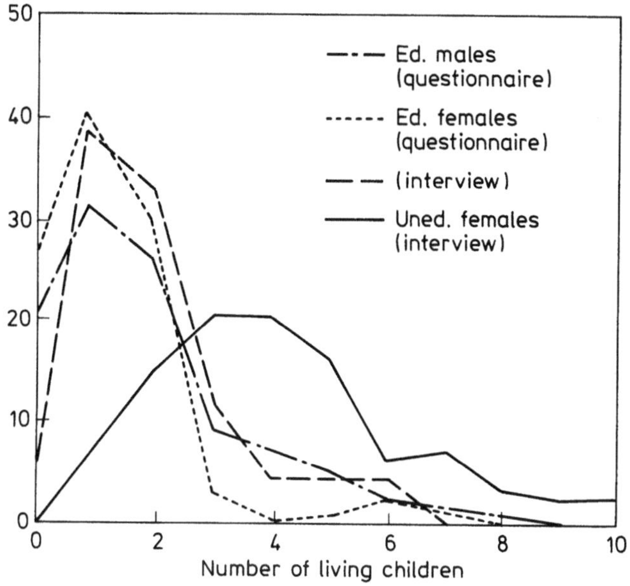

Fig. 1. Distribution of subjects of the three broad groups by number of living children

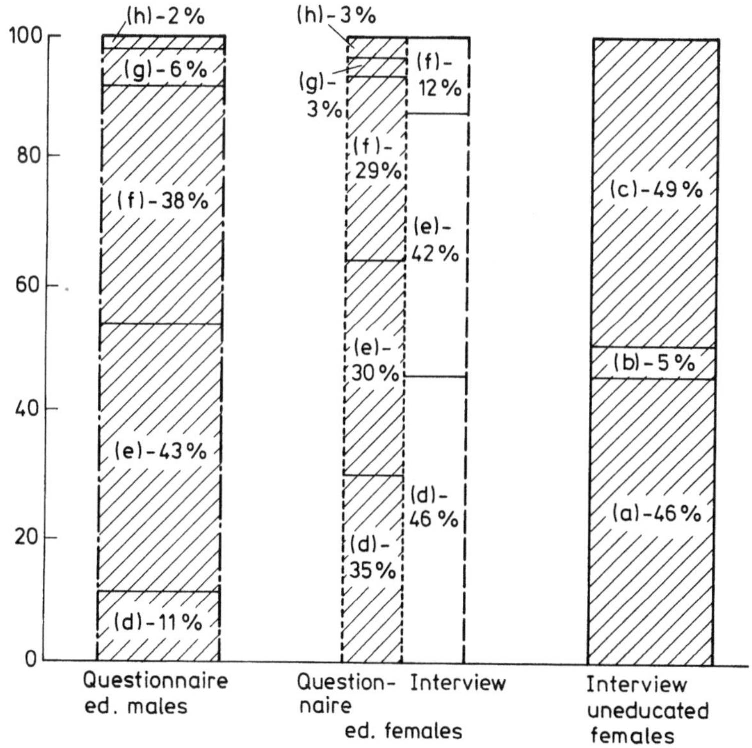

Fig. 2. Distribution of subjects of the three broad groups by educational level (A) illiterate, (B) literate, (C) school level, (D) undergraduate, (E) graduate, (F) postgraduate, (G) doctorate, (H) not stated

Table 1. Acceptance of family planning

	Educated		Un-educated
	Men	Women	Women
Percentage fully in support of family planning	94	95 (24)[a]	32
Percentage supporting family planning under circumstances	3	1 (0)	46
Percentage fully against family planning	2	3 (0)	19
Nonresponse	1	1 (0)	3

[a] Parentheses indicate interviewed data of educated women

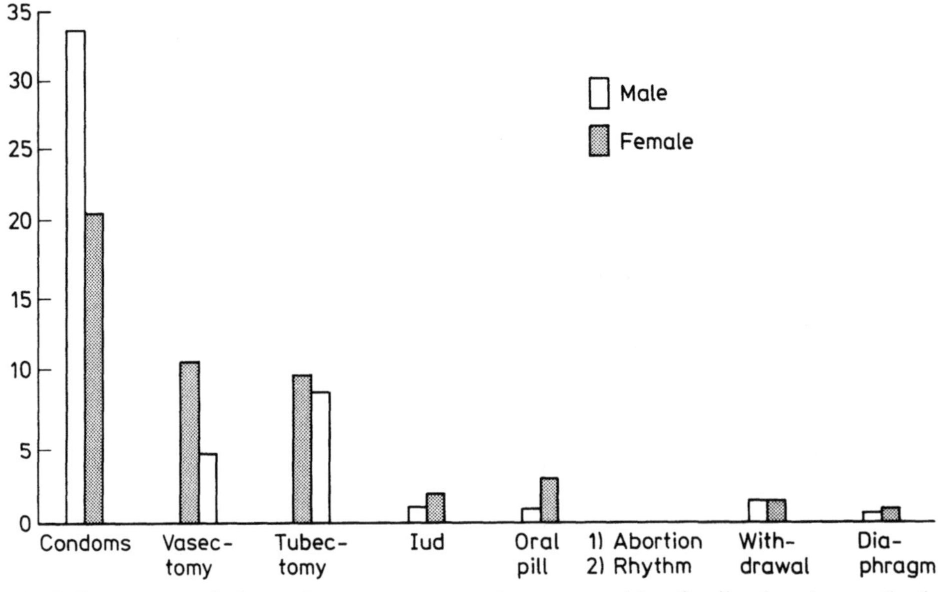

Fig. 3. Percentage of educated government employees practising family planning methods along with spouses

Name of contraceptive	Hindu	Muslim	Christian
Tablets	27%	30%	28%
Vasectomy Tubectomy	28%	20%	28%
Nirodh (indian condom)	12%	15%	10%
Loop	19%	19%	24%

Fig. 4. Practice of contraceptives among 1000 uneducated females in Calcutta on the basis of religion (1980–1985)

Table 2. Attitudes of educated men, women, and uneducated women toward the contraceptives

Q. no.	Text as in questionnaire	Possible answers	Number of subjects			χ^2	
			Ed. male	Ed. female	Uned. female	Value (d.f.)	Significance
13(i)	Do you consider that the use of contraceptives should be prevented for any or more of the following reasons? Check the reasons	(a) Yes	47	65 (5)	52	11.82 (2)	1%
		(i) From the moral point of view	10	12 (2)	33	38.44 (2)	0.1%
		(ii) From the religious point of view	3	8 (1)	36	72.38 (2)	0.1%
		(iii) For the sake of health	32	45 (2)	36	4.88 (2)	Ns
		(iv) For the mental discomfort	25	31 (3)	32	6.09 (2)	5%
		(v) From the cultural point of view	8	14 (1)	16	6.09 (2)	5%
		(b) No	32	19 (16)	10	6.09 (2)	5%
		(c) No response	21	16 (3)	38		

Table 3. Choices of contraceptives

Q. no.	Question item		Number of subjects giving each answer		
	Text as in questionnaire	Possible answers	Educated males	Educated females	Uneducated females
0 1	2	3	4	5	6
16	What do you consider to be the best method against conception?	a) Abstinence	17	12 (0)	2
		b) Rhythm method	18	17 (3)	2
		c) Withdrawal method	14	30 (6)	7
		d) Condom	8	1 (5)	5
		e) Diaphragm	31	18 (4)	13
		f) Jelly	13	11 (3)	7
		g) Foam tablets	5	2 (0)	39
		h) Vasectomy	9	4 (3)	13
		i) Salphingectomy	2	4 (2)	24
		j) Oral tablet	0	6 (2)	3
		k) Indifferent (no idea)	0	0 (2)	0
		l) None	0	2 (2)	19
		m) No response	8	13 (0)	9

arose, the same majority of people did not exhibit the positive attitude as shown in Table 2.

Choices of contraceptives were given to them as in in Table 3.

The 1980–1985 survey was undertaken by the author to assess the change of attitudes in the main religions of India, viz., Hindu, Muslim, and Christian.

Table 4. Use of contraceptives among 1000 uneducated females in Calcutta on the basis of religion (1980–1985)

Contraceptive	Religion		
	Hindu	Muslim	Christian
Tablets	27%	30%	28%
Vasectomy and tubectomy	28%	20%	28%
Nirodh (indian condom)	12%	15%	10%
Loop	19%	19%	24%

Table 5. Percentage of government employees practising family planning methods

Method	Male	Female[a]
Condom	34.2	0.6
Diaphragm	0.2	0.6
Jelly, foam tablet	–	–
Vasectomy	10.6	4.6
Tubectomy	9.3	8.8
IUD	1.7	3.4
Oral pill	1.2	4.9
Abstinence/rhythm	–	–
Withdrawal	2.4	2.4

[a] Practising family planning methods along with their spouses (Fig. 4)

Psychological Interpretation

Apart from the religious and social reasons *against the use of contraceptives*, there were certain underlying resistances. When analyzed, it was found:

1. Narcissism stands in the way of use of contraceptives. The majority of educated women accepting family planning still oppose the use of contraceptives mainly due to the fear of injury to body and mind ("health and mental dissatisfaction"). Even uneducated women are afraid of practising contraception due to the fear of sterility and infertility. Fear of mechanical and chemical methods of contraceptives leads the educated class to take recourse to abstinence, rhythm, and withdrawal methods.
2. The ambivalence of emotions is the characteristic of all kinds of emotions not excluding also love for children. The feeling of hatred toward the children when anthropologically probed gives evidence of widespread practice of killing the child, infanticide, child sacrifice, and abortion by either crude or surgical methods. Due to the educational attainment and moral development this kind of emotion, i.e., hatred, has been repressed. Flugel (1960) is of the opinion that if psychologically considered the abstention from conception is a certain extent equal to a series of actions expressed through infanticide or abortion. Uneducated women consider contraception as being against God's

desire of procreation; therefore abortion is a kind of sin. God gives the power of fertility and that should not be controlled.

3. The rejection of contraceptives expresses a primitive pride for sexual fertility and sexual potency. Some of the interviewers of the author (uneducated women) told her that "one should not spoil the tree which bears fruits." It is a common pride in rural India especially for the woman for her fecundity and if a woman has a large number of children she enjoys a higher status than others by virtue of her power for fecundity. Among educated classes the mother of one issue or having no issue is proud of her musical or literary talents; the transference of emotion has been done to this object.
4. Some of the happy couples, in spite of being sufficiently reasonable, could not accept contraceptives wholeheartedly for the reason that during coitus they do not get sufficient orgasm if they use contraceptives.
   a) Many happily married women have stated that during the sexual act they get a "heavenly pleasure," which emphasizes Helen Deutsch's opinion (1947): that in the ecstasy of the sexual act "the emotional barriers between the I and you disappear." The men sometimes forget to take contraceptives at the moment of tumescence immediately before the sexual intercourse.
   b) As the women generally play a passive role in the sexual field if their husbands do not take initiative for taking contraceptive measures, in spite of their ardent desire they cannot use contraceptives.
   c) The sexual act assumes an immense dramatic and cathartic significance not for men alone but especially also for women.
5. A psychological repression does exist in the sexual field and any intrusion into it by an external force cannot be accepted easily by many. The use of contraceptives is also a kind of intrusion into a "forbidden" area of married life, which in our country is considered to take a purity and sanctity in itself. In this reference, my case No. 12[1] (married educated woman) is a glaring example. She was not only happy in married life but also possessed an extreme form of motherliness.
6. Objection to contraceptives especially female methods is probably based on the fact that they will decontrol the male's authority over the female and even dominance over the sexual sphere which has so long been enjoyed by the male partner. On the other hand, the objection against the male method is mainly due to the fear of losing virility or sexual strength on the part of males.
7. Fear of sterility due to mechanical and chemical methods leads mainly the educated and uneducated women to take recourse of oral tablets. They think anything taken by mouth is not so injurious as the child takes mother's milk, which initially in his life nourishes him. Fear of oral tablet is less in comparison with other contraceptives.

---

[1] Case No. 12: She was 32 years of age (at the time of data collection) and highly educated. Her husband's age was 45. She had two children aged 14 and 9, and had enjoyed a happy married life of 18 years. She had a strong sexual life and was still stating that they were both responsive to each other. Before both her conceptions she took a bath, purified her soul by a prayer to God, and made herself ready to meet her partner.

8. The author agrees with J. M. Stycose, regarding an unknown fear for contraceptives about which uneducated women's knowledge is meager.
9. Some of the persons including women also felt that by using contraceptives they will become shameless. A small percentage of people still believe that people will exploit the practice of contraceptives, in premarital and extramarital relations.
10. Even many educated persons think that contraceptives are only some of the measures by which one wants to enjoy the sexual pleasure without incurring the "penalty of parenthood," so it is a violation of moral law.
11. Religious opposition sometimes stands in the way of using contraceptives.
12. Desire for male offspring leads to repeated pregnancy, and stands in the way of using contraceptives.

Motives for the Use of Contraceptives

These depend mainly on:

1. Happy married life and showing an equal responsibility between partners, and the desire for giving proper facilities to children motivate people to use contraceptives.
2. Sometimes children of a large family are deprived of the parental love especially the mother's care and attention in the distressed period of her childhood, which motivates her strongly to have a small family.
3. The more career-oriented women strongly believe in small families and the strict use of contraceptives; these Borgatte and Westerff regarded as "less community minded," "more emancipated," and interested in extrafamilial leisure activities.
4. Some educated men and women believe the birth of children interferes with personal freedom. So they answer question No. 3 of the author's study as "rather relieved," without children.
5. Some psychological difficulties, viz., losing her personality, fear of death, restrictions of movement during pregnancy, sexual frigidity, and lack of emotional warmth strongly motivate the use of contraceptives in educated women.
6. "Sibling rivalry" leads to contraceptive use. If a woman in her childhood is deprived of parental love, after her marriage with an unconscious feeling of sibling rivalry she wants to identify herself with her mother and the rivalry situation is also transferred unconsciously to her own child, who according to her appears to be another sibling. All the mechanisms act unconsciously in her mind and she consciously rejects motherhood.
7. The sense of duty and responsibility toward children, family, etc., lead them to use contraceptives for a small family. In conclusion, it may be said that there are two groups who support family planning: One group, generally the educated males and females, support family planning as they are more conscious about the future of the family not only in the struggle for existence but to increase their standard of living. The other group (uneducated females) want a

small family due to overburden, health grounds, and mainly economic reasons in order to provide a better standard of life for their children.

References

Deutsch H (1947) (The) Psychology of women, vol 2, "motherhood." Research Book, London, p 92

Flugel JC (1960) The psycho-analytic study of the family. Hogarth Press and Institute of Psycho-analysis, London

Sexual Satisfaction: Diaphragm Versus Cervical Cap

C. C. Wheeler[1] and H. Lehfeldt[2]

[1] 310 East 46th Street Suite 12-H New York, NY 10017, USA
[2] 110 East 82nd St., New York, NY 10128, USA

This is the first report of an ongoing study carried out jointly by a clinical psychotherapist and a gynecologist investigating an erotogenic zone, the so-called Grafenberg spot (G-spot) in the anterior wall along the urethra, its occurrence, and its frequency. There is still uncertainty about the existence, or nonexistence, of the G-spot today, more than 40 years after the original publication on the subject.

These doubts may be due, in part, to contradictory statements in the medical literature. The first mention of such an erotogenic zone appeared in an article coauthored by Grafenberg and Dickinson in 1944, in which the authors assumed that this zone was present in only *some* women:

> Occasionally a patient has reported failure to reach orgasm when wearing a vaginal diaphragm, due to the principal or only zone of erogenous feeling being located along the suburethral surface of the anterior wall – an area *sometimes* [our italics] carrying prominent rugae. Because the cervix cap leaves the anterior wall uncovered, whereas the diaphragm covers it, these patients can obtain orgasm after the change is made.

By contrast, in two articles published by Grafenberg alone (1950, 1953), it is implied that this erotogenic zone is present in *every* woman:

"There is, however, a small erotogenic zone along the anterior vaginal wall corresponding to the course of the urethra."

Another contradiction with the Grafenberg-Dickinson first-published mention of this zone appears in the second edition of Dickinson's atlas *Human Sex Anatomy* (1949), accompanied by the author's detailed drawings of the text: in the illustrations of the female urethra and of the anterior vaginal wall no erotogenic zones are depicted.

This investigation was conducted to resolve whether or not reported increase in sexual satisfaction experienced by former diaphragm users who had changed to the cervical cap was in fact due to the exposure of the anterior vaginal wall which is left uncovered by the cap. For our research we devised a special questionnaire designed to compare sexual satisfaction experienced by cap wearers who had formerly used the diaphragm method. The sex history interviews included questions about the number of years of cap and diaphragm use, sexual arousal, and frequency of intercourse and of orgasm.

In addition, questions were asked concerning masturbation, primarily to identify knowledge of the impact of stimulation on arousal and orgasm, awareness of sexual functioning, range of sexual experience, and self-diagnosis of the anatomical location of erotogenic areas. Respondents were asked to list, in order of importance, their preference for sexual stimulation to orgasm from the following six anatomical genital sites: external genitals including clitoris, inside the vagina,

Sexology
Eds.: W. Eicher, G. Kockott

Table 1. Frequency of orgasm: diaphragm versus cap

	100%	75%	50%	25%	0%
Diaphragm ($N=32$):	7	8	5	1	11
Cervical cap ($N=44$):	20	13	2	0	9

anterior (front) vaginal wall, posterior (back) vaginal wall, lateral (side) vaginal walls, or simultaneous stimulation of external and internal genitals.

From a total population of 420 women fitted with the Prentif cervical cap in the clinical investigation conducted under United States Food and Drug Administration supervision (HL), 125 former diaphragm users were selected for testing. Our special questionnaire was sent to this target group: 44 women replied, 59 did not reply, and 22 questionnaires were returned because of no forewarding address.

Our sample ($N=44$) were middle-income, college-educated women seen in private practice in New York City. They were highly motivated to avoid unplanned pregnancy. Ages ranged from 23 to 42 years, with a mean of 32 years.

Findings

Contraceptive experience with the diaphragm ranged from 1 month to 12 years, with a mean of 5 years. For the cervical cap, experience ranged from 6 months to 7 years, with a mean of 4 years. Frequency of intercourse during use of the diaphragm as well as during use of the cervical cap was equally reported as one to three times per week. Sexual satisfaction with the diaphragm was stated by 47% of the respondents as ranging from "moderately dissatisfied" to "neither satisfied nor dissatisfied;" 66% of the cap users said they were "extremely satisfied." Greater sexual arousal was reported by 22 cap wearers; 14 women reported no difference in arousal observed between the two contraceptive methods; one woman reported greater arousal with the diaphragm, attributed by her to "cervical stimulation."

Only 7 women reported orgasm every time when using the diaphragm, while 20 cap users reported achieving orgasm every time when using their contraceptive. Failure to achieve orgasm while wearing either one of the two contraceptives was reported by 11 women with the diaphragm and by 9 with the cervical cap. Twelve of the respondents failed to specify orgasmic experience with the diaphragm.

Age at first orgasm through masturbation was reported as ranging from age 4 to 22, with an average at 16 years. Of the women having reported that they never achieved orgasm through masturbation, two nevertheless continued to masturbate regularly. Frequency of masturbation was reported as one to six times/week, with 40 women reporting masturbation leading to orgasm more than 90% of the time.

Within our sample of 44, a special group of 9 women reported no orgasmic experience during intercourse using either diaphragm or cap, while *always* achieving orgasm when masturbating. Not one of these nine women reported the anterior vaginal wall as the site for stimulation. Frequency of masturbation varied between daily to once per month. It is remarkable that most women in this group expressed extreme sexual satisfaction with the cervical cap, in spite of the fact that they failed to reach orgasm during intercourse. This finding regarding sexual functioning may be interesting for the physician but is familiar to the psychotherapist.

Discussion

The fact that 47% of the respondents reported moderate dissatisfaction with the diaphragm compared with 66% reporting extreme satisfaction with the cervical cap is explained by sample bias: women who were dissatisfied with the diaphragm wanted a different contraceptive and changed to the cap.

Explanations offered by the respondents for reported increased sexual arousal using the cap were: the convenience of prolonged protection, no necessity for repeatedly using chemical spermicides, less interference for the sex partner, better separation between contraception and coitus, thus increased spontaneity and uninterrupted sex, and less frequent bladder irritation.

Some women attributed their improved sexual satisfaction to factors other than change in contraceptive technique, such as choice of a different partner, improved relationship, better sexual self-awareness, and pleasuring.

Our poll of women who prefer the cap to the diaphragm as a barrier contraceptive does not indicate that this choice is due to the presence of an erotogenic zone in the anterior vaginal wall. The respondents' designation of anatomical sites in the genital area for masturbation failed to show that this zone was selected by any of the 44 women whose questionnaires were evaluated in our investigation. Additional research, including comparative sex histories and clinical observation, is needed to document the existence or nonexistence of an erotogenic area in the anterior vaginal wall along the urethra.

References

Dickinson RL (1949) Human sex anatomy, 2nd edn. Williams & Wilkins, Baltimore

Grafenberg E (1950) The role of urethra in female orgasm. Int J Sexol 3:145

Grafenberg E (1953) The role of urethra in female orgasm. In: Pillay AP, Ellis A (eds) Sex, society and the individual. Int J Sexol

Grafenberg E, Dickinson RL (1944) Conception control by plastic cervix cap. West J Surg 52:335

Barrier Contraception: A Reevaluation

J. A. Goldman

Department of Obstetrics and Gynecology, Golda Meir Medical Center, Petah-Tikva, Israel

The "pill" and IUD have been the contraceptives of choice for millions of women all over the world in recent years. The advent of these methods signaled a decline in the use of barrier methods. In view of numerous serious adverse and medical complications reported with the pill, such as the increased risk of thromboembolic disease and other side effects, as well as those associated with the IUD, many women have been deterred from their use. Furthermore, it seems that the era of the IUD, initiated by Gräfenberg and revived by Oppenheimer in the late 1950s, is unfortunately approaching its end. One of these devices, the Dalcon shield, caused problems and was consequently voluntarily removed from the market, after the manufacturers faced skyrocketing legal costs and filed a bankruptcy action in 1985 (14000 women brought suits for damages allegedly caused by this device). Unfortunately, the production of other IUDs, such as the Lippes loop, Tatum T, and Copper T has now been suspended in the United States.

In view of the foregoing, as well as the recent AIDS epidemic, it seems that the "almost forgotten" barrier methods of contraception may become popular again. We have consequently decided to reevaluate the vaginal diaphragm as well as the condom.

Material

Between 1976 and 1986, 183 women attending a family planning outpatient clinic were advised on contraception.

Table 1. Age distribution of 247 women using barrier and rhythm method contraception

Age group (years)	Total	Diaphragm	Condom	Rhythm
Below 19	54	9	27	18
20–25	61	26	24	11
26–30	53	21	20	12
31–35	44	19	15	10
36–40	23	6	9	8
42–45	12	4	3	5
Total	247	85	98	64

Sexology
Eds.: W. Eicher, G. Kockott

Table 2. Family situation of 247 women using barrier and rhythm contraception

Family situation	Total	Diaphragm		Condom		Rhythm	
		No.	%	No.	%	No.	%
Unmarried	66	22	25.9	26	26.5	18	28.1
Married	148	55	64.7	61	62.2	32	50.0
Divorced	20	5	5.9	7	7.2	8	12.5
Widowed	13	3	3.5	4	4.1	6	9.4
Total	247	85	100.0	98	100.0	64	100.0

All were highly motivated patients. Two methods of barrier contraception were studied, 85 using the diaphragm and 98 the condom. These two groups were compared with a group of 64 using the rhythm method (Tables 1, 2).

Women were seen 4–6 weeks after they began to use contraception, and at 6-month intervals during a 2-year follow-up period, unless complications or side-effects developed and checkup was necessary. The study covered a total of 5570 woman-months: diaphragm 1938 woman-months, condom 2244 woman-months, and rhythm method 1388 woman-months.

Results

Continuation rates of usage at 12 and 24 months for all three methods of contraception are as follows (Table 3): in the group using a diaphragm, 91.4% were still taking them after 12 months and 87.1% after 24 months.

In the condom group, the continuation rate after 1 year was 94.9%, and after 2 years, 87.9%. Among couples using the rhythm method, 90.6% and 79.7% reported continuation of usage after 12 and 24 months respectively. There were no statistically significant differences between the three groups.

There were rare complications (Table 4).

A small number of patients stopped using the method of contraception because of medical reasons. Eighteen women discontinued the chosen contraceptive method for unknown reasons (they failed to return for follow-up), or in order to

Table 3. Continuation rates in women using the diaphragm, condom, and rhythm method

Months	Diaphragm		Condom		Rhythm	
	No.	%	No.	%	No.	%
1	85	100	98	100	64	100
6	84	98.8	96	98.0	61	95.3
12	80	94.1	93	94.9	58	90.6
18	77	90.6	92	93.9	54	84.4
24	74	87.1	86	87.8	51	79.7

Table 4. Cumulative events during a 24-month period in 247 women using two barrier methods (diaphragm and condom) as compared with the rhythm method

Event	Total	Diaphragm	Condom	Rhythm
Urinary tract infection	2	1	–	1
Vaginitis	6	2	1	3
Pelvic inflammatory disease	–	–	–	–
Other side effects	3	1	2	–
Reported cessation of contraception				
Medical reasons	2	1	1	–
Personal reasons	18	6	5	7
Pregnancy	16	4	6	6
Woman-months of use	5570	1938	2244	1388
Failure rate (PEARL index)	–	2.48	3.21	5.19

use a different method. Nevertheless, most women were disciplined and well motivated.

Pregnancies occurred in 16 women during 5570 woman-months. There were four in the diaphragm group, six in the condom group, and six in the group of the couples not using any contraceptive.

The Pearl Index was:

Diaphragm	–	2.48
Condom	–	3.21
Rhythm methods	–	5.19

Comment

Vaginal barrier contraceptives are among the oldest forms of birth control, which have been partially abandoned since the introduction of the pill and IUD.

The advent of the latter signaled a decline in the use of barrier methods and growing popularity of the newer methods. Of 52% of married women in the United States reporting use of either diaphragm or condom in 1955, the figure dropped to 32% in 1965, 20% in 1970, and 15% in 1975. Nevertheless, the barrier methods will become more popular as contraindications and complications of the pill and IUD become obvious, and are the concern of the public. The former are not associated with any serious side effects. In spite of their reduced effectiveness, they appear to offer a number of significant advantages, such as their ease of use and lack of intervention in the biological processes. In addition, they achieve a degree of protection against some sexually transmitted diseases, especially gonorrhea, herpes virus, *Chlamydia trachomatis*, and AIDS. Furthermore, the barrier methods of contraception are apparently still widely used, despite the fact that their use-effectiveness does not reach the level of the pill and IUD. The inconvenience of the former may be more acceptable to many couples than the unwanted risks to health or fertility associated with the more effective contraceptive methods. They are, in fact, most suitable for youngsters who are not yet ready to commit themselves to a continuous method of contraception, as well as to the group of women approaching their forties and unwilling to use the pill or IUD.

While none of the two prescribed methods of contraception, as well as the control group of rhythm users proved to be ideal, results are good, most probably due to the fact that all our patients were well motivated and cooperative, and were counseled on the use of contraceptive at their own request. The popularity of the condom in the Federal Republic of Germany comes only after the pill, with 26% users, and with identical use in the United States. In Japan 70% of men use the condom.

Conclusion

1. Barrier methods of contraception are reasonably effective, acceptable, and safe methods of contraception in all age groups.
2. Couples who are established users of barrier methods, especially youngsters and those approaching middle age, should not be encouraged to change to a more modern method of birth control with its attendant risks.
3. These means of birth control have no systemic side effects, and have no medical contraindications to their use.
4. The trend toward barrier method is extremely important given the current disenchantment with other techniques. In view of the present state of affairs with the IUD, it is important that public education campaigns be carried out, pointing out the safety of these agents, and the relatively high rates of effectiveness, such as in this series of highly motivated patients, that can be attained when they are properly and consistently used.
5. Finally, in view of the AIDS scare, the condom will no doubt regain its popularity!

The Contraceptive Effectiveness of the Diaphragm and Its Effect on the Sexual Relationship

R. Schicketanz [1] and G. Döring [2]

[1] Gerlichstr. 12, 8000 München 60, FRG
[2] Hechendorf Seeleite 9, 8031 Seefeld 2, FRG

The data about the contraceptive effectiveness of the diaphragm vary widely within the medical literature. The combination of a diaphragm with a spermicide increases the effectiveness. Therefore most publications deal with this combination. Contraceptive effectiveness with the use of the diaphragm (in combination with a spermicide) depends greatly on the method of data collection and on the chosen population. Socioeconomic as well as educational factors influence the application and handling of this contraceptive method.

Therefore widely varying factors of contraceptive effectiveness result from different studies. Long-term studies on a large scale have been conducted especially in Great Britain, Sweden, and the United States. They show failure rates of 1.9–34. The number of unintentional pregnancies on a 100 years application base varies between 2 and 3 according to more recent publications. Vessey and Wiggins (UK, 1974) report a failure rate of 2.4. The study by Lane, Arceo, and Sobrero (USA, 1976) finds contraceptive effectiveness to range between 1.9 and 2.2. In this study 80% of the women were under 30. The lack of such data from the Federal Republic of Germany initiated this study.

Acquirement of Method and Material

A questionnaire concerning the use and effect of diaphragms resulted from data gained in Pro Familia (Munich), a Family Planning Clinic. Pro Familia is a member of International Planned Parenthood Federation (IPPF). The questionnaire contains the following subjects: the previous contraceptive career of the clients, getting to know and using the diaphragm method. The study also deals with the reported experiences and effects whether positive or negative. It also indicates the months of exposure and the number of unintentional pregnancies. An attempt has been made to record in detail application and the method of handling in the month when unintentional conception occurred. Also questions were asked concerning the experience of the partners with this kind of contraception, concerning the man's, woman's, as well as both partners' future desire for children, etc.

The study was advertised in woman's lib journals, in Pro Familia magazines, and in local papers in Munich. In addition branches of Pro Familia distributed questionnaires all over the Federal Republic of Germany. It was also laid out in some libraries within the FRG as well as in some pharmacies and doctor's offices in Munich.

Sexology
Eds.: W. Eicher, G. Kockott

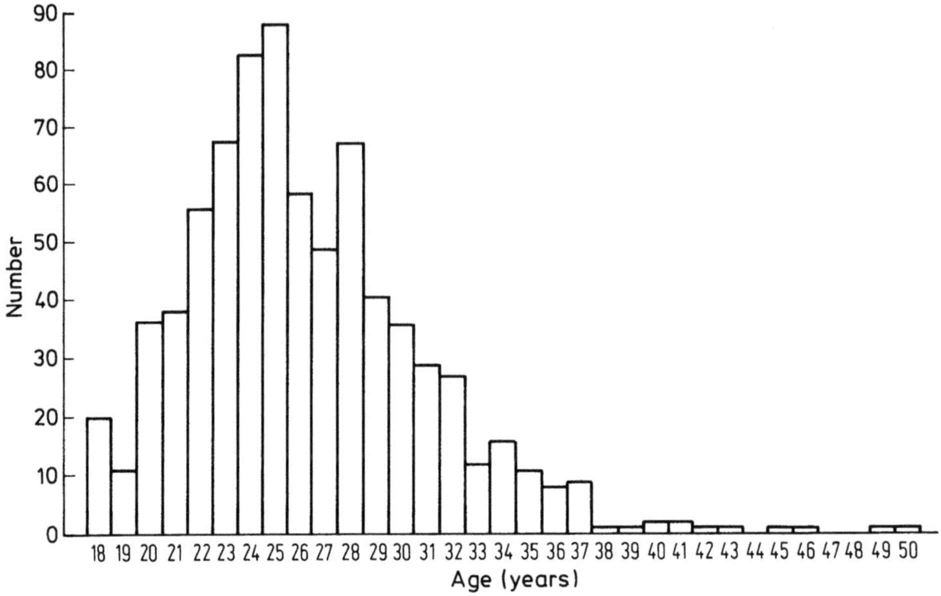

Fig. 1. Age distribution among 778 diaphragm users

Table 1. The education level among diaphragm users ($n=778$)

Education	Number of women	Percentage
School	12	1.54
High School	132	16.97
College	363	46.66
Studied	268	34.45
Not specified	3	0.39

Table 2. Marital status of the diaphragm users ($n=778$)

Status	Number of women	Percentage
Not married	643	82.65
Married	99	12.72
Divorced	34	4.34
Widowed	1	0.13
Not specified	1	0.13

A total of 3000 questionnaires were distributed from spring 1984 through the end of the year. Eight hundred and nine questionnaires were returned of which 31 could not be evaluated. They had been uncompletely answered or they described less than 5 months of application. Following the paper of Vessey and Wiggins the period of application was limited to a minimum of five menstrual cycles. The age of the participants had to be more than 18 years. The questionnaires could be returned anonymously to Pro Familia, Munich. Questionnaires were available for statistical evaluation from 778 women whose age ranged from 18 to 50 years. Figure 1 shows the age distribution, Table 1 shows the education of the diaphragm users, and Table 2 shows their personal status.

According to Fig. 1, the age-group of 22–28 years was most frequent, and 79.43% of the women were under 30 years of age.

There are some striking characteristics among the diaphragm users in this study: 81.11% of the women have a higher education, 82.65% are not married. (89.20% live in a stable partnership, and only 10.80% live as singles.)

Only 37.15% live together as a couple sharing one home. In total, 778 women had 151 children and there were 73 miscarriages.

Acceptability of the Contraceptive Diaphragm in Combination with a Spermicide from the Random Sample ($n=778$)

Six hundred and forty-seven women (83.16% of the random sample) reported to be content with the contraceptive diaphragm; 96.14% of the women declared the insertion of the diaphragm and the touching of their own genitals as positive; 95.76% of the partners accept this kind of contraception within the random sample; and 66.45% of the partners had been involved in applying this method.

The high acceptability concerning the use of diaphragms combined with a spermicide, with the positive attitudes of the male partners toward this contraception, indicates that this factor itself is a prior condition for using the contraceptive diaphragm at all, so as in other contraceptive methods.

Contraceptive Effectiveness of the Diaphragm

The Pearl index reflects the failure rate per 100 woman-years of use of a contraceptive method, i.e., the number of pregnancies in 100 woman-years at risk. We counted all conceptions as failures when caused by improper use. The diaphragm in combination with a spermicide was applied during 19101 cycles (months of exposure) with 69 pregnancies. The Pearl formula in this case $= \frac{69 \times 12 \times 100}{19101} = 4.33$. We obtained a failure rate of 4.33 from a total of 778 women, diaphragm users aged from 18 to 50 years.

Influence on Failure Rate

Table 4 shows two age groups: 18–29 years and 30–50 years. The failure rate among older women is lower than that among younger women. There is an influence on age.

Further splitting of age groups does not report the influence of age more clearly among these diaphragm users.

Table 3. Dependence of the failure rate on age ($n=778$)

Age groups	Number of women	Months of exposure	Pregnancies at risk	Failure rate per 100 woman-years
1–29	618	13167	52	4.74
30–50	160	5934	17	3.43

Table 4. Quality of information concerning the diaphragm and its failure rate ($n=768$)

Quality of information	Number of women	Months of exposure	Number of pregnancies	Failure rate per 100 woman-years
Good	592	14069	44	3.75
Satisfying	126	2924	14	5.74
Nonsatisfying	50	1678	10	7.14

Table 5. Presentation of the failure rate depending on user instruction being available or not ($n=778$)

Instruction	Number of women	Months of exposure	Number of pregnancies	Failure rate per 100 woman-years
Instruction available	678	16217	55	4.07
No instruction available	91	2622	12	5.48
Not specified	9	262	2	–

Quality of Information and Instruction, How To Use the Diaphragm

It was necessary to eliminate 10 diaphragm users with 430 months of exposure and 1 pregnancy. They did not respond distinctively. The information about application of the diaphragm could be rated as "good," "satisfying," or "nonsatisfying."

This partition of the sample into three different groups shows a significant decrease in failure rate depending on the quality of given instruction on how to use the diaphragm. It had been suspected that there was an influence on proper application of the diaphragm whether user instructions were available or not.

The data in Table 5 show clearly that the failure rate for women having "no instruction available" is higher than for well-informed women.

Women Who Had Achieved Their Desired Family Size Compared with Those Who Wanted To Get Pregnant in the Future

Table 6 presents the failure rates in women who had achieved their desired family size and those women who wanted more children in the future or did not know how to decide.

The data in Table 6 show a low failure rate in diaphragm users with completed family planning. Women among the diaphragm users who have future intentions of becoming pregnant have a higher failure rate per 100 woman-years of use.

Table 6. Failure rate depending on whether diaphragm users had their completed family planning

Family planning	Number of women	Months of exposure	Number of pregnancies	Failure rate per 100 woman-years
Completed	109	3285	8	2.92
Perhaps	284	7073	25	4.22
Want to get pregnant in future	372	8048	35	5.22
Not specified	13	695	1	–

Table 7. Failure rate of diaphragm depending on the partner's desire to have children ($n = 778$)

Family planning	Number of partners of the diaphragm users	Months of use of the diaphragm	Number of pregnancies	Failure rate per 100 woman-years
Completed	267	7142	18	3.03
Perhaps	226	5320	22	4.97
Wants to have a child more	201	4346	16	4.42
Not specified	84	2293	13	–

Couples in which the partner does not want children in the future, prevent pregnancies most effectively. Where the partner is undecided there is a negative effect on the failure rate.

Failure Rate and Duration of Use of the Diaphragm

In examining the relationship between failure rate and duration of use, the latter has been subdivided into a duration of use of 5 months to 2 years, 2–5 years, and more than 5 years.

Table 8. Failure rate of the diaphragm depending on use and duration ($n = 778$)

Duration of diaphragm use	Number of women	Months of exposure	Number of pregnancies	Failure rate per 100 woman-years
5–23 months	464	5349	28	6.28
24–59 months	257	9115	35	4.61
60 months and more	57	4637	6	1.55

Analysis of our random sample shows that application safety of the diaphragm increases with duration of use. The Pearl index of women having used the diaphragm for more than 5 years is only 1.55. This result represents the lowest failure rate per 100 woman-years of the whole study.

Summary

Seven hundred and seventy-eight women participated in our study using the diaphragm with spermicide as their contraceptive method through a total of 19101 months of exposure. Sixty-nine unintended pregnancies occurred during that period. This results in a Pearl index of 4.33. According to the details provided about the circumstances during the cycle of conception, only 26 unintended pregnancies occurred when the diaphragm with spermicide was properly used. Thirty-nine women reported improper use during the cycle of conception: for example, they did not use a spermicide, they left the diaphragm for less than 6 h after sexual intercourse in the vagina, or they had unprotected intercourse (not using any contraceptive method) on one or more days in the middle of the cycle. A more proper use and fit may cause a higher contraceptive effectiveness so that a failure rate per 100 woman-years lower than 4.33 Pearl index of this study should be expected.

The different detailed examinations demonstrate that certain factors influence the reliability of the diaphragm.

Advantages concerning a low failure rate are:

- Higher age
- Detailed information and instruction on proper use
- Family completion
- Long duration of using the diaphragm

Taking into account the factors which could be influenced by doctors – information and instruction – the failure rate in using the diaphragm should be less than given in this study.

With a failure rate of 2 to 4 – confirmed also by other publications – the contraceptive effectiveness of the diaphragm with spermicide is of the same order as that of the condom.

Doctors should mention and recommend this alternative as being a completely risk-free method concerning health which is used only when needed – especially for persons who cannot use hormonal contraception or where IUDs are declined or contraindicated.

References

Balog J, Langhauser C, Rhine I (1977) Recent trend in preference of contraceptive methods: pills down, diaphragm on rise. Contraception 15:553

Bernstein GS (1974) Use of diaphragm with spermicidal agent. Med Asp Hum Sex 8:187

Döring GK (1983) Empfängnisverhütung, 9th edn. Thieme, Stuttgart

Döring GK, Schicketanz R (1986) Über die Zuverlässigkeit des Scheidendiaphragma als kontrazeptive Methode. Geburtshilfe u. Frauenheilkunde 46:33

Herms V (1984) Nicht hormonale Kontrazeption. Sexualmedizin 13/5:248, 13/6:343
Huggins GR (1977) Contraceptive use and subsequent fertility. Fert Steril 28:603
Lane ME, Arceo R, Sobrero AJ (1976) Successful use of diaphragm and jelly in a young population. Fam Plan Perspect 8:81
Population Reports (1976) Barrier methods, the diaphragm and other intravaginal barriers. Pop Inform Program, Baltimore, Series H/4, p 57
Population Reports (1984) New developements in vaginal contraception. Pop Inform Program, Baltimore, Series H/7:157
Prill HJ (1968) Motivation und Einstellung der Frau zur Kontrazeption. In: Kepp R, Koester H (eds) Empfängnisverhütung aus Verantwortung. Thieme, Stuttgart, p 94
Schicketanz R (1985) Das Scheidendiaphragma – seine Wirksamkeit in der Anwendung – eine partnerschaftliche Methode der Empfängnisregelung. Inaug. Diss., München 1985
Sobrero AJ (1973) Vaginal diaphragms. Med Aspects Hum Sex 7/3:23
Tietze C, Lewit S (1967) Comparison of 3 contraceptive methods: diaphragm with jelly/cream, vaginal foam and jelly/cream alone. J Res 3:295
Tietze C (1971) Ranking of contraceptive methods by levels of effectiveness. Adv Planned Parenthood 6/1:117
Vessey M, Wiggins P (1974) Use-effectiveness of the diaphragm in a selected Family Planning Clinic Population in the United Kingdom. Contraception 9:15
Weiß S, Pavlat-Meier R (1985) Neue Erfahrungen mit einer alten Methode. Sexualmedizin 14/2:85, 14/3:135

Salivary Luteinizing Hormone Determination for Large-Scale Testing of the Validity of So-called Natural Family Planning Methods

K. Loewit [1], A. Ortlieb [1], G. Wolfram [2], and R. Widhalm [2]

[1] Institute for Medical Biology and Genetics, University of Innsbruck, Austria, Schöpfstraße 41, 6020 Innsbruck
[2] Institute for Marriage and Family, Spiegelgasse 3, 1010 Vienna

Introduction

So-called natural family planning methods (NFPs) – we prefer the less misleading and more descriptive term of "self-observation methods" (SOMs) – are still a matter of controversy (Döring 1985). Thus a more rational understanding and attitude regarding their physiological foundations, advantages, and disadvantages seems desirable. For this purpose we have introduced a noninvasive method of hormonal ovulation detection, the radioimmunological determination of salivary luteinizing hormone (LH), in order to enable more large-scale studies to be carried out without putting an undue burden upon the volunteering women. It was also shown that the salivary LH peak may serve as a suitable indicator of ovulation. The overall correlation of salivary LH to serum LH was found to be highly significant ($r=0.788$, $n=60$, $P<0.0001$) (Loewit et al. 1985) and the salivary LH peak was centered ± 0.5 days around the time of ovulation in 9/15 (60%) and ± 1.5 days in all of 15 sonographically monitored ovulations (Loewit et al. 1987). With this methodology at hand we have started to evaluate the theoretical reliability of SOM parameters and rules. Preliminary results concerning the correlation of cervical mucus pattern and basal body temperature (BBT) with the salivary LH peak in around 270 cycles so far and of the respective variations of the cervix uteri in 115 cycles are reported here.

Participants and Methods

As shown in Table 1, 75 healthy women aged between 21 and 42 years, mean 28.1 ± 5.3 years, supplied 273 cycles of an average length of 28.0 ± 3.8 days. The relevant salivary LH peak occurred between the 9th and 23rd day of the cycles with a mean of 14.6 ± 3.6 days. Thirty percent of the women participated with only 1 cycle, 60% with 2–6 cycles, individual women, however, with 12, 17, 18, and even 33 cycles. All participants were either already experienced in SOM or were especially instructed for the study. They recorded and charted cervical mu-

Table 1. Participants and cycles

No. of volunteers	Age (years)	No. of cycles	Cycle length	Day of salivary LH peak
75	28.1 ± 5.3 (21–42)	273	28.0 ± 3.8 (16–37)	14.6 ± 3.6 (9–23)

cus quality and BBT, measured rectally with a mercury thermometer, in the usual way. Some also examined their cervix for cyclic changes according to the criteria of "soft and open" (s/o), "hard and closed" (h/c), or intermediate states respectively. In addition, right after taking BBT, all of the volunteers collected daily samples of 3–5 ml of so-called early morning saliva during the midfollicular to the early luteal phase of the cycle and kept them frozen in household refrigerators until delivery to the laboratory. From these samples LH was determined after the end of the cycle by a modification of a serum-LH-radioimmunoassay yielding a tenfold increase in sensitivity as described earlier (Kraft et al. 1984). LH values exceeding the mean + one standard deviation (SD) were tentatively considered as peaks and correlated with SOM data.

Results and Discussion

Cervical Mucus Pattern

In 270 cycles with the mucus symptom present the beginning of mucus secretion as judged from either a feeling of moisture in the genital region instead of dryness or from the appearance of mucus at the vaginal opening was noted between 10 days before and 2 days after the salivary LH peak (day 0), without a clear maximum on any day as shown in Fig. 1. Thus, the beginning of mucus secretion or its first observation respectively show great individual variations, the bulk of the observations (73%) occurring on days −7 to −2 in almost equal percentages. Considering the 7 days preceding ovulation as potentially fertile, the beginning of the mucus symptom cannot serve as a marker for the beginning of the fertile period, occurring too late in 86% of the cycles. This is even more true for the beginning of "fertile-type mucus," which appeared or was recorded between 8 days before and 5 days after the LH peak, showing maximum values between days −3 and 0, as is well known from the literature (for review see Frank and Raith 1985). The wide range in noticing such first mucus symptoms not only reflects a great physiological variability but also problems of interpretation, which obviously do not exist to the same extent in recognizing the peak symptom or maximum *Spinnbarkeit* of the mucus around the time of ovulation. Maximum *Spinnbarkeit* peaks at day 0, and 80% of all peak symptoms were observed within ±2 days of the salivary LH peak, thus confirming the close parallelism of this symptom with the LH peak (Billings et al. 1980; Billings 1981; Freundl et al. 1984; Moghissi et al. 1972; Moghissi 1980; Morishita et al. 1979; Templeton et al. 1982). Nevertheless in 31 out of 222 cycles (14%) the peak symptom occurred 3–6 days after day 0, thus eventually postponing the 1st day of elevated BBT, which by definition excludes the presence of fertile-type mucus. The last day of cervical mucus observation, occurring in 40% of the cycles in the still fertile time, ranges from day −6 to day +10, with a small maximum 2 and 3 days after the LH peak, and thus is not a helpful sign in any way.

Cyclic Changes of the Cervix Uteri

Self-examination of the cervix reveals a characteristic pattern of changes which like the corresponding changes of the cervical mucus depend on estrogen and ges-

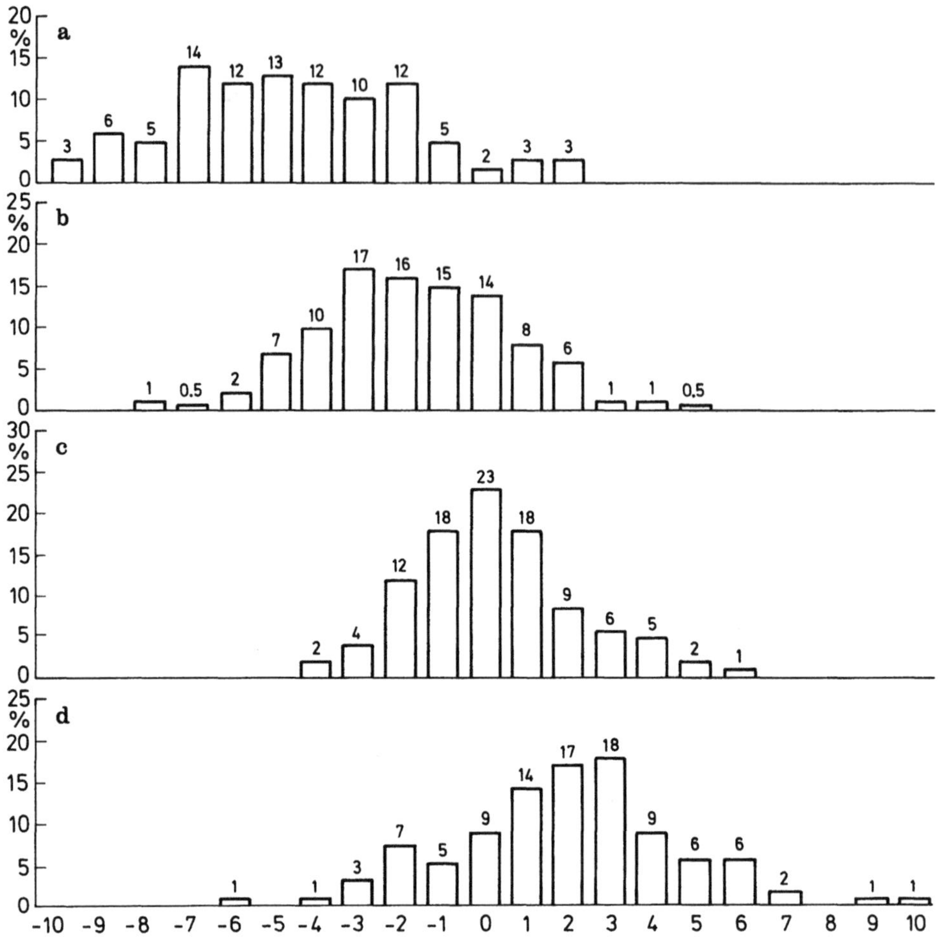

Fig. 1. Cervical mucus pattern in comparison with the salivary LH peak (day 0). *A*, first day of mucus observation (wet days) ($n=270$); *B*, first day of fertile-type mucus (*Spinnbarkeit*) ($n=222$); *C*, peak symptom of fertile-type mucus ($n=222$); *D*, last day of mucus observation ($n=270$)

tagen levels. Thus, the cervix is in a low position and feels hard with its orifice closed in the early follicular phase of the cycle. Toward ovulation with rising amounts of estrogen it becomes softer, and the os cervicis opens up slowly and becomes more difficult to reach, because of a higher position of the cervix. After the estrogens have fallen and gestagens increase, i.e., normally after ovulation, the cervix changes back to hard and closed and low within 1–2 days. This change is more pronounced and easier to recognize than the preovulatory transition (Frank and Raith 1985; Keefe 1962; Loewit et al. to be published; Rötzer 1978). Figure 2 shows this metamorphosis of the cervix in relation to the salivary LH peak.

The first observation of a fertile-type (s/o) cervix including intermediate stages shows a wide range from day −10 to +2 with only a small maximum 3 and 4 days before the LH peak. In over 90% of all cycles this symptom occurred during the possibly fertile time and thus cannot serve as an indicator of the beginning

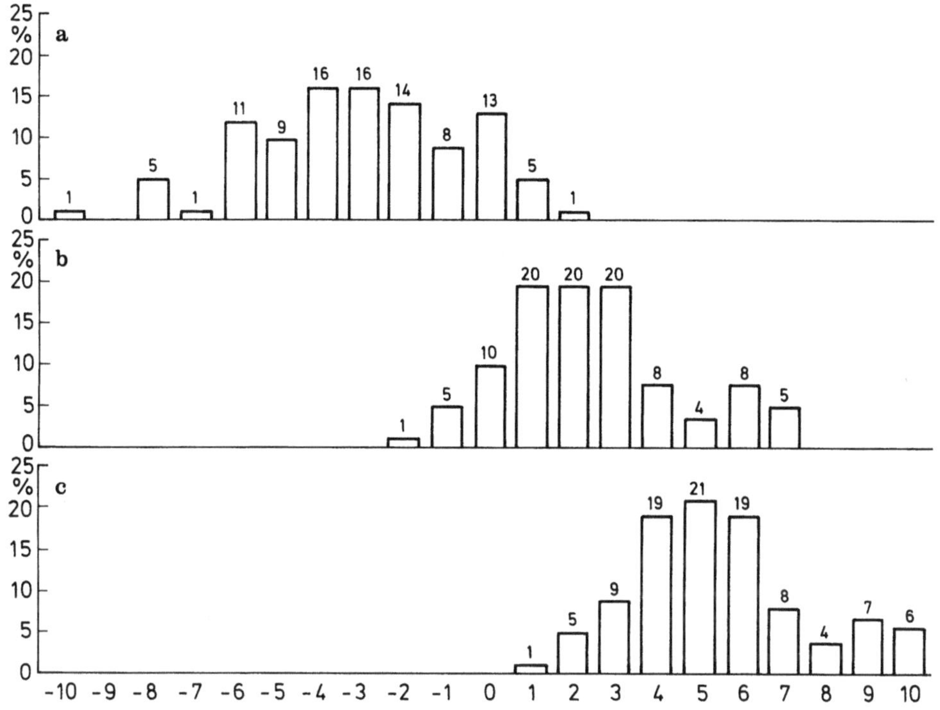

Fig. 2. Cyclic changes of the cervix uteri compared with the salivary LH peak (day 0). *A*, first day of soft/open cervix ($n=86$); *B*, first day (again) of hard/closed cervix ($n=10$); *C*, fourth day of hard/closed cervix ($n=108$)

of the fertile period. The 1st day of hard and closed cervix after ovulation – not including intermediate stages – occurred between days -2 and $+7$, showing maximum values 1–3 days after the LH peak in 60% of the cycles but delayed beyond day $+4$ in 25%.

Basal Body Temperature

As can be seen from Fig. 3 the dip or nadir of BBT reaches its maximum values at day 0 occurring in 60% of the cycles within ± 1 day and in 80% within ± 2 days of the salivary LH peak. It ranges however from day -6 to day $+4$ and therefore can serve as hint to the time of ovulation, but can not pinpoint this event, as is well known from the literature (Baumann 1981; Döring 1967, 1985, 1986; Moghissi et al. 1972; Moghissi 1976; Morris et al. 1976; Templeton et al. 1982). The 1st day of elevated BBT, i.e., a temperature reading above the six preceding ones with no more mucus of the fertile type present (Rötzer 1968, 1986), occurred between days -2 and $+7$ as did the first hard and closed cervix. Maximum values were found at days $+1$ and $+2$ in accordance with the fact that the typical and sudden rise in BBT takes place 1–2 days after ovulation (Döring 1986). However, in 42% of the cycles the first rise in BBT occurred between 3 and

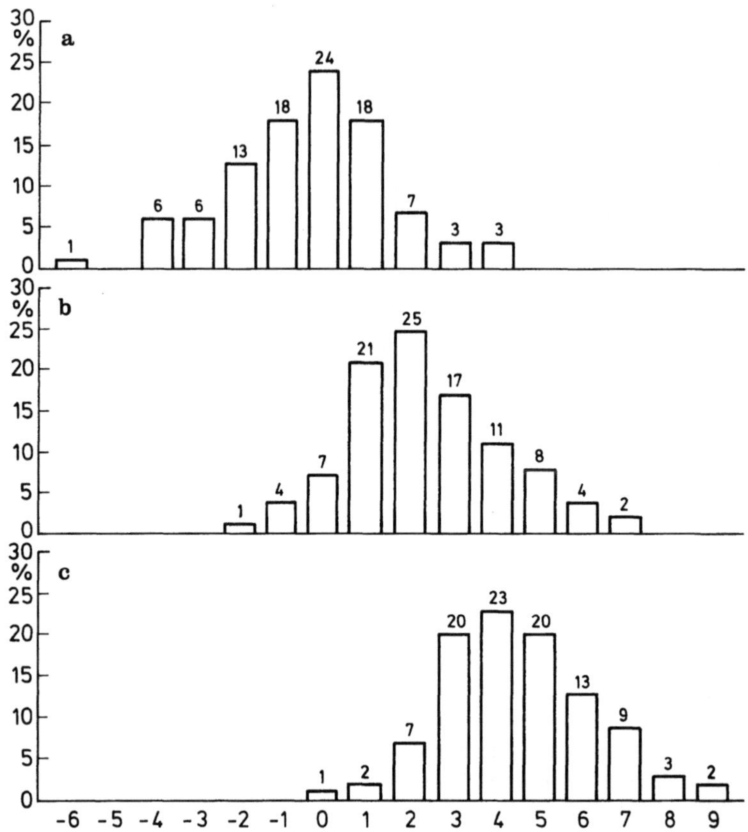

Fig. 3. Cyclic variation of body temperature in comparison with salivary LH peak (day 0). *A*, nadir of BBT ($n=269$); *B*, first day of elevated BBT ($n=273$); *C*, third day of elevated BBT ($n=264$)

7 days after the salivary LH peak, thus again demonstrating the interindividual variability of endocrine functions and their interrelation with external influences in seemingly healthy women.

Indicators of the Postovulatory Infertile Period

As has been shown SOMs are unable to indicate the beginning of the preovulatory fertile time early enough for contraceptive purposes. They enable us, however, to recognize the beginning of the postovulatory safe period. According to SOM rules infertility begins on the 4th day (or the evening of the 4th day) after the mucus peak symptom (M4) (Billings 1981; Billings et al. 1980; Rötzer 1978, 1986) or on the 4th day of hard and closed cervix (C4), as we have recently reported (Loewit et al. 1987, to be published), or on the 3rd day or evening of the 3rd day of elevated BBT (BBT3) as has long been established and empirically proven (Döring 1954, 1983; Population Reports 1981; Rötzer 1968, 1986). Figure 4 relates these rules to the salivary LH peak: M4 occurred in 6% (13/222 cycles) on the fertile days 0 and +1, C4 in only 1% (1/108 cycles) and BBT3 in

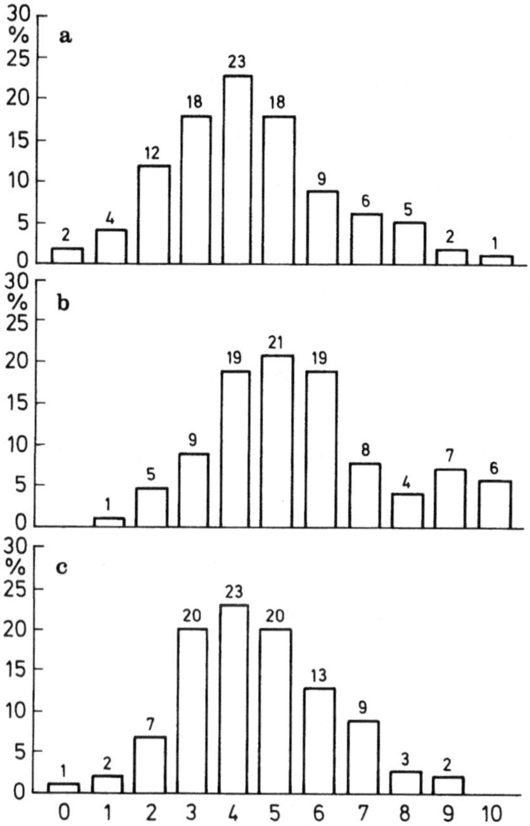

Fig. 4. Indications of the postovulatory infertile period in comparison with the salivary LH peak (day 0). *A*, fourth day after the peak – symptom of cervical mucus ($n = 222$); *B*, fourth day of hard/closed cervix uteri ($n = 108$); *C*, third day of elevated BBT ($n = 264$)

3% (9/264 cycles) in this study. Also the 2nd day after the salivary LH peak, theoretically, still has a remote possibility of being fertile. M4 occurs on day +2 in 12%, C4 in 5%, and BBT3 in 7%, thus reaching theoretical reliabilities of 82% for M4, 94% for C4, and of at least 90% for BBT3 as in the study by Freundl et al. (1984). C4 therefore is as reliable an indicator of infertility as is BBT3, while the 3rd day of hard and closed cervix would have a similar theoretical risk of 6% +9% as has M4 (6% + 12%), which of course cannot be directly translated into unwanted pregnancies. Unfortunately, high reliability is still paid for by an undue extention of the seemingly fertile period: M4 in 41% of 222 cycles occurred beyond day +4, C4 in 65% of 108 cycles and BBT3 in 47% of 264 cycles, in some cases even as late as days 9 and 10.

This study shows that M4 is the least reliable marker of the beginning of the postovulatory infertile period. It confirms again the reliability of BBT3 and introduces as a new "rule of thumb" the 4th day of hard and closed cervix in double control with BBT3, whatever comes first.

References

Baumann JE (1981) Basal body temperature: unreliable method of ovulation detection. Fertil Steril 36:729–733

Billings JJ, Billings EL, Catarinich M (1980) Atlas of the ovulation method, 4th edn. Advocate, Melbourne
Billings JJ (1981) Cervical mucus: the biological marker of fertility and infertility. Int J Fertil 26:182–195
Döring GK (1986) Die Temperaturmethode zur Empfängnisverhütung, 1st edn, Thieme, Stuttgart
Döring GK (1985) Physiologie und Pathologie der Basaltemperatur bei der Frau und ihre diagnostische Bedeutung. Fortschr Med 83:885–887
Döring GK (1967) Über die Zuverlässigkeit der Temperaturmethode zur Empfängnisverhütung. Dtsch Med Wochensch 92:1055–1061
Döring GK (1983) Empfängnisverhütung, 9th edn. Thieme, Stuttgart
Döring GK (1985) Foreword. In: Frank P, Raith E (eds) Natürliche Familienplanung. Springer, Berlin Heidelberg New York Tokyo
Frank P, Raith E (1985) Natürliche Familienplanung. Springer, Berlin Heidelberg New York Tokyo
Freundl G, Suberg D, Flynn AM, Diemer HP (1984) Natürliche Familienplanung (Symptothermale Methode) und objektive Ovulationsparameter – eine Pilotstudie. Geburtshilfe Frauenheilkd 44:368–374
Keefe EF (1962) Self-observation of the cervix to distinguish days of possible fertility. Bull Sloane Hosp Wom 8:129–136
Keefe EF (1979) The cervix as a guide to control of conception. Int symp on natural family planning. Tokyo 1979
Kraft HG, Fischer-Korp C, Loewit K (1984) A radioimmunological method for LH measurement in saliva. Contraceptive Delivery Systems 5:99
Loewit K, Kraft HG, Ortlieb A (1985) Measurement of LH in saliva: a new approach to ovulation detection. In: Runnebaum B, Rabe T, Kiesel L (eds) Future aspects in contraception, part 2. MTP Press, Boston The Hague Dordrecht Lancaster 1985
Loewit K, Ortlieb A, Kraft HG, Widhalm R, Wolfram G (1987) Wie erkennt man die „sicheren“ Tage? Sexualmedizin 16:52–57
Loewit K, Huber J, Ortlieb A, Widhalm R, Wolfram G (to be published) Speichel LH als Ovulationsindikator: Vergleich zwischen Speichel-LH, Serum-LH und Ultraschallbefund. Geburtshilfe Frauenheilkd
Loewit K, Wolfram G, Ortlieb A, Widhalm R (to be published) Speichel-LH als Ovulationsindikator: zur Wertigkeit der Autopalpation der Zervix uteri für die Erkennung der fruchtbaren und unfruchtbaren Zyklustage. Geburtshilfe Frauenheilkd
Moghissi KS, Syner FN, Evans TN (1972) A composite picture of the menstrual cycle. Am J Obstet Gynecol 114:405–418
Moghissi KS (1976) Accuracy of basal body temperature for ovulation detection. Fertil Steril 27:1415–1421
Moghissi KS (1980) Prediction and detection of ovulation. Fertil Steril 34:89–98
Morishita H, Hashimoto T, Mitani H, Tanaka T, Higuchi K, Ozasa T (1979) Cervical mucus and prediction of the time of ovulation. Gynecol Obstet Invest 10:157–162
Morris NM, Underwood LE, Easterling WJR (1976) Temporal relationship between basal body temperature nadir and luteinizing hormone surge in normal women. Fertil Steril 27:780–783
Population Reports (1981) Periodic abstinence: how well do new approaches work? Series I, No. 3. Population information program. Johns Hopkins University, Baltimore
Rötzer J (1968) Erweiterte Basaltemperaturmessung und Empfängnisregelung. Arch Gynäkol 206:195–214
Rötzer J (1978) Sympto-thermal method and family planning. Acta Med Rom 16:339–348
Rötzer J (1986) Natürliche Geburtenregelung, 16th edn. Herder, Vienna
Templeton AA, Penney GC, Lees MM (1982) Relation between the luteinizing hormone peak, the nadir of the basal body temperature and the cervical mucus score. Br J Obstet Gynecol 89:985–988
WHO (1983) Temporal relationship between indices of the fertile period. Fertil Steril 39:647–655

Temperature Computers

K. Loewit [1], H. G. Kraft [1], A. Ortlieb [1], and G. Wolfram [2]

[1] Institute for Medical Biology and Genetics, University of Innsbruck, Austria, Schöpfstraße 41, 6020 Innsbruck
[2] Institute for Marriage and Family, Spiegelgasse 3, 1010, Vienna

Introduction

Behavioral methods of conception control or contraception are being met with increasing interest (WHO 1981) and constitute a growing – though still very small – segment of family planning methods: In recent surveys in Austria and the Federal Republic of Germany, 2.8% reported the use of basal body temperature (BBT) (Münz 1987) and 3.9% the use of natural family planning (NFP), with 14% stating their intention to practise such methods in the future (Döring 1986 b). Contrary to previous calendar methods (Knaus 1933; Ogino 1932), modern self-observation methods (SOM) like the symptothermal method (STM) (Rötzer 1986) are safe and reliable (Döring 1986 a; Frank and Raith 1985; Rice 1981; Rötzer 1968, 1978 a, 1978 b, 1986).

However, they still suffer from two major handicaps: their generally bad reputation within the medical profession dating from former unreliable attempts of calculating the fertile days of the cycle and intrinsic methodological problems, especially regarding large-scale practicability and acceptability, in particular concerning sexual abstinence. Therefore in regard to professional confidence in SOM, basic research into their theoretical foundations is still necessary to arrive at a more knowledgeable and rational approach and, in regard to their practicability, methodological improvements would be highly desirable. Thus, several devices have been designed using computer technology in order to facilitate the practicability of SOM in relieving women or couples from reading thermometers, drawing and interpreting graphs and charts, calculating fertile days, observing and correlating various symptoms of fertility, etc. Only some of these fertility indicators are temperature computers. Lately, two of them, "Anne" and "Rite Time," have been criticized for poor performance by Döring and Daucher (1986). Recently, "baby comp," a promising temperature computer with a unique mathematical program, has been introduced (Dtsch. Apoth. Z. 1987) and is currently being tested. Other instruments measure tissue (e.g., vaginal) impedance, cervical mucus viscosity, or salivary electrical resistance in order to detect or even to predict ovulation (Rabe 1985; Schenker 1985; Albrecht 1985).

In an attempt to further study the physiological foundations of SOM, we have introduced a noninvasive method of hormonal ovulation detection by measuring luteinizing hormone (LH) in saliva (Kraft 1984) in order to accumulate a large body of data without putting an undue burden upon the volunteers. These studies showed that salivary LH was significantly correlated with serum LH ($r = 0.788$, $n = 60$, $P < 0.0001$) (Loewit 1985) and that it was also a suitable indicator of ovu-

Sexology
Eds.: W. Eicher, G. Kockott

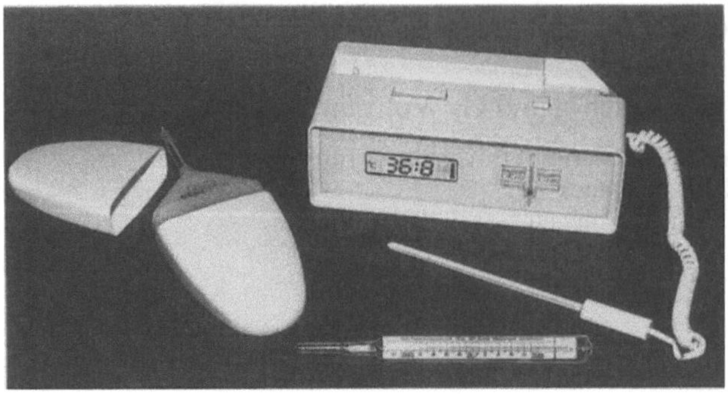

Fig. 1. The temperature computers "Rite Time" and "Bioself 110"

lation, as judged from simultaneous determination of serum LH and sonography of the maturing and rupturing follicle in 15 cycles: all salivary LH peaks were found ±1.5 days (60% ±0.5 days) around the time of ovulation (Loewit 1987).

Within the framework of these studies two temperature computers, "Rite Time" (RT) and "Bioself 110" (BS), were tested for their performance and reliability (Fig. 1).

Participants, Methods, and Devices

Participants

Twenty-three women, 16 nulliparae and 7 parae, average age 27.0±5.7 years, range 22–42 years, volunteered for this study and each contributed between 1 and 17, on average 3, of the 84 cycles studied. The participants were either already experienced in SOM, mainly the STM, or individually instructed and were highly motivated. Almost two-thirds were either engaged in or had completed an academic training. Thus, this group is not representative of the population in general; however, it reflects the predominance of higher educated women in the small segment practising SOM in Austria and the Federal Republic of Germany (Münz 1987; Döring 1986b) and is considered very suitable for basic research purposes.

In addition to recording and charting their BBT and cervical mucus pattern in the usual way, the volunteers also used either one of the two temperature computers and kept records of the data displayed. Immediately afterwards (i.e., before tooth-brushing, eating, drinking, etc.) they collected several milliliters of so-called early morning saliva, starting with the beginning of the mucus symptom until the postovulatory higher level of BBT had been established. In this way usually between 10 and 15 samples of saliva were collected in small plastic tubes and stored frozen in a household refrigerator until delivery to the laboratory for LH determination.

Methods

Salivary LH has been determined radioimmunologically by modifying a commercially available LH-Ria kit, as previously described in detail (Kraft 1984; Loewit

1985). Luteinizing hormone values exceeding $\bar{x}_{LH}+1$ SD were tentatively regarded as LH peaks. The peak day was labeled day 0 and served as a reference point for ovulation detection. Cycle days were centered around day 0. According to well-established SOM rules [temperature method, STM (Döring 1986, 1986a; Rötzer 1986, 1968)], the postovulatory infertile period starts with the evening of the 3rd day of elevated BBT (BBT3), which therefore was used as a second reference point for the reliability of the temperature computers under examination. No essential additional information came from correlations with cervical mucus patterns in general, even though in individual cases they helped in detecting errors of the devices or in determining the first rise of BBT.

Devices

RT (Rite Time Ltd., POB C12, Chatham, England) is an electronic thermometer for oral measurement of BBT with a computer memory program for one cycle. It has a built-in time slot of 3 h during which measurements are registered in the memory of the device and, provided daily BBT measurements, it is able to detect the postovulatory rise in BBT, having a method of sorting out unphysiological temperature changes. Outside the time slot it may be used as a conventional thermometer. The time slot has to be set according to individual convenience but is not to be changed during a particular cycle. At the beginning of each menstrual cycle (day 1 of the monthly period) the computer memory has to be set for day 1. From day 4 on regular measurements of BBT are required, the temperature being displayed in degrees Celsius. The display window changes from blank (for the fertile time) to six bar lines at the beginning of the postovulatory infertile period. Thus RT only indicates infertility. The time of high fertility must be calculated from previous experience.

The device can also be used as an ordinary clock or alarm clock. Experience with RT dates from a long-term case study, with 17 of the 20 cycles studied being contributed by one 23-year-old nulliparous woman over a period of 2½ years. The average duration of the 20 cycles was 26.4 ± 1.9 (23–29) days.

BS (Bioself Distribution S.A., 7, avenue de Thônex, CH 1226, Thônex-Geneva), too, is an electronic temperature-recording device for oral, rectal or vaginal measurement of BBT. It is equipped with a microprocessor, calculating the fertile period of the cycle by subtracting 18 from the shortest and 9 from the longest cycle recorded according to the calendar method (Ogino 1932; Knaus 1933) and detecting the BBT shift by comparing each measurement with the eight previous ones according to the temperature method. Again, rises in temperature exceeding those typical for ovulation are rejected by the program. BS starts out from a hypothetical 28-day cycle and adjusts to the individual cycle pattern by storing the length of the last six menstrual cycles. It does not accept cycles longer than 39 or shorter than 19 days. Also a time slot of ± 2 h is set automatically at the time of the first temperature recording. Thereafter measurements are only accepted within this time slot, as indicated by a yellow light signal. The beginning of each cycle is recorded by pressing a special button. BBT is not shown; instead, light signals indicate the state of fertility; a constant red light signals possible fertility (from day 5 to the beginning of flashing red and again thereafter until "BBT3");

flashing red indicates the most fertile period as calculated from the longest and shortest cycle; constant green light is displayed during the infertile phase (from "BBT3" for maximally 16 days during the luteal phase and again during the first 5 days of the following cycle. The memory of BS stores the temperature and light signals of the last 64 days, the length of the last six cycles, and the remaining battery capacity. These data may be retrieved in graphic form by inserting the temperature probe of BS into a special printer. BS has been studied during 64 cycles of 22 women, the average cycle length being 28.3 ± 3.2 (23–27) days.

Results and Discussion

Reliability in Comparison to the Salivary LH Peak

As can be seen from Table 1, RT signaled infertility in 2 out of 19 (2/19) cycles at days +1 and +2, i.e., on probably or possibly fertile days. However, on day +1 cervical mucus of the fertile type was still present, the cervix was soft and open, and thus the error of the device was obvious for someone experienced in SOM. On the other hand, on day +3, a certainly infertile day, infertility was signaled only in about one-fourth of the cycles in accordance with the manufacturer's intention that RT "is cautious and errs on the safe side." In 58% of all cycles the infertile period was indicated after day +4, thus designating up to five infertile days as fertile. Figure 2 illustrates that even by day +5 fertility is still indicated in almost one-third of the cycles, the last signals changing to "infertile"

Table 1. First indication of infertility by two temperature computers in comparison with the salivary LH peak (day 0)

1. Infertility signal		Rite time (n=19)		Bioself 110 (n=63)	
Before LH peak	3 days	–		1	1.6%
	2 days	–		2	3.2%
	1 day	–		–	
Simultaneously	0	–		1	1.6%
After LH peak	1 day	1	5.3%	–	
	2 days	1	5.3%	1	1.6%
	3 days	3	15.8%	5	7.9%
	4 days	3	15.8%	9	14.3%
	5 days	5	26.3%	8	12.7%
	6 days	2	10.5%	2	3.2%
	7 days	2	10.5%	7	11.0%
	8 days	–		3	4.8%
	9 days	2	10.5%	5	7.9%
	10 days	–		1	1.6%
	11 days	–		1	1.6%
Never appeared		–		17	27.0%
Appeared too early		2	10.6%	5	8.0%
Appeared after day +4		11	57.8%	27	42.8%[a]

[a] 58.5% of 46 cycles with green display (see Fig. 2).

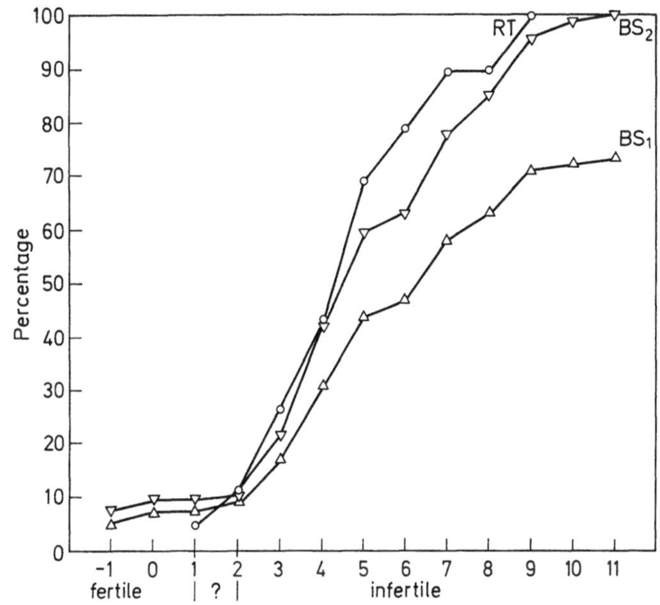

Fig. 2. Cumulative incidence of indication of infertility by two temperature computers in comparison with the salivary LH peak (day 0). *RT*, Rite time, 19 cycles; *BS*, Bioself 110; BS_1, 63 cycles, no infertility indication in 17 cycles; BS_2, 46 cycles with infertility display

as late as day +9. In accordance with a study by Royston (1984), correlating RT data with ovarian ultrasonography in 14 cycles or with the serum LH peak in 13 cycles of 6 women, also in this study, the RT signal indicating infertility occurred in all cases after the salivary LH peak, mean $= 4.9 \pm 2.1$ days ($n = 19$), the corresponding values in Royston's study being 5.2 for the day of maximum follicular development and 4.3 for the day of the serum LH peak, range 1–7 days. However, without hormonal control, a premature signal was suggested in only 2/73 cycles (3%).

The data for BS show that the green light appeared too early in 5/63 cycles. In all of these cases fertility was indicated by the appearance of the cervix or cervical mucus and the first green display occurred before the 14th day of the cycle. Thus, the error of the device could be realized. Again, by day +3, infertility was signaled in only 16%, the latest green-display occurring at day +11. Thus, in 43% of all cases, the green light appears after day +4 and the BS estimate of the infertile period is even somewhat more conservative than that of RT. In this way, errors implying the danger of unwanted pregnancy are kept low (2.6% less than RT), but up to 7 infertile days are not recognized as such. However, in this study, due to the more sophisticated program of BS which requires at least eight measurements before it can detect the BBT rise and due to the fact that 34% of all cycles were first recordings for the device, the green light did not appear at all in 27% of the cycles. If only those cycles are compared, where the green light was present, RT and BS closely parallel each other, as depicted in Fig. 2. In contrast to RT, BS does indicate the most fertile time by flashing red signals. But even though BS adjusts to the individual cycle length after 6 months, it brings no advantage over conventional observation of the cervix or cervical mucus in recognizing the optimal time for conception.

Reliability in Comparison to BBT3

In 15/20 RT cycles, complete oral and rectal temperature records were available. In two-thirds of the cases (10/15) the first rise in BBT was recorded on the same day, in one-third it differed by ±1 day, RT showing the first rise in temperature 2 times 1 day before and 3 times 1 day after the respective rectal measurements. Thus, in this longitudinal study, the oral measurements were in better agreement with rectal BBT than in a recent report on 15 cycles of five women, which described opposite findings (Döring 1986c).

As shown in Table 2, on the day of BBT3 simultaneity was reduced to less than one-third (6/20) of the cases. In over two-thirds RT signaled infertility 1–4 days earlier (40%), or later (30%), than conventional BBT. In the study by Döring (1986c) the variation was between 4 days earlier and 6 days later than BBT. The results of this longitudinal study, however, are in perfect agreement with data on 38 cycles of 20 women, showing that RT's signal occurred within 2 days of the user's own estimate in 82% of the cycles (Royston 1984) as compared with 80% (16/20) in this study. Most of the BS measurements were taken rectally. Since, however, the temperature is not displayed and also the printed graphs show only relative values, a direct comparison with conventionally taken BBT is not possible. BS, also, indicated infertility only in about one-third of the cases at the day of BBT3. However, in distinction from RT, the green light preceded BBT3 only in 20% of the cycles by 1 (15%) or 2 (5%) days. Thus, also in comparison to the empirically well established beginning of the infertile time after ovulation, BS seems to be the more reliable instrument.

Table 2. Indication of infertility by two temperature computers in comparison with the 3rd day of elevated basal body temperature (BBT3, day 0)

1. Infertility signal		Rite time ($n=20$)		Bioself 110 ($n=40$)	
Before BBT3[a]	4 days	1	5.0%	–	
	3 days	–		–	
	2 days	2	10.0%	2	5.0%
	1 day	5	25.0%	6	15.0%
Simultaneously	0	6	30.0%	13	32.5%
After BBT3	1 day	2	10.0%	8	20.0%
	2 days	1	5.0%	5	12.5%
	3 days	2	10.0%	3	7.5%
	4 days	1	5.0%	1	2.5%
	5 days	–		1	2.5%
	6 days	–		1	2.5%
Appeared too early		8	40.0%	8	20.0%
Appeared late		6	30.0%	19	47.5%

[a] BBT was measured rectally with a mercury thermometer.

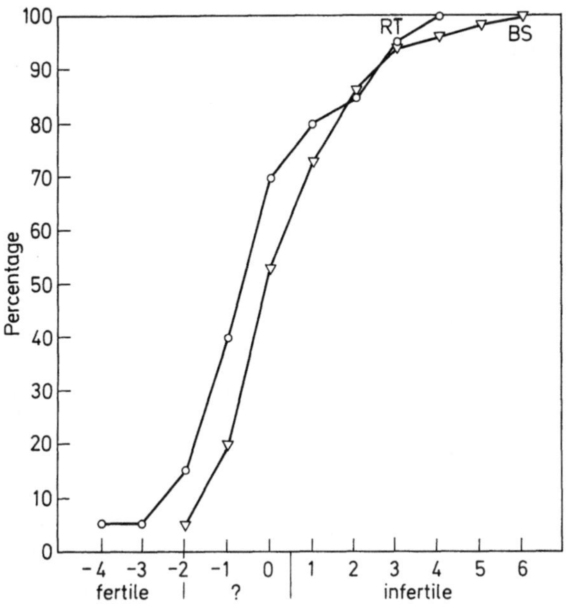

Fig. 3. Cumulative incidence of indication of infertility by two temperature computers in comparison with the 3rd day of elevated basal body temperature (BBT3, day 0). *RT*, Rite Time, 20 cycles; *BS*, Bioself 110, 40 cycles

These data conflict with the observation of only about 8%–11% of false infertility indications (Fig. 2) compared with the LH peak. This discrepancy is explained by and hints to the time lag of BBT in regard to the LH peak. As we have shown, BBT3 was delayed in 58% of 60 BS cycles or 52% of 194 cycles beyond day +4, thus occurring in these cases from 5 to even 10 days after the salivary LH peak (Loewit 1987).

Indeed, checking the relation to the LH peak in individual cycles where RT or BS infertility signals occurred before BBT3 reveals that only about one-fourth of the cases fell on the possibly fertile days +1 and +2, the rest occurring between 3 and 7 days after the LH peak, though still before BBT3. This explains the high reliability of BBT3, which more often than not comes much too late. On the other hand it underlines the need for a better marker of infertility. At the moment, however, BBT3 cannot be dispensed with. As shown in Table 2 and Fig. 3, RT infertility display and BS-green lag behind BBT3 in 30% and 48% of the cycles, BS reaching 100% of infertility display 2 days later than RT. Thus, the reliability of BS again is paid for by a shortening of the infertile period. This is once more born out by the number of infertile days for each instrument as summarized in Table 3. While in the RT study the average number of postovulatory infertile days is practically the same whether indicated by RT or taken from BBT [as in the study by Royston (1984) even though absolute values differ], it is almost 1 day shorter for BS as compared with BBT3. However, the standard deviation is larger for the instruments than for BBT3. Thus, the shortest periods of infertility from 3–7 days/cycle occur almost twice as often with the instruments as with conventional BBT readings. These, in turn, comprise to a greater extent the longer infertility period

Table 3. Postovulatory infertile days per cycle as indicated by RT and BS in comparison with conventional BBT interpretation

No. of infertile days per cycle	Rite time ($n=20$)				Bioself 110 ($n=40$)			
	RT display		BBT3 interpretation		BS display		BBT3 interpretation	
	(n)	(%)	(n)	(%)	(n)	(%)	(n)	(%)
3	1	5.0	–		1	2.5	–	
4	1	5.0	1	5.0	1	2.5	–	
5	–		–		1	2.5	–	
6	2	10.0	2	10.0	2	5.0	–	
7	4	20.0	2	10.0	1	2.5	3	7.5
8	3	15.0	7	35.0	5	12.5	5	12.5
9	5	25.0	7	35.0	9	22.5	7	17.5
10	2	10.0	–		7	17.5	10	25.0
11	1	5.0	1	5.0	11	27.5	8	20.0
12	1	5.0	–		2	5.0	4	10.0
13	–		–		–		3	7.5
Average	7.9 ± 2.2		8.0 ± 1.5		9.2 ± 2.1		10.0 ± 1.6	
Cycle length	26.4 ± 1.9				28.9 ± 3.1			

$\chi^2 = 6.6 < 15.51$ $(= \chi^2_{2;\,0.05})$
$P > 0.05$

$\chi^2 = 10.92 < 18.31$ $(= \chi^2_{2;\,0.05})$

of 8–12 days (75% vs. 60% of the cycles in the RT group) and of 8–13 days (92% vs. 85% of the BS cases).

Finally, it should be remarked that in principle both instruments were well accepted by their users. In the study by Royston (1984), 48% of the participants were willing to replace their usual methods with RT, although 55% stated they were "not very confident" at the start of the infertile period as given by RT. In this study, most of the volunteers of the BS group would not rely solely on the instrument unless they could read the temperature themselves. This was the strongest criticism made. A thorough instruction of the user is an indispensable prerequisite of high use-effectiveness, as is a basic understanding of SOM or cycle physiology in order to be able to detect possible errors of the device.

Thus, both instruments cannot replace the user's own know-how in SOM, if they are to be used in a critical and safe way with confidence. Furthermore, neither the beginning of the fertile and infertile periods nor the optimal time for conception can be better recognized by using the temperature computers than from conventional SOM. In our limited experience – the results of BS may become better in longitudinal studies, those of RT may show greater variation in cross-sectional ones – the devices allow for an easier and more convenient way of practising SOM for already experienced or specially instructed people. They still do not overcome the principal obstacles to large-scale use of SOM in the general population. Future instruments should be able to predict ovulation in good time and to detect its occurrence earlier than BBT in order to extend the pre- and postovulatory infertile periods, without jeopardizing the reliability and handling practicability of the devices. From past and present efforts it becomes obvious that this goal is still very difficult to reach.

Acknowledgments. The technical assistance of Mr. A. Friedl and Mr. S. Zennebe and the financial support granted to the first author by the Dr. Legerlotz foundation are gratefully acknowledged.

References

Albrecht BH, Fernando RS, Regas J, Betz G (1985) A new method for predicting and confirming ovulation. Fertil Steril 44:200–205

Baby comp (1987) Dtsch Apothek Z 127

Döring GK (1986) Die Temperaturmethode zur Empfängnisverhütung (1st edn, 9th edn 1954). Thieme, Stuttgart

Döring GK (1986a) Empfängnisverhütung, 10th edn. Thieme, Stuttgart

Döring GK, Baur S, Frank P, Freundl G, Sottong G (1986b) Ergebnisse einer repräsentativen Umfrage zum Familienplanungsverhalten in der Bundesrepublik Deutschland 1985. Geburtsh Frauenheilk 46:892–897

Döring GK, Daucher HK (1986c) Bestimmung der unfruchtbaren Tage im Zyklus der Frau. Fortschr Med 104:941–942

Frank P, Raith E (1985) Natürliche Familienplanung. Springer, Berlin Heidelberg New York Tokyo

Knaus H (1933) Die periodische Frucht- und Unfruchtbarkeit des Weibes. Zentralbl Gynäkol 57:1393–1408

Kraft HG, Fischer-Korp C, Loewit K (1984) A radioimmunological method for LH measurements in saliva. Contraceptive Delivery System 5:99

Loewit K, Kraft HG, Ortlieb A (1985) Measurement of LH in saliva: a new approach to ovulation detection. In: Runnebaum et al. (eds) Future aspects in contraception. MTP, Boston, pp 31–47

Loewit K, Ortlieb A, Kraft HG, Widhalm R, Wolfram G (1987) Wie erkennt man die „sicheren" Tage? Sexualmedizin 16:52–57

Loewit K, Huber J, Ortlieb A, Kraft HG, Widhalm R, Wolfram G (to be published) Speichel-LH als Ovulationsindikator: Vergleich zwischen Speichel-LH, Serum-LH und Ultraschallbefund. Geburtsh Frauenheilk

Münz R (1987) Empfängnisverhütung und Familienplanung. Prakt Arzt 41:11–30

Ogino K (1932) Über den Konzeptionstermin des Weibes und seine Anwendung in der Praxis. Zentralbl Gynäkol 12:721–732

Rabe T, Kiesel L, Runnebaum B (1985) Future aspects in contraception: an overview. In: Runnebaum B, Rabe T, Kiesel L (eds) Future aspects in contraception, part 1. MTP, Boston

Rice FJ, Lanctôt ClA, Garcia-Devesa C (1981) Effectiveness of the sympto-thermal method of natural family planning: an international study. Int J Fertil 26:222–230

Rötzer J (1968) Erweiterte Basaltemperaturmessung und Empfängnisregelung. Arch Gynäkol 206:195–214

Rötzer J (1978a) The symptothermal method: ten years of change. Linacre Quart 45:358–374

Rötzer J (1978b) Sympto-thermal method and family planning. Acta Med Rom 16:339–348

Rötzer J (1986) Natürliche Geburtenregelung, 16th edn. Herder, Vienna

Royston JP, Humphrey SJE, Flynn AM, Marshall J, Zarzosa-Perez A (1984) An automatic electronic device (Rite Time) to detect the onset of the infertile period by basal body temperature measurements. Br J Obstet Gynaecol 91:565–573

Schenker JG, Mor-Yosef S (1985) Natural family planning. In: Runnebaum B, Rabe T, Kiesel L (eds) Future aspects in contraception, part 2. MTP, Boston

WHO (1981) A prospective multicentre trial of the ovulation method of NFP. I The teaching phase. Fertil Steril 36:152–158

Contraception with the Diaphragm: A 2-Year Follow-up Study

T. G. Schätzler

Arbeiterwohlfahrt Beratungszentrum Lore-Agnes-Haus, Lützowstraße 32, 4300 Essen 1, FRG

The use of the diaphragm and spermicide as an intravaginal barrier-method of contraception was investigated at the West German family-planning center of the Arbeiterwohlfahrt. The follow-up study was based upon the application of a semistandardized method of learning how to handle the diaphragm and spermicide by step-by-step instructions for 158 women and investigated their early and later experiences by questionnaires in two follow-ups after a mean observation period of 2 years and 4 months.

According to the theoretical concept that the method is a combined mechanical and chemical barrier at the cervix uteri, its functioning is demonstrated to the woman on a pelvic model. After contraceptive counselling the gynecological examination is carried out, to exclude any contraindications and to estimate the size of the test diaphragm. The cervix uteri is demonstrated to the patient through the speculum by a mirror, so that she is orientated with regard to the anatomical structures in her vagina, when she performs the vaginal self-examination. This procedure gives her a visual and palpable feedback to apply the diaphragm and spermicide in the next step correctly. Corresponding to the gynecological findings the woman tries to insert a test diaphragm with the dome of the membrane pointing at the cervix. Using the dome-like technique, two laps of the rubber membrane cover a pouch filled with spermicide guaranteeing its transport at the entrance of the cervical canal and a good adherence to the vaginal vault. The correct intravaginal position and size of the contraceptive device is confirmed by gynecological reexamination and demonstrated to the patient. With a final vaginal self-examination the woman learns to be sure of her cervix uteri being covered by the rubber membrane before every use of the diaphragm.

This method of fitting a diaphragm was performed with a clientele of 158 women and had the following objectives:

1. To improve knowledge about conception and contraception
2. To reduce apprehensions, anxieties, or reservations against intravaginal contraceptive devices
3. To allow somatic self-experience by genital self-examination
4. To ensure the correct handling of the diaphragm and spermicide theoretically and practically

The follow-up study investigated the effectiveness of the aims and the patterns of the users' sexual and contraceptive behavior. The computer analysis was performed at the University of Freiburg, Department of Medical Sociology, the assistance of which I appreciate very much, with the Statistical Package for the So-

Sexology
Eds.: W. Eicher, G. Kockott

cial Sciences (SPSS). The corrected response rate was 64% after 4 months and 48% after 2 years.

About 80% of the 158 sexually active women had been students or graduates, 75% unmarried, 75% childless, and 70% 20–29 years old. The social data of the follow-ups showed no significant differences. The sizes of the ORTHO-coil-spring-diaphragms ranged from 65 to 75 mm in diameter for nulliparous and from 75 to 85 mm for parous women. Octoxynol, a jelly of citric acid, and nonoxynol-9 were the spermicidal agents being used. Twenty-five percent of all patients had deviations from the common genital anatomy; in 27% the gynecological findings needed to be checked. Forty percent of the women were experienced with oral contraceptives and 21% with different methods of natural family planning (NFP) before they tried the diaphragm. Ninety-nine percent of the clientele accepted the way the instructions were given and 92% thought positively about the gynecological examination. Ninety-one percent emphasized the experience of self-examination and 77% the visual control of their intravaginal anatomy. Half of the women had no problems of handling the diaphragm at all, 45% only had difficulties with the contraceptive discipline of regular application, and 6% had factual difficulties in handling it.

The personal motivation for the use was classified according to the frequency of the answers in the first follow-up:

- That the diaphragm has no health hazards (93%)
- That it maintains the physiological menstrual cycle (91%)
- That it protects safely from unwanted pregnancy (83%)
- That it does not interfere with sexual feelings (65%)
- That it is not detrimental to fertility (65%)
- That it improves communication with the sexual partner (60%)
- That it makes more conscious of sexuality and fertility (50%)

In the second follow-up 27% used the diaphragm before every sexual intercourse, 28% every time but not during the period of menstrual bleeding, and 32% in combination with different NFP methods. None of the users had difficulties checking the correct intravaginal position of the diaphragm by self-examination. Questioned about the changes of sexual feelings by using the method, the women showed:

- No change in 50%
- An improvement in 32%
- A disturbance in only 12%.

The mean frequency of sexual intercourse was 9.85 times/month in the second follow-up, and the diaphragm was applied 6.8 times/month due to the use of NFP methods, condoms, or discontinual application. The continuation rate was 76% after a mean period of use of 19.4 months. During 1300 months overall nine pregnancies occured due to:

- Discontinual application (3)
- Application of diaphragm without spermicide (1)
- Combination with the rhythm method (1)
- Wrong size of diaphragm being fitted elsewhere (1)
- Method failure in spite of correct application (3)

According to Pearl and Tietze the use-effectiveness in this follow-up study was 8.31 pregnancies in 100 women-years and the method-effectiveness was 2.77.

In 1986, Döring and Schicketanz stated in their retrospective study that the method and quality of instructions given for the combined use of diaphragm and spermicide determine whether the user will succeed with the method or not. But the results of several retrospective and follow-up studies cannot be compared because of different or undefined starting conditions. Our well-defined method of learning step-by-step instructions tries to ease the somatic and emotional approach toward the application and is comparable with exercises for the enhancement of psychosexual self-experience, described by Kaplan or Barbach. Using the diaphragm and spermicide by the patient it is not possible to delegate contraceptive competence to an expert like the doctor, who inserts an IUD or prescribes oral contraceptives. On the contrary, as with all local barrier methods it is necessary that experts in contraceptive knowledge delegate their competence to the client.

The social data in the present follow-up study show a special group of mainly independent, sexually experienced women of high educational standard, who are motivated to contracept with the diaphragm. Their incidence of gynecological disorders and deviations is in the normal range. The contraceptive preexperiences in our study are the same as in representative studies about female contraceptive behavior in the Federal Republic of Germany, carried out by Oeter and Wilken in 1977 and by the EMNID institute in 1985. The acceptance and the efficiency of our method of teaching the application of diaphragm and spermicide are very high, so that the effectiveness of the four objectives could be verified. The main problems of handling were not the application itself but the contraceptive discipline of regular use. The apprehensions of health hazards or somatic and psychological side effects of other contraceptive methods were the main motivations to change for the diaphragm. Many women want to get back physiological menstrual functions and authentic sexual feelings, which they think to be disturbed by the application of sexual hormones or the implantation of IUDs. This is underlined by the improvement of sexual feelings, which one-third of the women report in the second follow-up.

About 40% of the users tried to limit the frequency of application by omitting the diaphragm and spermicide during their supposed infertile period of the menstrual cycle. This risky contraceptive behavior leads to the use-effectiveness of 8.31 pregnancies in 100 woman-years. It must be underlined here that this use-effectiveness is not improved by secondary selection of the clientele. Vessey stated in 1974 that the use-effectiveness is much better for women who are experienced with the diaphragm for more than 6 months than for women who are starting with the method. But an elimination of "beginners" in our study would give an unrealistic impression of contraceptive security, because every experienced woman once had to start and could have failed with the method. With a Pearl index of 2.77, the theoretical method-effectiveness of the diaphragm and spermicide is not much different to the effectiveness of IUDs and could be reached by improved contraceptive discipline.

Conclusions must be drawn with reserve: the present study is very small and the clientele is not representative for the normal population. But the women in our investigation could be a pilot study group for future contraceptive behavior as students and graduates had been in the 1960s for oral steroid contraceptives. They have an increasing interest in traditional and natural methods of contraception. The use of diaphragm and spermicide is an alternative for women, who cannot apply oral contraceptives or IUDs due to medical reasons or do not want to do so. This reflects the increasing reservations against high-standard contraceptive technology and changing patterns of sexual and contraceptive behavior. The application of the diaphragm method means contraception only when required and needs high motivation and contraceptive discipline of the user to be successful. The method of learning by step-by-step instructions is highly effective and supportive for the user in her sexual relationship with her partner.

A Study of The Acceptability of Vasectomy in India

P. Kothari, D. Pardanani, B. Parulkar, R. Patel, A. Sheth, and N. Parekh
203 A Sukhsagar, N.S. Patkar Marg., Bombay 400 007, India

Introduction

Despite the advantage of the availability of a vast budget and necessary propaganda facilities by all media, the concept of vasectomy as a contraceptive procedure is still not well accepted by the Indian masses. With a view to understanding the prevalent methods and the reasons for nonacceptability of vasectomy, a survey was carried out recently in Bombay. Two hundred married couples with no marital discord were studied in detail.

Aim of the Study

The survey was carried out to study the factors which preclude males from undergoing vasectomy.

Materials and Methods

Two hundred married couples were selected and parameters like age group, socioeconomic background, educational status, religion, and number of children were considered. The study was carried out in the Out Patients' Department of K.E.M. Hospital, Bombay. The subjects were divided into two groups. Group 1 consisted of 100 vasectomized males whose attitude toward vasectomy was evaluated. The second group consisted of 100 males who refused vasectomy, and their attitude toward vasectomy and reasons for refusal were evaluated.

In individual interviews it was noted that most people accepted vasectomy mainly because of financial and other difficulties in bringing up more children. They accepted vasectomy as they thought it to be a rational decision. Some men chose vasectomy as IUDs did not suit their spouses. It is surprising to note that none of them were counselled together about the vasectomy procedure, the intraoperative risks, and the possible outcome prior to surgery. They were also not informed clearly that vasectomy does not affect the sexual desire, the performance of an individual, or the volume of ejaculate. Most of them admitted that if all these details had been explained to them prior to the procedure, they would have accepted vasectomy much earlier.

Sexology
Eds.: W. Eicher, G. Kockott

Table 1. Group 1

Age group			
18–25 years	26–35 years	36–42 years	
35	45	20	
Education			
Illiterate	High school education	College education	
10	40	50	
Socio economic status			
Lower class (income less than Rs. 500 per month)	Middle class (income Rs. 500–2500 per month)	Upper class (income Rs. 2500 and above per month)	
5	60	35	
Religion			
Hindu	Christian	Zoroastrian	Muslim
65	15	5	15
No. of children	Individuals		
1	2		
2	34		
3 or more	64		

Table 2. Single most important reason for accepting vasectomy

	No.
1. Financial difficulty in bringing up more children	28
2. Difficulty in bringing up children because of working situations	10
3. Difficulty in bringing up more children because of unfavorable family constraints	6
4. Awareness of population hazard	18
5. Knowledge about reversal of the procedure	7
6. Incentives offered	23
7. Better sex life	4
8. Medical reasons which prevent wife from further pregnancies	2
9. Unsuitability of other contraceptive methods	2

Conclusion

It is of the utmost importance that both the partners are counselled prior to surgery about the operative procedure, the intraoperative risks, and the possible outcome. The fact needs to be emphasized that sterility and virility are two entirely different things and depend upon the different types of cells present in the testes. Tying or ligation of the vas will have no effect on virility. These myths were prevalent not only among the uneducated but also among the highly educated ones. Christians and Muslims had strong religious reasons against adopting contraceptive procedures.

It was inferred from the personal interrogation that the illiterate lower class people did not pay much attention toward the need for contraception and consid-

Table 3. Group 2

Age group			
18–25 years	26–35 years	36–45 years	
40	35	25	
Education			
Illiterate	School education	College education	
70	20	10	
Economic status			
Lower class (income less than Rs. 500 per month)	Middle class (income Rs. 500–2500 per month)	Upper class (income Rs. 2500 and above per month)	
50	42	8	
Religion			
Hindu	Christian	Zoroastrian	Muslim
30	15	1	54
No. of children	Individuals		
2	60		
3 or more	40		

Table 4. Reasons for refusal

	No.
1. Sexual life	
a) Fear of decreased sexual pleasure after vasectomy	30
b) Apprehension about absence of ejaculation after vasectomy and as a result spouse may not have "that" sexual pleasure as before. (Myth – after vasectomy the quantity of ejaculate is reduced considerably or may be totally absent and this may lead to dissatisfaction of the partner)	10
c) Equating vasectomy to loss of manhood	14
2. Because of religious reasons (Christians and Muslims)	25
3. Only daughters and expecting a male child	12
4. Fear of social security in old age	8
5. Vasectomized individuals have increased incidence of heart attacks (myth)	1

ered vasectomy an offence against Nature. The educated class planned for proper spacing and the number of children. Some of the persons from lower economic groups were aware about their own financial position and the difficulties with increased number of children. However, the majority of the subjects were not certain about the simplicity of the vasectomy procedure. It will be better accepted if the misconceptions regarding vasectomy are cleared. It should be explained that sexual life after vasectomy would be the same as before. It needs to be cleared that live sperms may be present in the semen above the point of vasectomy. On average, after about 10–12 ejaculates and/or until two semen reports are sperm negative, one should perform sexual activity with contraceptive protection. Omitting this fact from the patient's information can lead to severe marital discord arising out of an unexpected pregnancy.

It should also be pointed out that vasectomy is relatively simple as compared with ligature and if reversal is needed vasectomy stands a much higher percentage of success of the fallopian tubes. As it is a simple procedure, mass vasectomies can be more easily organized. Public education eradicating the myths and fears and establishing goals would be a primary step toward making vasectomy more acceptable.

II. Sterility and Sexuality

Sexual Behavior and Female Fertility

J. Kremer

University Hospital, 9724 Groningen, The Netherlands

Influence of Libido, Coitus and Orgasm on Female Fertility During the Preovulatory Phase of the Menstrual Cycle

In a number of mammals ovulation only occurs after mating or after artificial insemination, due to tactile stimulation of the upper part of the vagina to which the female animal reacts with a behavior pattern which has orgasmic characteristics. Examples of these so-called reflex ovulators are the cat, the rabbit, and the camel. In rodents mating is necessary, not for ovulation but for the formation of a corpus luteum. There is no clear proof that such mechanisms occur in the human. Much has been written on the possible effects of female orgasm upon the incidence and time of ovulation, in particular by German gynecologists, but the theory has never been adequately confirmed or refuted. Ovulation or the formation of a corpus luteum is probably rarely induced by coitus in the human and it is the exception that would prove the overall rule.

Another obsolete theory is the so-called insuck theory, stating that the woman's orgasm aspirates the spermatozoa out of the vagina during coitus. Sobrero and MacLeod (1962) and later on Masters and Johnson (1966) proved that insuck of spermatozoa into the uterine cervix by female orgasm does not occur.

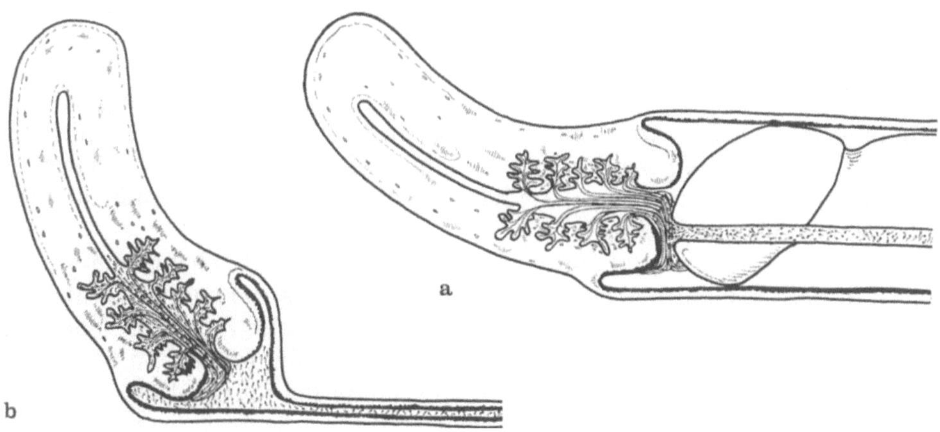

Fig. 1. A Situation in the vagina during the ejaculation process; contact between semen and preovulatory cervical mucus results in penetration of spermatozoa into the ectocervical mucus. **B** Situation in the vagina after withdrawal of the penis. The cervical crypts are colonized with spermatozoa

Sexology
Eds.: W. Eicher, G. Kockott

Spermatozoa swim into and through the cervical mucus with the velocity of $^1/_2$–1 cm/min and so can reach the uterine cavity 3 min after coitus (Fig. 1). The sperm transport through the uterine cavity into the fallopian tubes occurs, however, much more quickly. It is quite possible that specific contractions of the uterine muscles effect this transport, because spermatozoa can reach the fallopian tubes within 5 min of an intravaginal semen application. The possibility of a complete intrauterine sperm transport within seconds was demonstrated by Fischel et al. in 1978 in sheep and 7 years earlier (1971) in women by Kremer and Blickman in Groningen, using a small quantity of an oil-soluble X-ray contrast medium. Naaktgeboren and Bontekoe (1976) in the Netherlands demonstrated that fright can disturb the contraction patterns of the uterine muscle in sheep. This phenomenon is supposed to be mediated by the release of epinephrine from the adrenal glands into the circulation. It is possible that psychological stress in women can also cause a disturbed pattern of uterine contractions which may be one of the causes of so-called unexplained infertility.

Influence of Libido, Coitus, and Orgasm on Female Fertility During the Postovulatory Period of the Menstrual Cycle

Sexual desire in nonprimate female mammals is restricted to the preovulatory period and is caused by the high level of estrogenic hormones in the blood. Sexual desire strongly decreases after ovulation due to the influence of progesterone, produced by the corpus luteum (Everett and Herbert 1972).

Sexual desire in female monkeys is much more androgen dependent than estrogen dependent. A female rhesus monkey whose ovaries have been removed surgically maintains her sexual desire thanks to the production of androgenic hormones by the adrenal glands. Her sexual desire disappears completely, however, if the adrenal glands are also removed (Waxenberg et al. 1959). Her sexual attractiveness for the male monkey but not her sexual desire returns after estrogen administration (Herbert 1966). But after an injection with testosterone she wants to copulate. The androgenic hormones, produced by the ovaries and the adrenals, also increase the sexual desire of women. An injection of testosterone also has a libido-increasing effect which can be noticed in female transsexuals. As member of the Genderteam Groningen I noticed that they often report an abnormally strong sexual desire, resulting in frequent masturbation during the initial period of treatment with androgens.

In order to obtain insight into a possible influence of the changing hormone levels during the menstrual cycle in women, I had a personal interview with each of 156 fertile, healthy women between 20 and 40 years old (Fig. 2); 75% of these women noticed such an influence and 25% did not. Almost 50% of the women in the group with a change of sexual desire during the course of the menstrual cycle mentioned that their desire was stronger during the week directly after the end of menstruation than during any other phase of the cycle. It is remarkable that in a relatively small group the sexual desire was the strongest during the ovulation phase, this being the phase with the highest estrogen concentration in the blood. It is likely therefore that the 34% of women with the strongest sexual desire

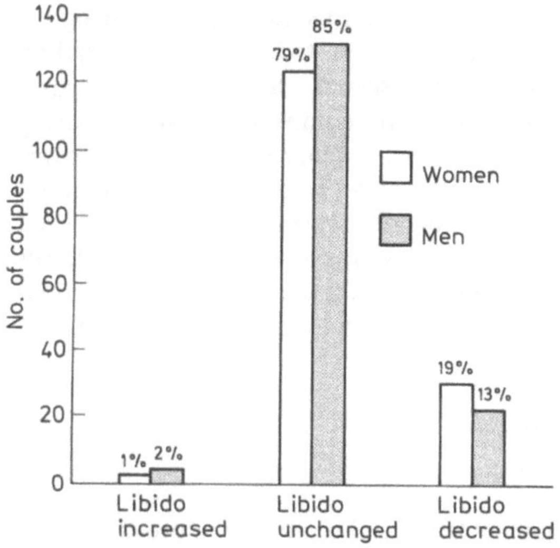

Fig. 2. Period of strongest sexual desire during the menstrual cycle in 117 women

after menstruation owe the increase to the period of abstinence during the menstruation period and not to a high estrogenic hormone level in the blood, because after menstruation the estrogen concentration in the blood is relatively low. Moreover, many of the women mentioned the abstinence during menstruation as an explanation of their increased libido after menstruation.

The human being is the only mammal where coitus also occurs after ovulation during the existence of the progesterone-producing corpus luteum. From a teleological point of view, coitus during the luteal phase of the cycle might be dangerous for the preembryo and that therefore nature took measures to prevent coitus during the period in which the preembryo has not yet been implanted into the uterine wall. One can imagine that uterine contractions due to an orgastic coitus disturb the intrauterine preembryo transport and the nidation process, not only in mammals but also in women. One can, however, also defend the opinion that coitus and orgasm during the luteal phase are harmless in women and they may even have a positive influence on the nidation process in the human through a better blood flow in the uterine wall due to frequent periods of sexual excitement.

Table 1. Pregnancies in 28 women related to number of orgastic coitus during the luteal phase of the menstrual cycle. Pregnancies were obtained by AID

Number of orgastic coitus	Number of cycles	Number of pregnancies	Percentage of pregnancies
0	30	15	50
1	6	4	66
2 or 3	9	5	56
4 or more	14	4	29

To find out more about the possible effect of coitus and orgasm during the luteal phase of the menstrual cycle I asked 48 women, treated with artificial insemination by donor (AID), to alternate frequent sexual intercourse with orgasm during the luteal phase of one menstrual cycle with complete abstinence during the luteal phase of the following cycle, and so on. Twenty-eight women became pregnant with AID during a treatment of 59 cycles (Table 1). Table 1 demonstrates that there was no influence of the number of orgastic coitus during the 1st week of the luteal phase when this number of coitus was lower than four. If coitus and female orgasm occurred at least four times during the 1st week after ovulation then the chance of achieving pregnancy showed a tendency to decrease.

Influence of Coitus Problems of Women on the Chance to Achieve Pregnancy

Depositing semen deeply into the vagina is beneficial to achieving pregnancy. In exceptional cases, however, a so-called coitus ante portas can result in the occurrence of pregnancy. This chance exists when much cervical mucus is produced and a thick thread of this mucus connects the cervical canal with the vulva. This thread can be used by spermatozoa to swim through and to reach the cervical canal in this way.

The most frequent cause of coitus ante portas is vaginismus. In some cases the vaginistic defence is so strong that even a semen deposition on the vulva is not possible.

Vaginismus is a multicausal symptom, due to vaginal penetration phobia, a former psychic trauma, a disturbed relationship, dyspareunia (reflex vaginismus), or a poor coital technique. Vaginismus due to vaginal penetration phobia and reflex vaginismus are often insufficiently differentiated by the gynecologist and therefore often ill-treated. In cases of vaginal penetration phobia it can often be noticed that the vaginistic defence starts even before the penis comes into contact with the female genitals, whereas reflex vaginismus generally starts after contact of the penis with a painful abnormality of the vulva or the entrance of the vagina. Women with vaginal penetration phobia often suffer from other kinds of phobias. They are often characterized by an infantile behavior and are often afraid to undergo a vaginal examination to the extent of panicking. It is important to realize that a number of these women do not want to have their vaginismus treated but only to achieve pregnancy.

The gynecologist, however, often tells these women that this can only be effected if the vaginismus is treated. This is not always the correct approach, because treatment can sometimes disturb a psychological balance. The vaginismus disappears partly or completely but is replaced by another neurotic symptom which can harm the woman socially much more. This means that sometimes artificial insemination is the treatment of choice. In the majority of the cases of vaginism due to vaginal penetration phobia it is possible, however, to convince the woman that overcoming her vaginismus often results in an increase of her happiness and self-esteem. The basic principles which I have used for more than 20 years in the treatment of these women are: First make it clear to the woman and

Table 2. Results of exercises by means of plastic rods with increasing diameter in 18 women with phobic vaginismus

Characteristics	Data (range)
Age	20–35 years
Mean duration of vaginismus	4.5 years (1–12 years)
Orgasm by petting	17 women
Mean number of consultations	6 (2–11)
Mean duration of treatment	7 months (2–11 months)
Treatment resulting in coitus	16 women
Orgasm during coitus	4 women
Wish to become pregnant	14 women
Pregnant by coitus	10 women
Pregnant by AIH	2 women

her partner that vaginal penetration phobia is not caused by a narrow vagina, and second tell her that she has to train herself to overcome her handicap and that the task of the therapist is only to show her the way and to coach her. She has to perform a difficult physical feat and the therapist is her trainer. As in sports the best trainer is a person with patience, dominance, and a certain amount of paternalism. That does not mean of course that paternalistic behavior is always the best approach to a woman with phobic vaginismus. But in a certain number of women it really works. The use of hard plastic rods with increasing diameters, a sort of pseudopenis, can be useful, provided it is explained to the woman that these rods are not used to dilate her vagina but are a means of training the relaxation of her pelvic muscles and of getting these muscles under control. The results of this treatment are demonstrated in Table 2, which shows that this method resulted in coitus in 16 of the 18 women under treatment. Fourteen of the 18 treated women wanted to achieve pregnancy. In 12 of them coitus could be effected after the coaching treatment, and 10 of them became pregnant within 1 year. Two women in the group who had been treated in vain for vaginismus by psychologists and sexologists over a long period refused further treatment and asked for AIH. Both became pregnant and, astonishingly, the vaginismus of one of them disappeared after the birth of the child and she even enjoyed coitus.

Influence of Fertility Investigations on Sexual Desire

It is often postulated that the psychological stress of fertility investigations disturbs sexual life for many couples. That was my reason for carrying out an investigation to get an impression about the validity of this statement. A hundred and fifty six women who were under AID treatment were interviewed about their and their husbands' sexual desire during the foregoing period of fertility investigations. The majority of men and women had not experienced a negative effect of the fertility investigations on their sexual life (Fig. 3). It must be noted that in all these cases the period of investigation had lasted less than 1 year and in the majority less than 6 months.

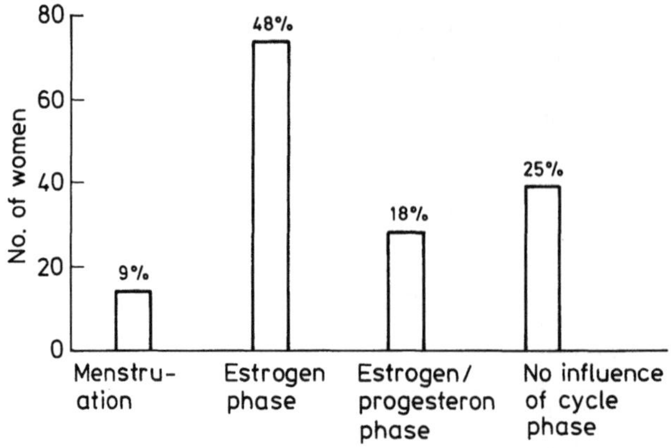

Fig. 3. Changes in sexual desire of wife and husband during the period of fertility investigations

Conclusion

There is a rather large overlap between the fields of sexology and fertility science. It is important that the fertility scientist knows the basic principles of sexology but also that the sexologist knows how a routine fertility investigation program works and what kinds of fertility treatment are available. During the gynecologist's training, both aspects, fertility science and sexology, must be taught. But it is also useful and desirable that during the sexologist's training knowledge of fertility science is gained. Prof. Musaph has been advocating the latter in the Netherlands and he has succeeded in arranging a training in fertility science for a number of his sexology students in Utrecht.

References

Everett BJ, Herbert J (1972) Hormonal correlates of sexual behavior in subhuman primates. Dan Med Bull 19:246–258
Fischel RE, Tadmor A, Lehrer AR, Schindler H (1978) Cineradiography of uterine mortality in the cycling ewe. Anim Reprod Sci 1:155–160
Herbert J (1966) The effect of estrogen applied directly to the genitalia upon sexual attractiveness of the female rhesus monkey. Excerpta Med In Cong Sex 3:212
Kremer J, Blickman J (1971) Het intra-uteriene transport en intra-tubaire transport van kleine hoeveelheden röntgencontrastvloeistof. Ned Tijdschr Geneesk 115:860
Masters WH, Johnson VE (1966) Human sexual response. Churchill, London
Naaktgeboren C, Bontekoe EHM (1976) Vergleichend-geburtskundliche Betrachtungen und experimentelle Untersuchungen über psychosomatische Störungen der Schwangerschaft und des Geburtsablaufes. Z Tierzüchtg Züchtgsbiol 93:264–320
Sobrero AJ, Mac Leod J (1962) The immediate Post Coital Test. Fertil Steril 13:184–188
Waxenberg SE, Drellich MG, Sutherland AM (1959) The role of hormones in human behaviour. I. Changes in female sexuality after adrenalectomy. J Clin Endocrinol Metabol 19:193–202

Sterility and Sexuality from the Andrologist's Standpoint

F. H. Comhaire, T. Farley, and P. Rowe

Department of International Medicine, Academisch Ziekenhuis, 135 de Pintelaan, 9000 Ghent, Belgium

Material and Methods

Investigations were carried out on 7781 couples consulting for infertility of at least 12 months duration using a standard protocol (WHO protocol 78923). This protocol included some questions about sexual and ejaculatory function in both the male and female partner. Data related to the latter were analyzed using the SPSS package and nonparametrical statistical methods (chi-square test).

Results and Discussion

Correlates of Inadequate Coital Erection

Relation Between Coital Erection and Erection upon Other Occasions

Only 15% of men with inadequate coital erection report never to have experienced early morning erections, and 38% never had erections during masturbation. In men with adequate coital erection these percentages were 1.0 and 5.4 respectively (Table 1). Almost 15% of 452 men who never had masturbatory erections, also report no early morning erections (Table 2). In contrast, 73% of 90 cases with no early morning erections never experienced masturbatory erections.

Hence, absence of early morning erections, suggesting organic impotence, is found in about the same proportion of men with inadequate coital or masturbatory erections. The remaining 85% of cases with inadequate coital erection have either early morning erections or masturbatory erections, suggesting a predominantly psychogenic cause of their inadequate coital erection.

On the other hand, the absence of early morning erections does not exclude adequate coital or masturbatory erections.

Table 1. Coital erection by early morning or masturbatory erection

	Coital erection	
	Adequate ($n=7681$)	Inadequate ($n=100$)
Early morning erections absent (%)	1.0	15.0*
Masturbatory erections absent (%)	5.4	38.0**

* $P<0.05$; ** $P<0.01$.

Sexology
Eds.: W. Eicher, G. Kockott

Table 2. Coital erection by early morning erection

		n	Masturbatory erection	
			Never ($n=452$)	Always ($n=584$)
Early morning erection	Never	89	66	23
	Always	947	386	561*

* $P<0.01$.

Table 3. Type of ejaculatory disturbance

	Ejaculatory disturbances	
	Patients (n)	Percentage of total population
No ejaculation during intercourse	48	0.6
Painful ejaculation	39	0.5
Ejaculation before intromission	30	0.4
Other abnormalities	59	0.8

Correlates of Coital Anejaculation and Abnormal Ejaculation

Only 0.6% of men had no ejaculation during intercourse. Half of these had never experienced ejaculation (Table 3). The other half report to have had either nocturnal ejaculations or ejaculations during masturbation.

These data suggest that half the cases with anejaculation during intercourse suffer from organic causes whereas psychogenic factors may be involved in the other half.

Painful ejaculation was reported by 39 men, which is one-third of the cases with abnormal ejaculation and 0.5% of the total population (Table 3). Early ejaculation, occurring before intromission, was reported by another 30 men (0.4% of the total population) whereas 59 men (0.8% of all men) had other unspecified ejaculation disturbances, including late ejaculation or extravaginal ejaculation due to hypospadias.

Relation Between Inadequate Coital Erection and Abnormal Ejaculation

Abnormal ejaculation was reported by only 1.3% of men with adequate coital erection against 21% of men with inadequate coital erection (Table 4). Ejaculation occurred before intromission in 8% of men with inadequate coital erection against only 0.3% of men with adequate coital erection. On the other hand, one-fourth of men with ejaculation before intromission had inadequate coital erection.

These findings suggest a possible role of ejaculation abnormalities in the pathogenesis of inadequate coital erection.

Table 4. Coital erection by ejaculatory abnormalities

Coital erection	Patients (n)	Ejaculation	
		Abnormal (%)	Before intromission (%)
Adequate	7661	1.3*	0.3*
Inadequate	100	21.0*	8.0*

* $P<0.01$.

History

Age Distribution of Sexual and Ejaculatory Inadequacy

Data on the distribution of inadequate coital erection are plotted against age in Fig. 1 (top panel). There is a clear increase in erectile inadequacy with increasing age. Near 5% of male partners of infertile couples over 40 years of age have inadequate coital erection.

The distribution of anejaculation against age shows a nadir between 30 and 35 years with slightly higher occurrence in younger and clear increase in older men (Fig. 1, middle panel).

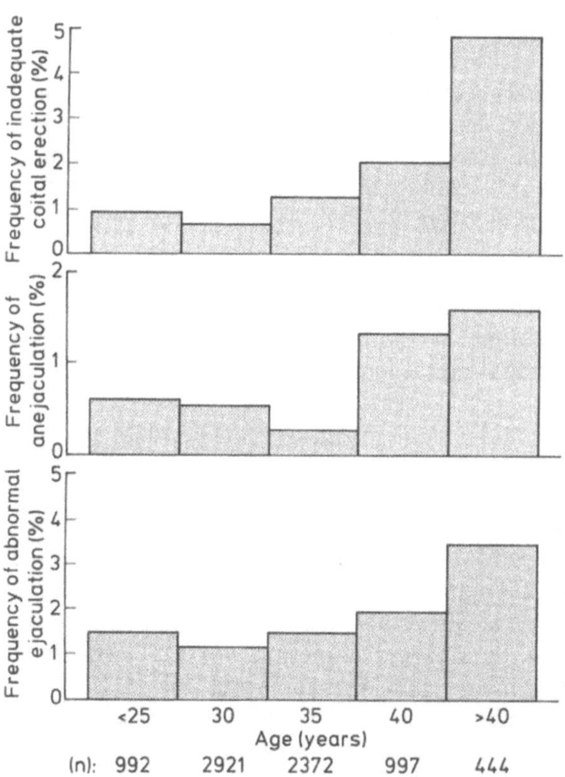

Fig. 1. Relation between age and inadequate coital erection (*top panel*), anejaculation (*middle panel*), and abnormal ejaculation (*bottom panel*)

Abnormal ejaculation presented a similar pattern as anejaculation with a nadir between 25 and 30 years (Fig. 1, bottom panel).

Discussion. Both erectile and ejaculatory function are more frequently impaired on men over 35 years of age. There seems to be some indication that men younger than 25 years of age may experience more frequent dysfunction.

Relation Between Erectile or Ejaculatory Abnormalities and Type of Infertility

Whereas anejaculation was less frequent in secondary infertility than in primary infertility, abnormal ejaculation and inadequate coital erection occurred somewhat more frequently in secondary than in primary infertility (Table 5). None of the differences were, however, significant.

Discussion. Although the observed differences are small, the contrast in the pattern between anejaculation and abnormal ejaculation is interesting. Since anejaculation is a major cause of infertility, one would expect it to occur less frequently in men who have fathered a pregnancy than in those with primary infertility. On the other hand, abnormal ejaculation and inadequate coital erection would be expected to occur more frequently in men with secondary infertility who, usually, are older than those with primary infertility.

Relation Between a History of Parotitis Infectiosa and Erectile or Ejaculatory Inadequacy

A history of infectious parotitis, occurring either before or after puberty, does not influence sexual or ejaculatory function. However, a history of orchitis associated with parotitis infectiosa is found to be associated with inadequate coital erection (Table 6). A history of orchitis was not related with anejaculation, but it had a borderline relation with abnormal ejaculation.

Discussion. The number of cases with a history of parotitis-associated orchitis is small and data must be interpreted with caution. A history of orchitis may be associated with increased prevalence of abnormal coital erection or abnormal ejaculation, which may both depend on impaired testicular function.

Relation Between Systemic Diseases and Erectile or Ejaculatory Inadequacy

Systemic diseases in general are associated with a significant increase in erectile and ejaculatory adequacy (Table 7). Diseases of the thyroid, adrenals, and respiratory or gastrointestinal tract are not found to interfere.

A history of diabetes mellitus is not significantly associated with erectile dysfunction but it is with anejaculation and abnormal ejaculation. The presence of glucose in urine was not correlated with erectile dysfunction, nor with abnormal ejaculation, while there was a borderline relation with anejaculation.

A history of neurological disease has a borderline relation with erectile dysfunction, and a significant relation with anejaculation and abnormal ejaculation. Data on physical examination confirm those findings.

Table 5. Type of infertility by erectile or ejaculatory dysfunction

Type of infertility	Patients (*n*)	Inadequate coital erection (%)	Anejaculation (%)	Abnormal ejaculation (%)
Primary	6332	1.2 (NS)	0.6 (NS)	1.4 (NS)
Secondary	1137	1.8 (NS)	0.3 (NS)	1.9 (NS)

NS, not significant.

Table 6. Parotitis-associated orchitis by erectile or ejaculatory dysfunction

Mumps orchitis	Patients (*n*)	Inadequate coital erection (%)	Anejaculation (%)	Abnormal ejaculation (%)
Absent	7654	1.2*	0.7 (NS)	1.5**
Present	109	3.7*	0.0 (NS)	3.7**

NS, not significant.
* $P<0.05$; ** $P<0.1$.

Table 7. Systemic disease by erectile and ejaculatory dysfunction

Factor	Absent (%)	Present (%)
Erectile inadequacy		
Diabetes		
History of diabetes	1.3	3.0 (NS)
Uridine glucose positive	1.6	3.6 (NS)
Neurological disease		
History of neurological disease	1.3	3.3*
Physical findings of neurological disease	1.3	0.0 (NS)
Anejaculation		
Diabetes		
History of diabetes	0.6	9.1**
Urine glucose positive	0.6	3.6*
Neurological disease		
History of neurological disease	0.6	8.2**
Physical findings of neurological disease	0.6	10.0**
Abnormal ejaculation		
Diabetes		
History of diabetes	1.5	12.1**
Urine glucose positive	1.6	7.1 (NS)
Neurological disease		
History of neurological disease	1.5	8.2**
Physical findings of neurological disease	1.5	10.0**

NS, not significant.
* $P<0.1$; ** $P<0.01$.

Table 8. History of testicular maldescent by sexual and ejaculatory dysfunction

History of testicular maldescent	Patients (*n*)	Inadequate coital erection (%)	Anejaculation (%)	Abnormal ejaculation (%)
Absent	7570	1.3 (NS)	0.6*	1.5 (NS)
Present	209	1.9 (NS)	1.9 (NS)*	1.9 (NS)

NS, not significant.
* $P<0.05$.

Table 9. History of testicular injury by sexual and ejaculatory dysfunction

History of testicular injury	Patients (*n*)	Inadequate coital erection (%)	Anejaculation (%)	Abnormal ejaculation (%)
Absent	7507	1.2*	0.5*	1.4*
Present	274	3.6*	2.6*	4.4*

* $P<0.01$.

Discussion. Most of the effects of systemic diseases on sexual and ejaculatory adequacy are related with diabetes and neurological diseases.

Testicular Characteristics and Sexual or Ejaculatory Adequacy

A history of testicular maldescent is not related to inadequacy of coital erection, nor to abnormal ejaculation. However, men with a history of testicular maldescent more frequently had anejaculation (Table 8). The type of treatment for the maldescent did not influence the ejaculatory function.

Discussion. Testicular maldescent was related with anejaculation; but this disease did not influence erectile adequacy.

Factors Causing Testicular Damage and Their Influence on Sexual and Ejaculatory Function

A history of testicular injury, severe enough to cause scrotal hematoma or hematuria, was reported by 274 men (Table 9). Such injury was significantly related with inadequate coital erection, anejaculation, and abnormal ejaculation.

Whereas the occurrence of post-traumatic testicular atrophy was related with more frequent erectile inadequacy (15%) as compared with cases with injury but without testicular atrophy (2.8%, $P<0.005$), this difference was not found for anejaculation or abnormal ejaculation.

There was no relation between a history of testicular torsion and sexual or ejaculatory inadequacy, but the number of cases is small ($n=11$).

Table 10. History of surgery with possible influence on fertility by sexual and ejaculatory dysfunction

History of surgery	Patients (*n*)	Inadequate coital erection (%)	Anejaculation (%)	Abnormal ejaculation (%)
Absent	7280	1.3 (NS)	0.6*	1.4**
Present	492	1.2 (NS)	1.4*	4.1**

NS, not significant.
* $P<0.05$; ** $P<0.01$.

Tabelle 11. History of intake of medication with possible influence of fertility by sexual and ejaculatory dysfunction

History of intake of medication	Patients (*n*)	Inadequate coital erection (%)	Anejaculation (%)	Abnormal ejaculation (%)
Absent	7590	1.2*	0.6*	1.5**
Present	188	5.3*	2.1*	3.2**

NS, not significant.
* $P<0.01$; ** $P<0.1$.

Table 12. History of excessive intake of alcohol by sexual and ejaculatory dysfunction

History of excessive intake of alcohol	Patients (*n*)	Inadequate coital erection (%)	Anejaculation (%)	Abnormal ejaculation (%)
Absent	7403	1.2*	0.6 (NS)	1.4*
Present	378	2.9*	0.0 (NS)	3.7*

NS, not significant.
* $P<0.05$.

Study of Other Factors with Possible Influence on Sexual and/or Ejaculatory Function

A history of *surgical procedures* in the urogenital region was reported by 492 patients. This history was not related with inadequate coital erection, but it was with ejaculation abnormalities and anejaculation (Table 10).

A history of *long-term intake of medication* with possible influence on fertility included medication which could interfere with sexual or ejaculatory adequacy was reported by 188 men. Indeed, such a history was significantly related with inadequacy of coital erection and ejaculation during intercourse, and with abnormal ejaculation (Table 11).

Excess alcohol consumption was recorded when a history revealed regular intake of more than 60 g alcohol/day. Men with excessive alcohol consumption more frequently had impaired erectile adequacy and abnormal ejaculation, but anejaculation did not occur among them (Table 12).

Discussion. The observed associations were expected since history taking concerning surgery and medication was aimed at the detection of factors which could impair reproductive function, including through provoking sexual or ejaculatory inadequacy.

The influence of excessive alcohol intake on erection is well known and may result from inhibition of testosterone synthesis in the testes, or from changes in androgen metabolism in the liver. The association of excessive alcohol intake and abnormal ejaculation is not readily explained by those mechanisms.

Role of Urinary Tract and Male Accessory Glands in Sexual and Ejaculatory Dysfunction

A history of urinary tract infection is indeed significantly related with inadequate coital erection and with abnormal ejaculation, and, to lesser extent, with anejaculation (Table 13). Specific urinary symptoms have a variable relation with sexual or ejaculatory disorders. A history of *sexually transmitted disease* is significantly correlated with inadequacy of coital erection and with abnormal ejaculation but not with anejaculation (Table 14).

A history of inflammatory disease of the scrotal content, other than orchitis related to parotitis infectiosa, was recorded as epididymo-orchitis. Such a history was not significantly related with inadequate coital erection, but it was related with abnormal ejaculation and had a borderline relation with anejaculation during intercourse (Table 15).

Abnormalities such as tenderness upon palpation of the scrotal content including testes, epididymides or vasa deferentia, were significantly associated with

Table 13. History of urinary symptoms by erectile and ejaculatory dysfunction

History of urinary symptoms	Coital erection		Regular ejaculation during intercourse		Ejaculation	
	Adequate (%)	Inadequate (%)	Yes (%)	No (%)	Normal (%)	Abnormal (%)
History of urinary symptoms	1.2	2.4*	0.6	1.1***	1.2	4.5*
Dysuria	1.2	2.3**	0.6	2.2 (NS)	1.3	5.4*
Urethral discharge	1.2	2.5***	0.6	0.9 (NS)	1.4	4.3*
Hematuria	1.3	1.1 (NS)	0.6	1.2 (NS)	1.4	1.1 (NS)
Frequency of urination	1.3	2.0 (NS)	0.6	1.0 (NS)	1.4	5.0*
Difficulty in voiding	1.3	2,8***	0.6	1.4 (NS)	1.4	7.8*

NS, not significant.
* $P<0.01$; ** $P<0.05$; *** $P<0.1$.

Table 14. History of sexually transmitted disease by sexual and ejaculatory dysfunction

History of sexually transmitted disease	Patients (*n*)	Inadequate coital erection (%)	Anejaculation (%)	Abnormal ejaculation (%)
Absent	6590	1.1*	0.6 (NS)	1.4**
Present	1181	2.1*	0.7 (NS)	2.5**

* $P<0.05$; ** $P<0.01$.

Table 15. History of epididymo-orchitis by sexual and ejaculatory dysfunction

History of epididymo-orchitis	Patients (*n*)	Inadequate coital erection (%)	Anejaculation (%)	Abnormal ejaculation (%)
Absent	7562	1.3 (NS)	0.6*	1.5**
Present	177	2.3 (NS)	1.7*	4.0**

NS, not significant.
* $P<0.01$; ** $P<0.1$.

Table 16. Physical findings of the scrotal content and accessory sex glands

History of urinary	Coital erection		Regular ejaculation during intercourse		Ejaculation	
	Adequate (%)	Inadequate (%)	Yes (%)	No (%)	Normal (%)	Abnormal (%)
Tenderness of the testes	1.8	5.8*	0.7	0.6 (NS)	1.9	1.9 (NS)
Abnormal epididymides	1.1	3.0*	0.6	0.8 (NS)	1.4	3.2*
Abnormal vasa deferentia	1.2	3.1**	0.6	2.1*	1.4	4.7*
Abnormal prostate	1.1	5.6*	0.6	0.8 (NS)	1.3	8.0*
Palpaple seminal vesicles	1.1	1.2 (NS)	0.6	0.2 (NS)	1.3	1.9***

NS, not significant.
* $P<0.01$; ** $P<0.05$; *** $P<0.1$.

inadequate coital erection (Table 16). Abnormalities of epididymides and vasa deferentia, but not tenderness of the testes, were related with abnormal ejaculation. Anejaculation was significantly related with palpable abnormalities of the vas deferens but not with tenderness of the testes or abnormal palpation of the epididymides.

Abnormal palpation of the prostate was significantly related with inadequate coital erection and abnormal ejaculation (Table 16). This was true for tenderness, and either soft or hard swelling of the prostate. There was no relation between the presence of palpable seminal vesicles and erectile dysfunction, but there was a borderline relation between the former and abnormal ejaculation. Anejaculation was not related with palpable abnormalities of the prostate or seminal vesicles.

Discussion. Clearly, there is a relation between a history of inflammation or infection of the urinary tract or of the scrotal content and sexual or ejaculatory dysfunction as well as with abnormal ejaculation, but not with anejaculation during intercourse.

Data on the physical examination of the scrotal content and accessory sex glands support the findings of the history, namely that there is a significant relationship between inadequate sexual or ejaculatory function and abnormalities which can be ascribed to (chronic) infection or inflammation. On the basis of the present data it is, however, impossible to decide whether the infection/inflammation is the cause or the result of the sexual or ejaculatory inadequacy.

Physical Examination

Relation Between Sexual and Ejaculatory Function and General Physical Examination and Examination of the Genital Region

Men with *abnormal signs of virilization*, in particular incomplete development of secondary sex characteristics as a sign of endocrine deficiency, had a higher frequency of sexual and ejaculatory inadequacy (Table 17). The same was true for gynecomastia, which was significantly associated with inadequate coital erection

Table 17. Secondary sexual characteristics by sexual and ejaculatory dysfunction

Secondary sexual characteristics	Patients (n)	Inadequate coital erection (%)	Anejaculation (%)	Abnormal ejaculation (%)
Normal	7655	1.2*	0.6*	1.5**
Abnormal	39	12.8*	5.1*	5.1**

* $P<0.01$; ** $P<0.1$.

Table 18. Gynecomastia by sexual and ejaculatory dysfunction

Gynecomastia	Patients (n)	Inadequate coital erection (%)	Anejaculation (%)	Abnormal ejaculation (%)
Absent	7614	1.3*	0.6**	1.5 (NS)
Present	48	4.2*	2.1**	4.2 (NS)

NS, not significant.
* $P<0.1$; ** $P<0.05$.

Table 19. Physical abnormalities of the penis by sexual and ejaculatory dysfunction

	Patients (*n*)	Inadequate coital erection (%)	Anejaculation (%)	Abnormal ejaculation (%)
Penis				
Normal	7609	1.2*	0.6***	1.4*
Abnormal	83	6.0*	2.4***	8.4*
Phimosis				
Absent	7662	1.3*	0.6**	1.5*
Present	30	6.7*	3.3**	10.0*
Hypospadias				
Absent	7672	1.3**	0.6 (NS)	1.5*
Present	15	6.7**	0.0 (NS)	20.0*

* $P<0.01$; ** $P<0.1$; *** $P<0.05$.

Table 20. Physical characteristics of the testes by sexual and ejaculatory dysfunction

	Patients (*n*)	Inadequate coital erection (%)	Anejaculation (%)	Abnormal ejaculation (%)
Testes				
Both present	7540	1.2*	0.6**	1.5 (NS)
At least one absent	163	3.1*	2.5**	3.1 (NS)
Testicular consistency				
Normal	2451	2.0 (NS)	0.6*	1.6*
At least one side abnormal	408	1.2 (NS)	1.5*	3.9**

NS, not significant.
* $P<0.05$; ** $P<0.01$.

(Table 18). Abnormalities of the penis were significantly associated with abnormal ejaculation and inadequate coital erection (Table 19).

The absence of one or both testes was recorded in 163 men and this was associated with increased prevalence of sexual and ejaculatory inadequacy. Abnormal consistency of at least one testis was associated with abnormal ejaculation but not inadequate erection (Table 20).

There is an inverse correlation between total testicular volume and prevalence of inadequate coital erection (Fig. 2, top panel). The same is true for abnormal ejaculation (Fig. 2, bottom panel), and – though less clearly – for anejaculation (Fig. 2, middle panel). Men with a total testicular volume less than 20/25 ml had a higher prevalence of sexual inadequacy (mean 2.7%) and abnormal ejaculation (mean 2.6%) than men with testicular volume in excess of this limit (1.0% for erectile inadequacy and 1.4% for abnormal ejaculation). This is confirmed by the

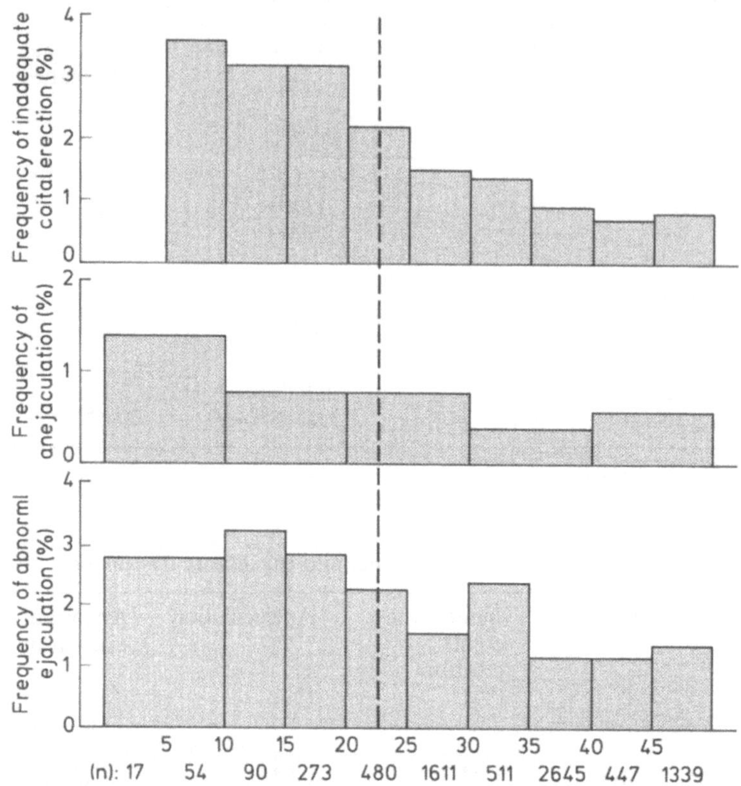

Fig. 2. Relation between total testicular volume and inadequate coital erection (*top panel*), anejaculation (*middle panel*), and abnormal ejaculation (*bottom panel*)

fact that men with adequate coital erection had a larger total testicular volume (37.13 ml $\pm$ 0.10 SEM) than men with erectile inadequacy (32.77 ml $\pm$ 1.11 SEM).

Discussion. Together with the data on secondary sex characteristics and gynecomastia, the data on testicular volume underscore the role of endocrine factors particularly in inadequate coital erection and abnormal ejaculation, whereas the influence on anejaculation seems to be less evident.

Scrotal Swelling and Hernia

The presence of scrotal swelling due to other causes than varicocele, which includes hydrocele and scrotal hernia, did not influence erectile adequacy (Table 21). On the other hand, patients with scrotal swelling more commonly had anejaculation, but this is not related with the presence of inguinal hernia. There is a borderline relation between abnormal ejaculation and scrotal swelling, particularly inguinal hernia ($P < 0.05$).

Table 21. Scrotal swelling by sexual and ejaculatory dysfunction

Scrotal swelling	Patients (*n*)	Inadequate coital erection (%)	Anejaculation (%)	Abnormal ejaculation (%)
Absent	7581	1.3 (NS)	0.6*	1.5**
Present	112	1.8 (NS)	3.5*	3.6**

* $P<0.01$; ** $P<0.1$.

Table 22. Varicocele by sexual and ejaculatory dysfunction

Varicocele	Patients (*n*)	Inadequate coital erection (%)	Anejaculation (%)	Abnormal ejaculation (%)
Absent	6318	1.2*	0.6 (NS)	1.5 (NS)
Present	1358	1.8*	0.8 (NS)	1.8 (NS)

* $P<0.1$.

Discussion. There are no arguments to lead us to believe that ejaculatory dysfunction may induce scrotal swelling. Therefore, it is reasonable to assume that scrotal swelling, including hernia, may cause ejaculatory inadequacy, both anejaculation and abnormal ejaculation. It remains to be studied whether this effect results from the scrotal swelling itself, or is mediated through possible influence on testicular function. The latter is suspected in the case of hernia, since these patients also have an increased prevalence of abnormal semen quality and lower testicular volume.

Varicocele

Men with either unilateral or bilateral varicocele presented a borderline increase in the frequency of inadequate coital erection. There is no relation between varicocele and impairment of ejaculation (Table 22).

Discussion. It has been shown that patients with varicocele and low serum testosterone concentration may suffer from inadequate coital erection. Furthermore it has been found that varicocele is associated with decreased testicular volume. These factors and the present findings support the hypothesis that varicocele may cause sexual inadequacy.

Laboratory Data

Urine Analysis in Sexual and/or Ejaculatory Inadequacy

A relation was found between abnormal urine analysis and inadequate coital erection, anejaculation, and abnormal ejaculation (Table 23). Proteinuria is re-

Table 23. Urine analysis by sexual and ejaculatory dysfunction

	Patients (n)	Inadequate coital erection (%)	Anejaculation (%)	Abnormal ejaculation (%)
Urine analysis				
Normal	6032	1.1*	0.6**	1.4**
Abnormal	253	2.4*	2.0**	5.5**
Proteine in urine				
No	6214	1.1 (NS)	0.6**	1.4**
Yes	71	2.8 (NS)	4.2**	5.6**
White blood cells				
Absent	6147	1.1 (NS)	0.6***	1.4**
Present	138	2.2 (NS)	2.2***	7.2**
Red blood cells				
Absent	6236	1.1 (NS)	0.6 (NS)	1.4 (NS)
Present	49	2.0 (NS)	2.0 (NS)	4.1 (NS)
Bacteriuria >100000/ml				
Absent	6038	1.2 (NS)	0.6***	1.6***
Present	160	0.0 (NS)	2.3***	4.6***

* $P<0.1$; ** $P<0.01$; *** $P<0.05$.

lated with anejaculation, whereas signs of infection and inflammation are related with abnormal ejaculation. The relation between inadequate coital erection and abnormal urine analysis was weak.

Discussion. These data confirm data of the history and physical examination and underscore the role of infection of the genitourethral region in ejaculatory inadequacy.

Relation Between Semen Analysis and Sexual and/or Ejaculatory Inadequacy

When semen quality is classified in order of severity of alteration (from normal semen to azoospermia), there is an increasing frequency of erectile and ejaculatory abnormalities with severity of semen alteration (Fig. 3). By definition, anejaculation and abnormal ejaculation are commonly associated with aspermia. Men with inadequate ejaculation more commonly had abnormal semen quality, including azoospermia (61.4%), than men with normal ejaculation (50.1%, $P<0.01$).

All semen quality data were impaired in patients with sexual or ejaculatory dysfunction, as compared with men without such alterations (Table 24, Fig. 4). In addition, men with abnormal ejaculation had an increased number of white blood cells in their semen.

Discussion The relation between erectile inadequacy and abnormal semen quality corresponds with the correlation between erectile inadequacy and decreased tes-

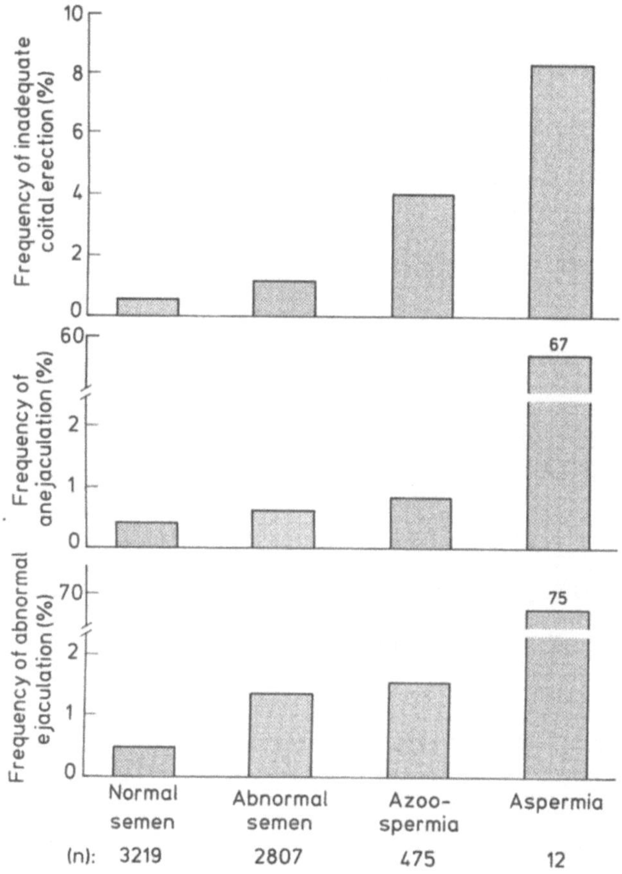

Fig. 3. Relation between semen classification and inadequate coital erection (*top panel*), anejaculation (*middle panel*), and abnormal ejaculation (*bottom panel*)

ticular volume, since testicular volume and semen quality are related. Since the present data were collected exclusively in couples consulting for infertility, it is improbable that differences in sexual adequacy among men with different degrees of severity of semen alteration result from the infertility problem itself. Hence, it should be accepted that the testicular abnormalities which cause abnormal semen equally result in increased prevalence of erectile inadequacy.

Endocrine Investigations

Endocrine results (Table 25, Fig. 5) suggest a tendency toward lower plasma testosterone concentrations in men with inadequate coital erection or anejaculation. FSH is significantly elevated in patients with anejaculation, and LH is elevated in men with erectile inadequacy. The serum prolactin level is not different in men with abnormal sexual or ejaculatory function from that in men with adequate function.

Table 24. Semen characteristics (mean ±SEM) by sexual and ejaculatory dysfunction

Semen characteristics by dysfunction	Absent	Present
Inadequate coital erection		
Ejaculate volume (ml)	3.20±0.02	2.96±0.18
Progressive motility (%)	44.7 ±0.3	37.0 ±3.3
Concentration (mill/ml)	60.8 ±0.8	50.7 ±7.0
Normal forms (%)	55.8 ±0.3	50.9 ±3.9
White blood cells (mill/ml)	0.58±0.03	0.76±0.36
Anejaculation		
Ejaculate volume (ml)	3.20±0.02	2.66±0.38
Progressive motility (%)	44.7 ±0.3	34.2 ±4.6
Concentration (mill/ml)	60.8 ±0.8	53.9 ±1.4
Normal forms (%)	55.8 ±0.3	51.8 ±4.9
White blood cells (mill/ml)	0.58±0.03	0.81±0.37
Abnormal ejaculation		
Ejaculate volume (ml)	3.20±0.02	2.84±0.28
Progressive motility (%)	44.8 ±0.3	36.9 ±2.6
Concentration (mill/ml)	60.8 ±0.8	57.3 ±6.7
Normal forms (%)	55.8 ±0.3	49.8 ±3.0
White blood cells (mill/ml)	0.57±0.03	1.60±0.50

Table 25. Endocrine investigation

Coital erection	Adequate	Inadequate
FSH (IU/liter)	5.77±0.14	6.48± 1.29
LH (IU/liter)	6.92±0.14	5.73± 0.79*
Testosterone (mmol/liter)	20.00±0.20	18.05± 1.93
Prolactin (mIU/liter)	280.6 ±3.4	281.9 ±21.3
Anejaculation	Absent	Present
FSH (IU/liter)	5.75±0.14	9.03± 1.97*
LH(IU/liter)	6.89±0.14	9.29± 2.50
Testosterone (mmol/liter)	20.00±0.20	17.73± 1.67*
Prolactin (mIU/liter)	281.0 ±3.4	218.6 ±24.3
Ejaculation	Normal	Abnormal
FSH (IU/liter)	5.79±0.14	5.35± 0.73
LH (IU/liter)	6.93±0.14	6.13± 0.58
Testosterone (mmol/liter)	19.96±0.20	19.08± 1.28
Prolactin (mIU/liter)	280.4 ±3.4	295.0 ±30.9

* $P<0.05$.

Discussion. The endocrine data do not suggest elevated prolactin to play a major role in sexual or ejaculatory dysfunction. A decreased plasma androgen concentration seems to be involved with anejaculation and with inadequate coital erection. In the latter the decreased androgen concentration coincides with a decreased mean concentration of LH in serum suggesting a central, hypothalamo-

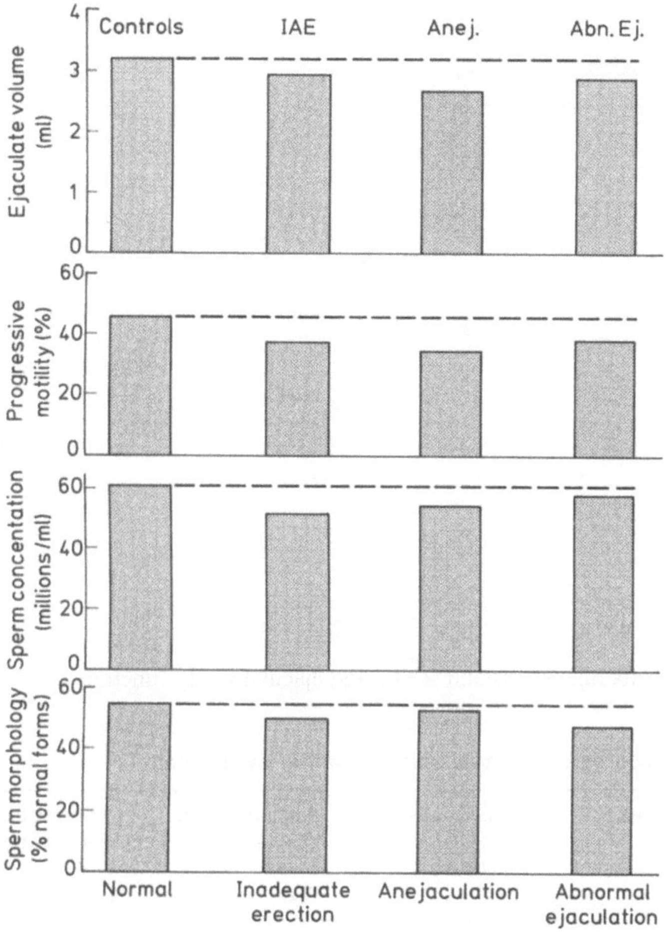

Fig. 4. Relation between semen characteristics and inadequate coital erection, anejaculation, and abnormal ejaculation

pituitary cause of the reduced testosterone level. The elevated concentration of serum FSH in patients with anejaculation suggests a primary testicular factor to be involved. Men with normal ejaculation have unremarkable endocrine results.

Testicular Biopsy

A testicular biopsy was performed in 298 patients. In 82 (27.5%), none of whom had erectile inadequacy, the histology was normal. In the remaining 216 cases, the biopsy showed hypospermatogenesis (82 cases), germ cell arrest (57 cases), Sertoli's cells only (38 cases), tubular hyalinization (36 cases), or an immature aspect (two cases). Of the patients with abnormal biopsies, three had erectile inadequacy, which is not significantly different from the group with normal histology. The prevalence of ejaculatory abnormalities was not different in men with normal or abnormal histology.

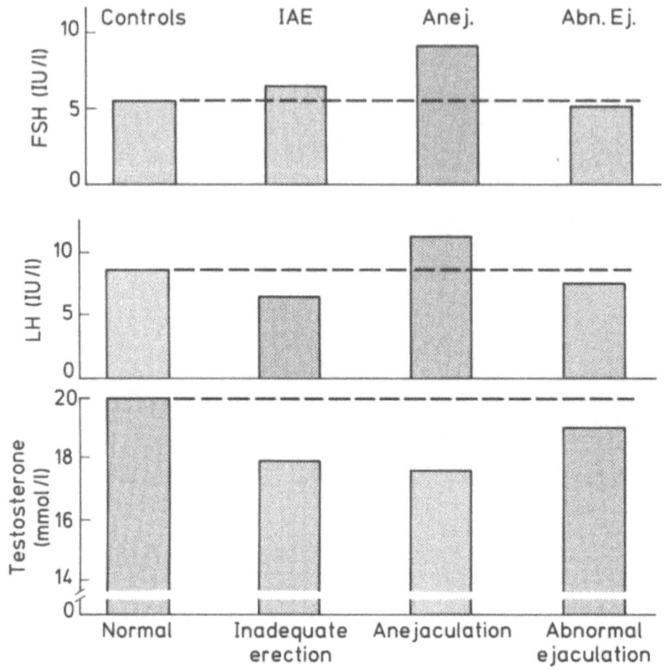

Fig. 5. Relation between endocrine results and sexual and ejaculatory dysfunction

Table 26. Prostatic expression fluid by sexual and ejaculatory dysfunction

	Patients (*n*)	Inadequate coital erection (%)	Anejaculation (%)	Abnormal ejaculation (%)
PEF culture				
Normal	710	1.0 (NS)	0.4 (NS)	1.3**
Abnormal	71	1.4 (NS)	1.4 (NS)	9.9**
PEF cytology				
Normal	612	0.5*	0.2**	1.0**
Abnormal	20	5.0*	5.0**	20.0.**

* $P<0.05$; ** $P<0.01$.

Discussion. A testicular biopsy was performed for the evaluation of infertility in men with extreme oligozoospermia or azoospermia. There was no relation between the histological findings and erectile or ejaculatory inadequacy.

Expressed Prostatic Fluid

Culture of expressed prostatic fluid was more frequently abnormal in men with abnormal ejaculation, but there was no relation with anejaculation or erectile inadequacy (Table 26). Abnormal prostatic cytology with an increased number of white blood cells in the expressed fluid, was significantly related with sexual and ejaculatory inadequacy.

Discussion. Culture of the expressed prostatic fluid was more commonly abnormal than prostatic cytology. Abnormal cytology was associated with abnormal erectile and ejaculatory function. This suggests prostatic inflammation rather than infection to be involved with erectile inadequacy. It is not clear from the present data whether the increased number of white blood cells in the expressed prostatic fluid is the cause or the result of inadequate coital erection or anejaculation. Abnormal ejaculation is significantly related with both signs of infection and inflammation of the prostate.

Interrelation Between Male and Female Factors

The frequency of vaginal intercourse, as recorded from female history taking, was significantly lower in couples where the man suffered from inadequate coital erection or ejaculatory disturbances (Table 27).

The frequency of noncoital sexual activity was similar in all groups.

Lubricants were more commonly used by couples where the men suffered from inadequate coital erection or abnormal ejaculation, but not in patients with anejaculation (Table 28).

Table 27. Mean frequency of vaginal intercourse per month (±SEM) by sexual and ejaculatory dysfunction

	Adequate or normal	Inadequate or abnormal
Coital erection	11.4±0.1	9.1±0.6
Ejaculation during intercourse	11.4±0.1	9.0±0.9
Ejaculation characteristics	11.4±0.1	9.6±0.5

Table 28. Female history of use of lubricants and systemic disease by sexual and ejaculatory dysfunction

	Patients (*n*)	Use of lubricants (%)	Systemic disease (%)
Coital erection			
Adequate	7632	7.1	7.8
Inadequate	99	3.2*	7.1 (NS)
Ejaculation during Intercourse			
Present	7687	3.3	6.4
Absent	47	4.2 (NS)	7.8 (NS)
Ejaculation			
Normal	7597	3.2	7.7
Abnormal	118	6.7**	12.7*

* $P<0.05$; ** $P<0.01$.

Table 29. Penile penetration, frequency of orgasm, dyspareunia, and vaginal discharge by sexual or ejaculatory dysfunction

	Patients (*n*)	Incomplete penile penetration (%)	Seldom or never orgasm (%)	Dyspareunia (deep and superficial) (%)	Excessive vaginal discharge (%)
Coital erection					
Adequate	7626	1.0	21.3	17.3	9.2
Inadequate	99	14.1*	39.4*	26.3*	23.2*
Ejaculation during intercourse					
Present	7682	1.1	21.4	17.4	9.4
Absent	47	10.6*	29.4 (NS)	19.1 (NS)	12.8 (NS)
Ejaculation					
Normal	7592	1.1	21.4	17.2	9.3
Abnormal	118	6.8*	27.3 (NS)	30.8*	13.6 (NS)

NS, not significant.
* $P<0.01$; ** $P<0.05$.

The degree of penile penetration (Table 29) was experienced as incomplete in a significantly higher number of female partners, if the male either had inadequate coital erection, or anejaculation, or abnormal ejaculation. However, the occurrence of female orgasm was only decreased if the partner had inadequate coital erection, but not if anejaculation or abnormal ejaculation were present.

Dyspareunia was related with inadequate coital erection and abnormal ejaculation, but not with anejaculation, whereas excessive vaginal discharge was related with inadequate coital erection only (Table 29).

Abnormal ejaculation and a female history of systemic disease were found to be significantly related. No relation was found between sexual and/or ejaculatory dysfunction in the male and pelvic inflammatory disease (PID) or Sexually Transmitted Disease (STD) in the female (Table 28).

Discussion. These data underscore the strong interrelation between erectile inadequacy and several aspects of female sexual experience. Anejaculation was related with the female experience of incomplete penile penetration, whereas abnormal ejaculation was related with both deep and superficial dyspareunia. The physiopathogenic mechanisms involved in the latter associations remain speculative.

Female Physical Characteristics and Male Sexual and Ejaculatory Function

Masculine hair distribution of the female partner was not significantly related with male sexual or ejaculatory dysfunction (Table 30). There was, however, a significant relation between incomplete breast development with Tanner stage 4 or less, and male sexual function. Indeed, male partners of females with incomplete breast development more frequently had inadequate coital erection, but less frequently presented ejaculatory dysfunction or abnormal ejaculation.

As expected, erectile inadequacy was related with increased prevalence of intact hymen. Abnormalities of the vulva and intact hymen were also related with

Table 30. Female physical findings by sexual or ejaculatory dysfunction

	Patients (*n*)	Masculine hair distribution	Incomplete breast development	Abnormal vulva	Intact hymen	Abnormal cervix	Abnormal adnexa
Coital erection							
Adequate	7540	4.8	27.4	0.7	0.1	11.6	7.7
Inadequate	98	4.1 (NS)	36.7*	1.0 (NS)	1.0**	12.4 (NS)	10.2 (NS)
Ejaculation during intercourse							
Present	7595	4.7	27.6	0.7	0.1	10.9	7.7
Absent	46	8.7 (NS)	12.8*	2.1 (NS)	0.0 (NS)	11.6 (NS)	6.4 (NS)
Ejaculation							
Normal	7511	4.7	28.6	0.7	0.1	11.5	7.6
Abnormal	115	7.0 (NS)	19.1*	2.6*	0.9**	21.1**	10.4 (NS)

NS, not significant.
* $P<0.05$; ** $P<0.01$.

abnormal ejaculation but not with anejaculation. There was no relation between abnormalities of the vagina or clitoris, or genital prolapse and male sexual dysfunction. However, abnormalities of the cervix were more common in the female partners of men with abnormal ejaculation.

Discussion. Considering the relation between specific physical appearances of the female and male sexual dysfunction is interesting but explanations are speculative. The coincidence of abnormal ejaculation and cervical abnormalities may be related to infection of the male accessory sex glands and transfer of bacteria into the cervical channel. No relation was found between abnormal adnexa and sexual or ejaculatory dysfunction, which is in agreement with the lack of coincidence of sexual and ejaculatory dysfunction and a history of STD or PID.

Female Endocrine and Ovulatory Data

Cycle length was similar in female partners of men with or without sexual or ejaculatory problems. Prolactin concentration in the female partners was not different if the male was sexually adequate or inadequate. Furthermore, the ovulatory status was not significantly different in female partners of men with erectile or ejaculatory inadequacy. The same was true for the frequency of tubal patency and endometriosis.

References

Comhaire FH, De Kretser DM, Farley TT, Rowe PJ (1987) Towards more objectivity in diagnosis and management of male infertility. Int J Androl [Suppl] 7:1–53

Diagnosis and Treatment of Marital Infertility Due To Sperm Antibodies

U. Deichert and W. Krause

Universitäts-Frauenklinik, Pilgrimstein 3, 3550 Marburg, FRG

In cases of marital infertility without definite findings in one of the partners (unexplained infertility), it is usual to assume immunological causes. In his investigations, Friberg (1981) showed that a long duration of unexplained infertility corresponds with so-called immunological incompatibility.

The term "disturbed cervix-sperm interaction" summarizes pathological findings of the seminal parameters and penetration disturbances, which are obviously caused by immunological factors or by the lack of cervical mucus. For these reasons, an insufficient number of motile sperms reaches the oozyte in the fallopian tube for fertilization.

For diagnosis we have to evaluate the relations in cervical mucus penetration. The first step is usually the in vivo test of sperm migration within the cervix mucus, i.e., the postcoital test according to Sims-Huhner or after artificial insemination the postinsemination test (PIT). When no motile spermatozoa are found, we test the sperm-mucus interactions by an in vitro test, the sperm-cervix-mucus contact test or SCMC test. It reveals information on the sperm quality in the native ejaculate and the motility score within the mucus. Firstly the SCMC test is performed in the homologous system with husband's sperm and wife's mucus. Secondly it is done in the heterologous system with the patient's mucus and husband's sperm against donor sperm and donor mucus respectively. A decrease of sperm motility in the mucus for 20% or more or a quotient of 1.2 of first percental motility and second motility after mucus contact is defined as pathological in both systems.

In addition and particularly in such cases, we determine the antispermatozoal activity in serum of both partners according to the method described by Kibrick.

In a retrospective study we were interested in the relationship between the results of the in vivo performed postcoital test, the SCMC test as an in vitro penetration test, and the titers of antispermatozoal activity in serum of the infertile couples. We examined a total number of 95 couples attending our clinic for diagnosis of sperm penetration disorders.

Twenty-five percent of their male partners showed a sperm count below 20 million/ml. In 52 cases the results of the homologous SCMS test were compared with those of the sperm-agglutination test for serum-sperm antibodies of the male partner. The lowest relative decrease of sperm motility was found in the group with negative antispermatozoal activity, but the highest decrease could be detected in the group with a titer of 8–32 and not of 64–128. So we do not see a real correlation between the outcome of the homologous SCMC test and male sperm antibodies in serum.

Sexology
Eds.: W. Eicher, G. Kockott

In 40 cases we compared the results of the SCMS test using donor spermatozoa with the titers of antispermatozoal activity in the serum of the female partner. Here we found the lowest relative decrease of sperm motility in the SCMC test in the groups with no and with low antibody titers and the highest decrease on average in the groups with high antibody titers.

When the number of speramtozoa in the postcoital test were compared with the antispermatozoal activity in female serum in 23 cases, we found a continuous decrease of the number of spermatozoa with rising antibody titers. For the same cases we saw the highest relative decrease of motility in the SCMC test with donor sperms with the lowest mean number of spermatozoa (the group of high antibody titers) in the postcoital test (PCT). At least for these results the outcome of the PCT corresponded with that of the SCMC test with donor sperms and the Kibrick test with female serum.

According to the literature, negative penetration tests (in vivo and in vitro) mostly show good correlations with positive antispermatozoal activity. Nevertheless there are case reports describing positive PCT in the presence of high antibody titers, as mentioned by Rümke et al. (1984).

We also observed some examples with similar findings followed by a pregnancy: In one of our patients with a positive antibody titer of 1:64 after AID, a pregnancy occurred, which ended in an abortion mens III. The question was whether the positive antibody titer influenced the abortion process. One other patient having a pathological SCMC test in the homologous and heterologous system, but negative antibody activity, became pregnant after diagnosis. Another patient with a negative PIT after AID became pregnant after cap insemination, showing a pathological heterologous SCMC test in the conception cycle.

These observations indicate that the presence of penetration disturbances or positive antibody titer do not absolutely contradict against pregnancy. Their occurrence, however, causes sterility problems, since Menge et al. (1982) found pregnancy rate significantly reduced when one or both partners showed antispermatozoal activity in serum or in other genital secretions. Thus in each case of immunological disturbances we see the necessity for adequate therapy of the couple.

The following methods have been used for treatment of infertility due to suspected immunological problems:

1. Corticoid medication
2. Intrauterine insemination (IUI) with washed spermatozoa
3. GIFT (Gamete intrafallopian transfer)/IVF
4. ZIFT (Zygote intrafallopian transfer)

Concerning IUI we prefer to perform the insemination with a filled bladder and ultrasound guided, and find it easy with this technique (Deichert et al. 1986). In a little study group with six pregnancies after IUI, one pregnancy occurred after IUI because of immunological factor. But in general the results with IUI in the case of immunological factor are poor rather than good. Better results are reported by IVF or GIFT. So we recently obtained a pregnancy after IVF in a woman with positive serum antibodies. But it ended in an early abortion.

The newest method is the transfer of fertilized ova at the prenuclear stage into the fallopian tube, called ZIFT. Devroey (1987, personal communication) reported a pregnancy rate about 40%, but in a very small group. Further investigations will show whether these optimistic results can be confirmed.

References

Deichert U, Klafki M, Brechnitz G, Daume E (1986) Vorteile der ultraschallgeführten hohen intracavitären Insemination. Ultraschall Klin Prax [Suppl 1]:8

Friberg J (1981) Postcoitaltests and sperm-agglutinating antibodies in men. Am J Obstet Gynecol 141:76–80

Rümke Ph, Renckens CNM, Bezemer PD, Amstel N van (1984) Prognosis of fertility in women with unexplained infertility and sperm agglutinins in the serum. Fertil Steril 42:561–567

Menge AC, Medley NE, Mangione CM, Dietrich JW (1982) The incidence and influence of antisperm antibodies in infertile human couples on sperm-cervical mucus interactions and subsequent fertility. Fertil Steril 38:439–447

The Influence of Sex Differences on the Acceptance of Infertility

H. J. Brand

Centre for Psychological Services, University of Stellenbosch, Stellenbosch, Republic of South Africa

The aim of this study was to investigate the influence of infertility on the relationship between husband and wife as well as the possible emotional reactions associated with the onset and development of a problem of this kind.

According to Bernard and Flapan (1963), all potential adoptive parents should be evaluated to determine the extent to which the presence of functional or psychogenic infertility has had a negative effect on the wife's self-image. It is obvious why a proposal like this should be taken seriously when the percentage of "problem" cases among adoptees is taken into account. Also, because the specific causes for these emotional and behavioral problems are not always clear. However, it is true that the success of the adoptive process depends far more on the behavior and qualities of the adoptive parents than on anything else (Jacka 1973).

Infertility in a marriage is an extremely sensitive matter as far as the married couple are concerned, and it is something which they find difficult to accept and come to terms with psychologically. According to a publication by The Group for the Advancement of Psychiatry (1973), infertility involves a kind of transformation of basic expectations in the personality. The knowledge that they cannot have their own children does not only mean initial emotional shock and disappointment for the married couple, but creates feelings of frustration, self-criticism, inferiority, and even guilt. This chronic emotional disillusionment can lead to aggression toward the marriage partner.

Terman (1938), on the other hand, found no relationship between absence of children and presence of marital unhappiness. These findings have been verified by the work of Hicks and Platt (1970). A corresponding view is to be found in Chester (1972), who found that the popular view that childless marriages more frequently lead to divorce is largely unfounded. The criticism regarding this research is that no differentiation was made between couples who voluntarily remained childless and those whose childlessness was involuntary, which complicates the attempts to interpret the findings.

Humphrey (1975) noted that couples who were involuntarily childless were more attuned to each other's thoughts and feelings than married couples with one or more children. Although the fact that they were childless was a painful experience for these married couples, it did not necessarily have a negative effect on their marital relationship. The finding of Boocock (1976), that childless married couples more frequently described their relationship with their marriage partner as satisfactory than a control group who had children, accords with this.

Sexology
Eds.: W. Eicher, G. Kockott

It appears, therefore, that there is no consensus on whether involuntary childlessness has a positive or a negative effect on the quality of a marital relationship. However, it is generally believed that if a married couple remains childless, while they do wish to conceive, the couple will face pressures which could eventually lead to friction in the relationship.

Method

Subjects

The subjects were 118 patients (59 married couples) from the Department of Spermatology and Infertility, Tygerberg Hospital. The ages of the women ranged from 269 to 442 months, with a mean age of 346 months. The minimum and maximum ages of the men were 301 and 564 months respectively, with a mean age of 384 months.

Seventy-five percent of the males and 69% of the females were Afrikaans speaking. The rest were English speaking.

Approximately half of the males (48%) had graduated from High School, while 16% had attended a university. Sixty-three percent of the female group had graduated from High School and 9% had completed a course at a university.

The couples had been married for between 1 and 17 years (mean = 6.3 years). Analysis of the period of treatment at the Infertility Clinic gave a positive skew distribution (index of skewness = 2894). The median value was 1.5 months.

Procedure

Since existing questionnaires concerned with determining the quality of a marital relationship [Marriage Adjustment Questionnaire, Locke and Wallace (1959); Two Person Adjustment Questionnaire, Spanier (1976); Marriage Index, Terman (1938)] were considered unsuitable for this study, a semistructured interview (Table 1) was used to obtain the required information. The questions consisted of 13 items with subsections, and were partly based on the work of Van Keep and Schmidt-Elmendorff (1974).

Results

The chi-square method was used to compare the responses of males and females ($2 \times n$ tables). According to Lewontin and Felsenstein (1965), the chi-square test is conservative at the 5%, 2%, and 1% levels when the expected frequency is one and the degrees of freedom is greater than four. The 2G statistic (Cilliers, 1972) was calculated only for those variables in which the theoretical frequency was smaller than one. In these cases the G test could be used since it is not bound to the minimum frequency requirement in the respective cells. For a contingency table with r rows and c coloumns, the following formula is used:

$$G=\sum_{1}^{r}\sum_{1}^{k}(2a\,1n\,a)-\sum_{1}^{r}(2R\,1n\,R)-\sum_{1}^{k}(2k\,1n\,k)+2N\,1n\,N \quad \text{(Wilks 1935)}$$

a = empirical frequency

R = row frequency

k = column frequency

N = total frequency

The obtained chi-square and $2G$ values are shown in Table 1. Eleven of these values were significant.

Inspection of the obtained frequencies revealed that:

Table 1. Differences between males and females on interview variables

Variables	χ^2	$2G$
Introduction		
1. How often do you talk about your childlessness? (Never) *1 2 3 4 5 6 7* (often)	15.6192*	–
2. Easy/Difficult to talk about it? Yes/no	0.9241	–
Marriage		
3. With whom do you discuss it mostly? Husband/friend/colleague/doctor/parents	14.9340**	–
4. How satisfied are you with your husband's (wife's) help? (Very dissatisfied with) *1 2 3 4 5 6 7* (very satisfied with)	12.7266*	–
5. Would you consider a divorce because of childlessness? Yes/no	0.5392	–
6. How "happy" was your marriage relationship:		
a) From the engagement until the marriage (Absolutely unhappy) *1 2 3 4 5 6 7* (absolutely happy)	3.8991	–
b) From the marriage until the decision to become pregnant	–	3.3500
c) From the decision to become pregnant until the time you began to realize that this does not happen	–	7.4962
d) From the time you began to think that something might be wrong until the first visit to a doctor	–	2.2979
e) From the first visit, until a diagnosis was made	–	6.6530
f) From hearing the diagnosis until now	–	10.4432
7. I want you to evaluate the degree of stress (tension) you have had experienced during the (previous) phases in your life:		
a) (Absolutely) no stress) *1 2 3 4 5 6 7* (extremely stressful) Phase 1	–	8.3556
b) Phase 2	4.6988	–
c) Phase 3	20.1853**	–
d) Phase 4	13.7220*	–
e) Phase 5	7.8473	–
f) Phase 6	21.1128**	–

Table 1. (continued)

Variables	χ^2	2G
Attitude towards infertility		
8. How did you *feel* when you realized that your marriage might be childless? Dreadfully disappointed/unhappy/no specific feeling/quietly happy (relieved)	29.5386**	–
9. How difficult a problem is childlessness for you now? Predominating (all-important)/intense/not of particular importance/of no importance	36.5020**	–
10. How did the fact of childlessness change your personality?		
Jealous	5.5326*	–
Inferior	1.3831	–
Incomplete	0.1092	–
No change	9.1957**	–
Positive change	0.319	–
11. For whom is the disappointment (over the inability for have children) greater? Yourself/husband (wife)/family	55.6054**	–
12. The behavior of people when in your presence: The try to avoid the subject of children/normal conversations/normally sympathize	1.3831	–
13. What/whom helped most to overcome the fact of childlessness? Husband (wife) encouragement/religious faith and acceptance of childlessness/friends – supporting of .../suppress thoughts	3.5068	–

* $P<0.05$
** $P<0.01$

- Females were more willing to discuss their infertility problem than males (item 1).
- The proportion of females who discussed the problem outside marriage was significantly larger than that of males (item 3).
- The women were more dissatisfied with the way their husbands treated them as a person, than were men with their wives (item 4).
- Females experienced more stress during certain phases of the treatment process than males (item 7).
- More females were extremely disappointed or unhappy at the realization that their marriage could remain childless than males (item 8).
- The majority of females described the emotional intensity of their infertility problem at present as intense or overwhelming whereas males did not (item 9).
- A significant proportion of females admitted that they had experienced feelings of envy toward people with children (item 10).
- More women than men disclosed that a personality change (relating to the infertility problem) had taken place (item 10).
- A considerable degree of consensus between males and females (that the disappointment about the possibility that the marriage could remain barren) was more intense for wives (item 11).

Discussion

The women not only discussed the infertility problem more frequently than their husbands, but also found it easier to talk about the subject (when the opportunity arose) with outsiders. This is consistent with the findings of Van Keep and Schmidt-Elmendorff (1974), who reported that women generally reacted positively to the postulation "I like to talk to someone about the fact that my marriage is childless," while most men reacted negatively.

The intensity of the initial disappointment (with the realization that the marriage would most likely be childless) was significantly greater for women than for men. This conclusion is directly supported by the research of Van Keep and Schmidt-Elmendorff (1974), who found that 57% of the infertile women in their study were extremely disappointed when pregnancy repeatedly failed to occur, while 41% of the men had a similar reaction.

Females also described the present intensity of the problem significantly more often as intense and/or completely overwhelming. There was also a significant consensus of opinion between groups that the psychological effect of the infertility problem was significantly greater for women than for men. In addition women experienced more envy and stress as a result of childlessness.

It seems that infertility not only evoked more intense emotional reactions initially, but that women, in comparison to their husbands, took longer to come to terms with the problem. Generally speaking, the negative effect of infertility on the behavior of women was greater than on that of men.

Consistent with these findings, women proved to be significantly more dissatisfied with the way in which their husbands dealt with their personal problems, than men were with their wives.

Bierkens (1973) showed that coming to terms with the idea of childlessness is an extremely painful process. Acceptance could be accelerated, however, if the problem was discussed with one another (especially the husband). The results of the present research indicate, however, that the patterns of communication between marriage partners were not satisfactory – a factor which would obviously hinder the course of a process of acceptance.

References

Bernard VW, Flapan M (1963) Psychogenic female infertility in relation to adoption. Community Psychiatry Research Unit, New York

Bierkens PB (1973) Psychologish aspecten van het kinderloze echtpaar. Nederlands Tÿdschrift voor Geneeskunde 117:770–776

Boocock SS (1976) The role of the parent: problems and prospects. In: Vaughan VC, Brazelton TB (eds) The family: can it be saved? Year Book Medical Publishers, Chicago

Chester R (1972) Is there a relationship between childlessness and marriage breakdown? J Biosoc Sci 4:443–454

Cilliers CA (1972) The Group-Rorschach and the gifted student. Doctoral dissertation, University of Stellenbosch

Group for the Advancement of Psychiatry (1973) The joys and sorrows of parenthood. Scriber's, New York

Hicks MW, Platt M (1970) Marital happiness and stability: a review of research in the sixties. J Marriage Family 32:553–574

Humphrey M (1975) The effect of children on the marriage relationship. Br J Med Psychol 48:273–279
Jacka AA (1973) Adoption in brief. NFER Publishing Co., Windsor
Lewontin RC, Felsenstein J (1965) The robustness of homogeneity tests in 2 × N tables. Biometrics 21:19–33
Lock HJ, Wallace KM (1959) Short marital-adjustment and prediction tests: their reliability and validity. Marriage Family Liv 21:251–255
Spanier GB (1976) Measuring dyadic adjustment: new scales for assessing the quality of marriage and similar dyads. J Marriage Family February:15–28
Terman LM (1938) Psychological factors in marital happiness. McGraw-Hill, New York
Van Keep PA, Schmidt-Elmendorff E (1974) Involuntary childlessness. J Biosoc Sci 7:37–48
Wilks SS (1935) The likelihood test of independence in contingency tables. Ann Mathemat Statist 6:190–196

III. Erectile Dysfunctions

Anatomy of the Penis and Physiology of Erection

U. Wetterauer

Department of Urology, University of Freiburg, Hugstetter Str. 55,
7800 Freiburg, FRG

Penile erection is the result of hemodynamic changes in the corpus cavernosum. Such changes include increased arterial influx in combination with sinusoid relaxation and venous drainage resistance. Without the latter only a tumescence can be achieved, but never rigidity (Table 1).

At rest, that is in the flaccid state, blood flow through the erectile system is so low that it can hardly be measured. For the induction of an erection, the blood flow must be increased 25 times to an average of 100 ml/min (Table 2). To maintain a rigid erection, a flow of 20–40 ml/min is necessary (Lue et al. 1984). This increase in blood flow necessary for erection explains why this mechanism is so sensitive to the smallest disturbances, even the slightest morphological defects.

Predisposing factors for arterial influx disturbances are arteriosclerotic vascular lesions, which occur in smokers, and in hypertensive and diabetic men. For this group, an ideal treatment is the intracorporeal injection of vasoactive drugs.

In contrast, still unsolved problems in terms of etiology and pathophysiology are the forms of erectile dysfunction where vasoactive substances are not effective and do not produce an erection. These patients, most of whom are young, complain of insufficient rigidity and only brief erections, which is probably caused by a cavernous or venous incompetence.

As a basis for understanding the clinical pictures, the radiological evaluation, and pharmacotherapy, I would like to discuss the anatomy and morphology of the corpus cavernosum and the functional changes during erection.

Corpus Cavernosum

The erectile system of the penis is made up of the pair of cavernous bodies with spongy tissue. Figure 1 shows an isolated corpus cavernosum in an erection artificially produced by the injection of saline solution (Tudoriu and Bourmer 1983). The spongy tissue is surrounded by a thick connective tissue membrane,

Table 1. Physiology of erection

Relaxation of sinusoids
Dilatation of arteries
Reduction of venous outflow
Closure of av-shunts

Table 2. Hemodynamic changes during erection

Blood flow through Corpus cavernosum	
– At rest	4 ml/min
– Induction of erection	80–120 ml/min
– Maintaining erection	20– 40 ml/min

Sexology
Eds.: W. Eicher, G. Kockott

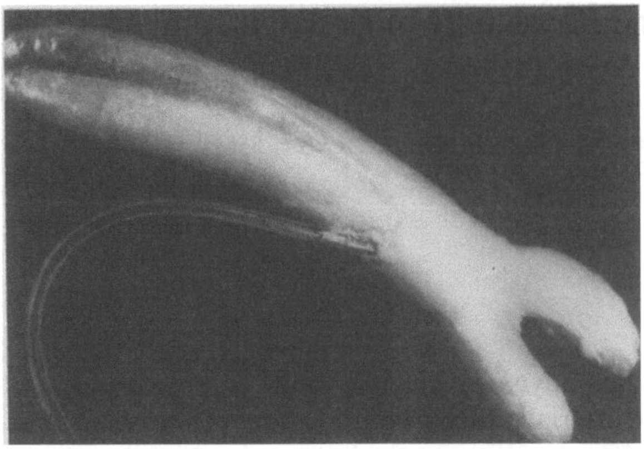

Fig. 1. Isolated cavernous body in artificial erection. (From Tudoriu and Bourmer 1983)

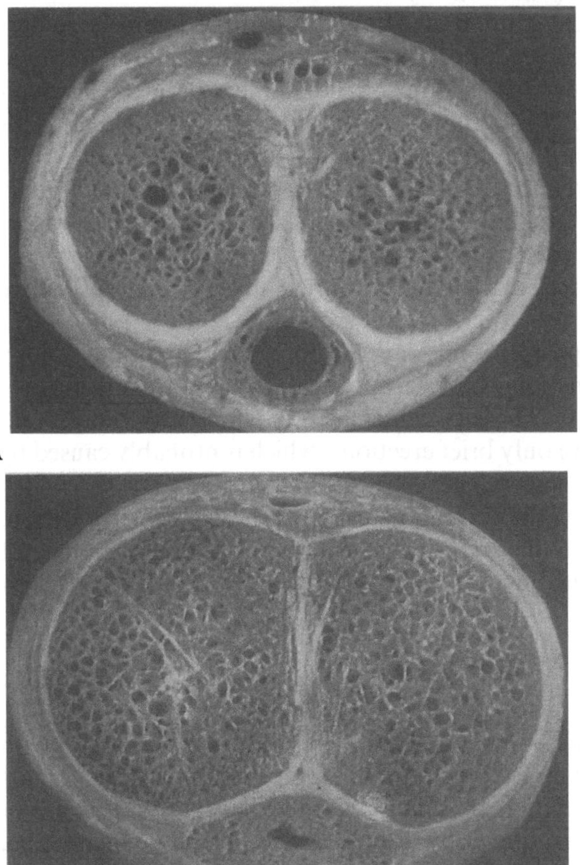

A

B

Fig. 2 A–B. Decrease of tunica albuginea thickness with erection. **A** flaccid penis; **B** cross section of erect penis. (From Tudoriu and Bourmer 1983)

the tunica albuginea. It consists of layers of collagenous and elastic fibers capable of withstanding blood pressure inside the spongy tissue.

In the flaccid state, the tunica is about 2–3 mm thick. During erection, the connective tissue is stretched, which causes the tunica albuginea thickness to decrease, as can be seen in Fig. 2 (Tudoriu and Bourmer 1983).

The stretching of the network of wavy collagenous fibers causes a decrease of the tunica thickness and a distension of the trabeculae that run into the spongy tissue. As a result, the veins lying inside the trabecular tissue are passively compressed during erection (Lierse 1982).

In the dorsal direction, the two cavernous bodies diverge to the side and form the crura of the penis, which are attached to the periost of the pubic arch and are covered by the ischiocavernous muscle. The septum between the cavernous bodies is incomplete in the mobile part of the penis so that both corpora form a functional unit.

Arterial Supply of the Penis

The arteries supplying the penis (Fig. 3) are normally arranged in pairs. The internal pudendal artery is a branch of the iliac artery, and after it gives off branches to the scrotal skin and to the bulbus and urethra, it divides into the deep artery and the dorsal artery of the penis. The dorsal artery runs along the dorsum penis on each side of the large dorsal vein under the Buck's fascia and provides the major supply to the glans penis. The main supply of the erectile tissue of the cavernous bodies is the deep artery that enters the corpus where the two crura merge.

The selective arteriography of the penile arteries using a DSA technique (Fig. 4) shows that the dorsal artery leads straight to the glans and provides no major branches to the cavernous tissue. The deep artery divides into multiple helical arteries, which in turn divide in a tree-like fashion into subdivisions opening finally in the cavernous spaces (Fig. 5). This is the main artery of the erectile tissue and causes a delayed X-ray, known as a "cavernosogram." The penile arteries have intravascular protrusions, which von Ebner has called polsters or cushions (von Ebner 1899) and are a major component of Conti's theory on the erectile mechanism (Conti 1952). These cushions, which consist of longitudinal smooth muscles and connective tissue fibers, are said to play an active part in the initiation of an erection, as when they relax the lumen of the arterial vessels widens and the blood flows more freely. Recent investigations in America, however, have cast doubt on the physiological function of these cushions, interpreting them as penile arteriosclerotic changes (Newman and Northup 1981).

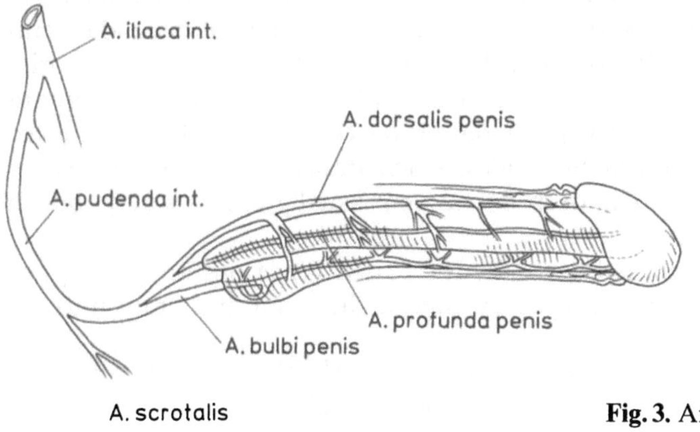

Fig. 3. Arterial supply of the penis

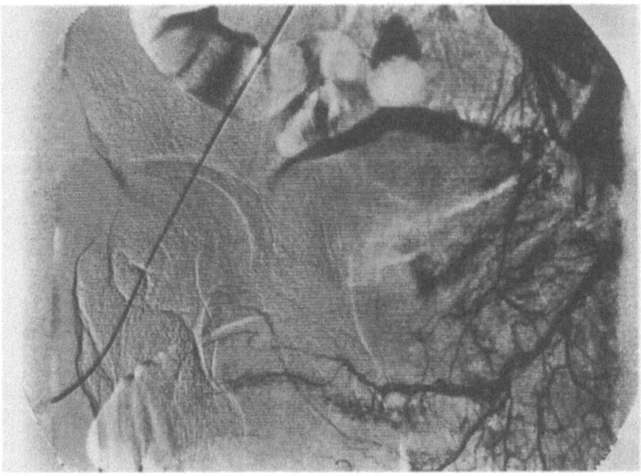

Fig. 4. Phalloarteriography: selective imaging of penile arteries in DSA technique

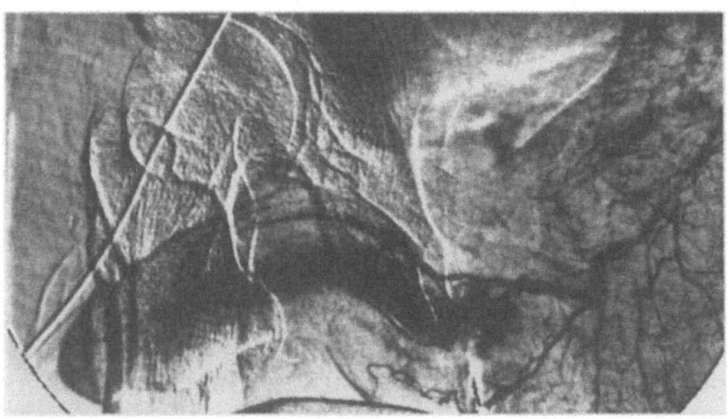

Fig. 5. Phalloarteriography: delayed X-ray of A. penis profunda, showing a "cavernosogram"

Venous Outflow

The venous outflow of the penis takes place through three different systems: (1) the superficial vein, (2) the deep dorsal vein, and (3) the venae profundae penis.

A network of subcutaneous veins merges to form the superficial dorsal veins, running between Colle's and Buck's fascia. They have multiple anastomoses to the deep dorsal vein. The superficial veins drain via the external pudendal veins to the saphena magna and, finally, to the femoral vein. The deep dorsal vein originates in a retrocoronal plexus and runs in the sulcus between the two corpora cavernosa to the pubis and to the pudendal plexus (Fig. 6). The deep vein is fed by 10 to 12 circumflex veins from both sides, which drain the cavernous body over the emissary veins (Fig. 7). The deep dorsal vein usually occurs singly, but in about 20% it can be double.

The third venous system is formed by the paired venae profundae penis or cavernous veins that leave the corpus by way of the crura and drain into the internal pudendal veins.

The deep dorsal vein characteristically has a remarkably thick muscular wall, so that it can easily be mistaken for an artery. Several valves are located at its base

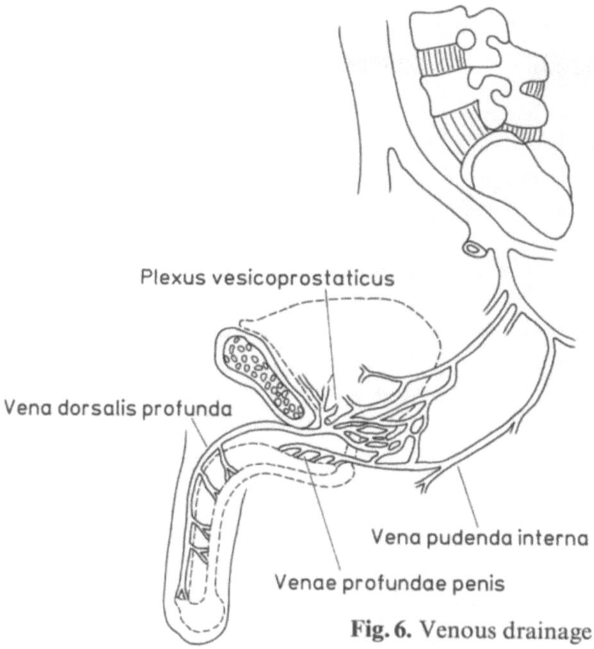

Fig. 6. Venous drainage of the penis. (From Porst 1987)

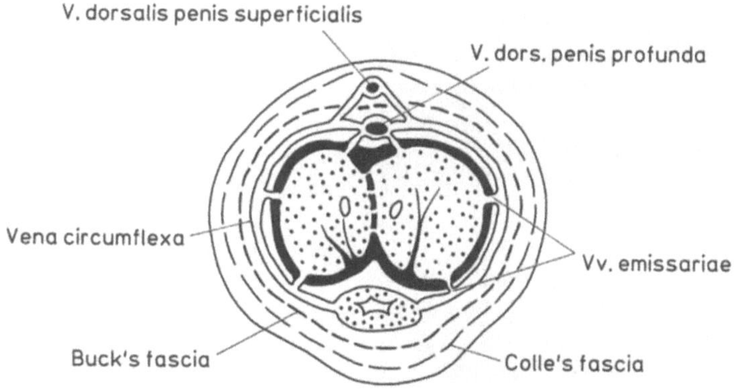

Fig. 7. Venous drainage of the penis, cross section

(Fitzpatrick 1982). The morphology of the deep dorsal vein alone is an indication of its active role in erection.

Using an infrapubic approach for dorsal penile vein ligature (Fig. 8), after the separation of Colle's fascia one can see large, superficial, pathologically draining veins in a 23-year-old man. After Buck's fascia has been incised from an infrapubic approach, the snared muscular deep dorsal vein appears, surrounded on both sides by the dorsal arteries and nerves (Fig. 9).

Under pathological conditions, cavernosography can demonstrate the course and the anatomical relationship of the draining veins. The radiogram in Fig. 10

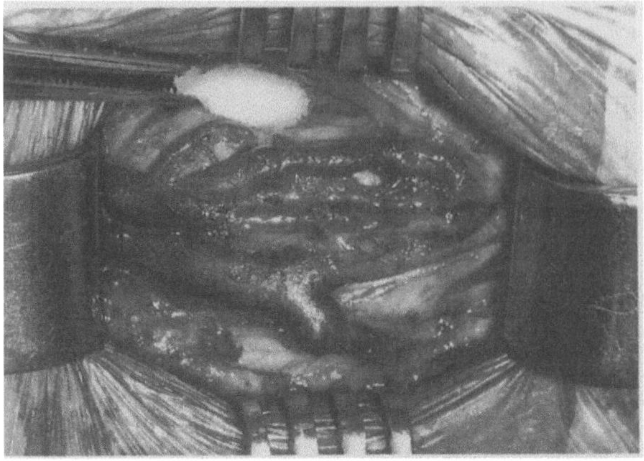

Fig. 8. Dilated superficial dorsal penile veins (infrapubic approach during dorsal penile vein ligature)

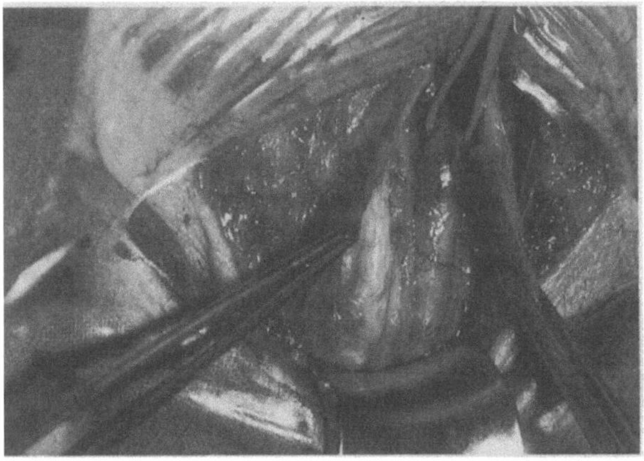

Fig. 9. Deep dorsal penile vein, snared

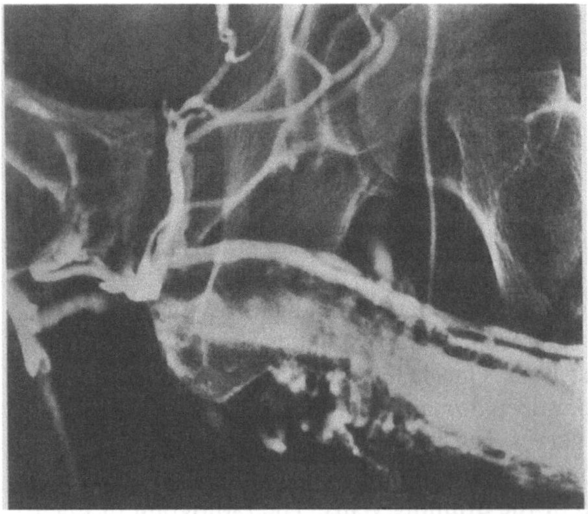

Fig. 10. Cavernosogram showing dorsal penile veins

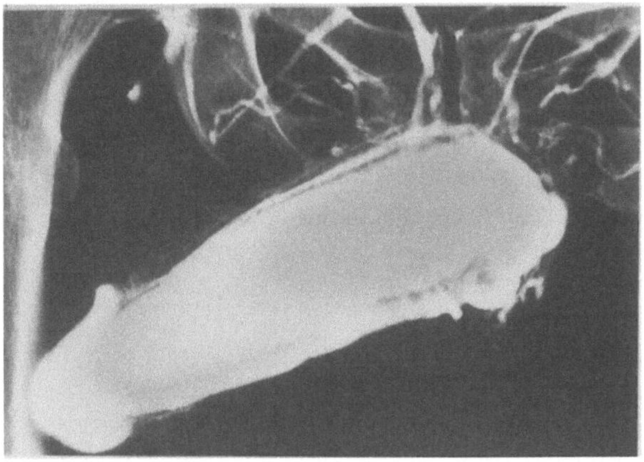

Fig. 11. Cavernosogram with opacification of glans and spongious body indicating venous fistulas

– the cavernous body is not completely filled yet – shows a thick vena profunda and superficial vein, which is partly projected above the former one. Both veins drain to the plexus vesicoprostaticus. On the right an ectopic vein makes the vena saphena magna opaque.

Venous anastomoses between the cavernous body and the glans and the corpus spongiosum are very faint, and the corpus spongiosum does not become opaque in cavernosography. Occasionally, however, these anastomoses are so distinct (Fig. 11) that they can be a major or concomitant cause of erectile dysfunction. The immediate opacity of the glans and corpus spongiosum is an indication that there are multiple venous shunts.

Innervation of the Penis

Clinical observations made in transverse lesions of the spinal cord have contributed to neurophysiological models for the erectile mechanism and have helped locate the so-called erection centers. At the spinal cord level a double representation of erection can be found (Fig. 12). The parasympathetic source of penile innervations has its origin in the spinal ganglia of the sacral root S2–S4. Sympathetic parts of the lateral horns of T_{10} to L_1 reach, via the sympathetic chain, the hypogastric plexus and the erectile tissue. The sensitive or somatic innervation runs via the pudendal nerve to the sacral root. A reflectorily provoked erection is mediated by the reflex arch of the sacral root. Reflex erections therefore occur in nearly all paraplegics with lesions above the sacral root.

Psychogenic erections, however, are mediated by sympathetic nerves and are found even in patients in whom the sacral region of the spinal cord has been completely destroyed. Recent experiments and animal models with the isolation of peripheral penile nerves and electrostimulation (e.g., Lue et al. 1984) were able to show that the innervation of the erectile tissue is much more complicated than is demonstrated in the model described above and that there are still many details that have to be elucidated.

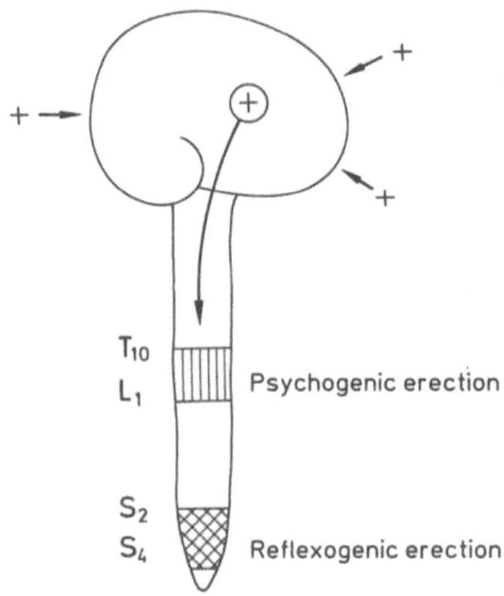

Fig. 12. Erection centers at spinal level

Neurotransmitters

Presently, research is focussing on the role of the neurotransmitters. These are the carrier substances that are released at the nerve endings and which call for an answer from the reacting organ, in this case, the smooth muscle cells of the sinusoids on the one hand, and the arterial walls on the other. The transmitter at the parasympathetic neuron is usually acetylcholine. But neither can the antidote atropine prevent an erection, nor does neostigmine, a cholinesterase inhibitor, induce an erection (Brindley 1986). Thus, cholinergic transmitters do not play a predominant role in erection, so that there must be other parasympathetic transmitters. To date it has not been conclusively determined which substance this is. There are indications, however, that vasoactive intestinal polypeptide (VIP) is one of the main cholinergic transmitters (Ottesen et al. 1984). During erection, this substance is found in the cavernous blood in concentrations much higher than in the flaccid state. When VIP is injected intracavernously a brief erection is produced.

Among the adrenergic receptors, a distinction is made between alpha- and beta-receptors. Experiments have shown that beta-adrenergic transmitters do not play a predominant role in erection. Neither does salbutamol provoke an erection, nor can beta-blocking agents (e.g., propanolol) – whether administered systematically or intracavernously – prevent an erection.

The alpha-receptors, on the other hand, are instrumental in the control of erection. A subclassification into alpha$_1$- and alpha$_2$-receptors has been proposed, which is based on the different reactions to different drugs (Starke 1981). Figure 13 lists the substances of this group assumed to be most important for erection. Today it is assumed that an erection is primarily mediated by the influence of the alpha$_1$-receptors. On the left in Fig. 13 you can see alpha-receptor-blocking substances of which phentolamine for pharmacodynamic reasons seems to be most suited for intracavernous injection.

Phenoxybenzamine, an alkylating drug, does irreversible damage to the receptors and remains active for a long time. It might also be cancerogenic and there-

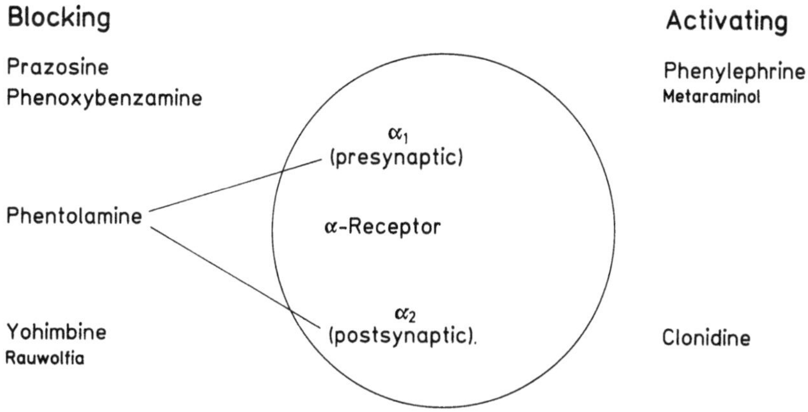

Fig. 13. Drugs influencing erection via alpha-adrenergic receptors

fore should not be used for therapeutic purposes. Yohimbine acts mainly on the alpha$_2$-receptors and has only a slight positive effect on erection.

The alpha-receptor-activating drugs are listed in Fig. 13 on the right. Of these, metaraminole has become important: on the one hand, as an antidote to phentolamine, it is able to interrupt pharmacologically prolonged erections (Stief et al. 1986 b), and, on the other, it has proved successful in the treatment of idiopathic priapism (Wetterauer et al. 1987).

Hemodynamic Models of Erection

In 1952 Conti proposed a model of the hemodynamic changes that occur during erection, which in part is still recognized today (Fig. 14). According to this model, in the flaccid state the arterial inflow is reduced to a minimum by the "polster arteries", which von Ebner described in 1899. The arteriovenous shunts are open; the blood runs past the erectile tissue.

In the erect state, however, the afferent arteries dilate with a relaxation of the muscular cushions and this results in maximum inflow into the sinusoids. At the same time, the collateral circulation via AV shunts and the venous outflow through emissary veins is reduced. These "throttle veins," which are also equipped with muscular pads, are said to be capable of active constriction.

Recent experiments and dynamic investigations, particularly by Wagner (1981), Lue (1983), and Jünemann (1986) have been able to demonstrate that the decisive control mechanism is located in the cavernous body itself.

Figure 15 illustrates a current concept of the physiology of erection. According to this concept, the penile veins are not sealed (or plugged), in other words the venous outflow is not reduced by the throttle veins outside the corpus cavernosum (the deep dorsal vein, for instance), but rather inside the wall of the tunica albuginea or by the subalbugineal venular plexus. On the one hand, the stretching of the collagenous fibers of the tunica leads to a compression and plugging of the emissary veins. On the other hand, the relaxation of the smooth

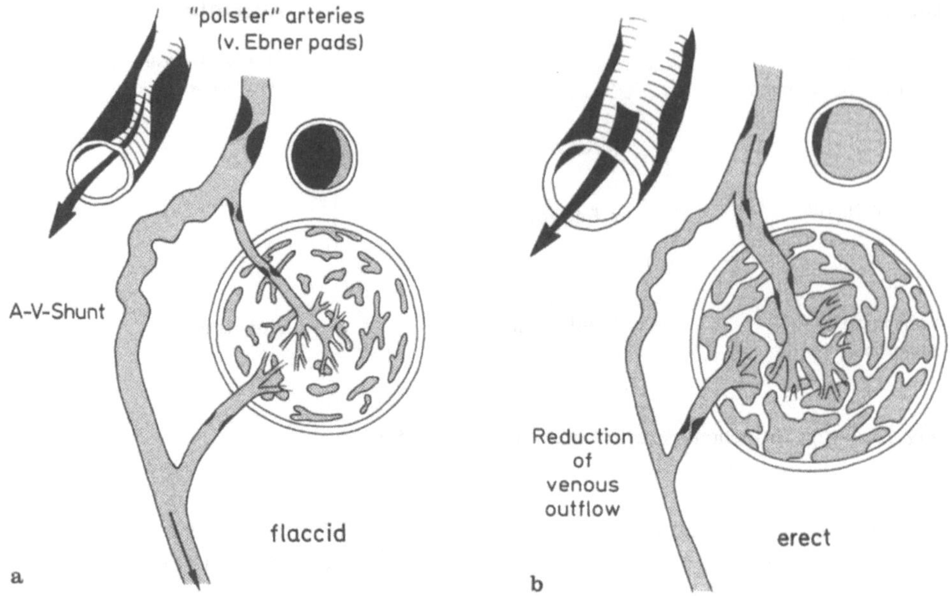

Fig. 14 A–B. Hemodynamic model of erection. **A** flaccid, **B** erect. (From Conti 1952)

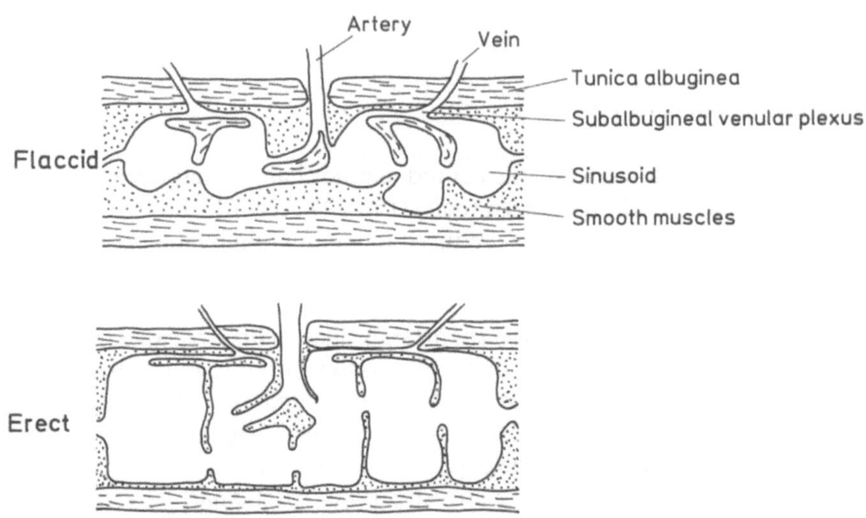

Fig. 15. Current concept of erection: passive venous outflow compression after relaxation of corpus cavernosum. (According to Jünemann 1987)

muscles of the sinusoids is instrumental in the compression of the subalbugineal venular plexus that is squeezed under the tunica albuginea, which is no longer extensible.

Wagner (1981) divided the functional changes that take place during an erection into different phases (Table 3): the first is the so-called sinusoidal phase in

Table 3. Sequence of erection

1. Sinusoidal phase
2. Tumescence or arterial phase
3. Erection or venous phase
4. Rigidity or muscular phase
5. Detumescence or resistance phase

which the smooth muscles of the cavernous spaces and the arterial system relax. At the same time the penis is elongated. In the second phase – referred to as tumescence or the arterial phase – the penile arterioles are widened and a maximum arterial inflow occurs. The increase in the volume of the cavernous spaces produces a passive occlusion of venous outflow. There is a moderate increase in intracavernous pressure, which results in an increased tumescence.

The erection or venous phase is characterized by a massive pressure increase. At this point the arterial inflow is already decreased and the outflow resistance is maximally increased. During rigidity or the muscular phase, in addition there is increased activity of the bulbocavernous and ischiocavernous muscles, which leads to an increase in pressure far beyond the systolic pressure. At this point the penis has reached maximum rigidity. The detumescence is characterized by a slowly increasing contraction of the sinusoid muscles and arterioles; the venous outflow is released. Further morphological and functional investigations are necessary to obtain information on the course of erection and on the underlying anatomical structures.

References

Brindley GS (1986) Pilot experiments on the actions of drugs injected into the human corpus cavernosum penis. Br J Pharmacol 87:495

Conti G (1952) L'érection du penis humain et ses bases morphologico-vasculaires. Acta Anat (Basel) 14:217

Fitzpatrick TJ (1982) The penile intercommunicating venous valvular system. J Urol 127:1099

Jünemann K-P, Lue TF, Fournier GR, Tanagho EA (1986) Hemodynamics of papaverine- and phentolamine-induced penile erection. J Urol 136:158

Lue TF, Takamura T, Schmidt RA, Palubinskas J, Tanagho EA (1983) Hemodynamics of erection in the monkey. J Urol 130:1237

Lue TF, Zeineh SJ, Schmidt RA, Tanagho EA (1984) Neuroanatomy of penile erection: its relevance to iatrogenic impotence. J Urol 131:273

Lue TF, Takamura T, Umraiya M, Schmidt RA, Tanagho EA (1984) Hemodynamics of canine corpora cavernosa during erection. Urology 24:347

Lierse W (1982) Blood vessels and nerves of the human penis. Urol Int 37:145

Newman HF, Northup JP (1981) Mechanism of human penile erection: an overview. Urology 5:399

Ottesen B, Wagner G, Virag R, Fahrenkrug J (1984) Penile erection: a possible role for vasoactive intestinal polypeptide as a neurotransmitter. Br Med J 1:9

Porst H (1987) Erektile Impotenz. Enke, Stuttgart

Starke K (1981) Alpha-Adrenoceptor subclassification. Rev Physiol Biochem Pharmacol 88:199

Stief CG, Bähren W, Gall H, Scherb W, Gallwitz A, Altwein JE (1986a) Schwellkörper-Autoinjektionstherapie (SKAT): erste Erfahrungen bei erektiler Dysfunktion. Urologe[A] 25:63
Stief CG, Gilbert P, Wetterauer U, Bähren W, Thon W, Altwein JE (1986b) Metaraminol – ein Antidot bei SKAT-bedingter prolongierter Erektion. Urologe[A] 25:164
Tudoriu T, Bourmer H (1983) The hemodynamics of erection at the level of the penis and its local deterioration. J Urol 129:741
Wagner G, Green R (1981) Impotence. Plenum, New York
Wetterauer U, Stief CG, Sommerkamp H (1987) Therapy of recurrent idiopathic priapism with intracavernosal metaraminol. 5th international forum of andrology, 15–17 June 1987. Paris
von Ebner V (1899) Über klappenartige Vorrichtungen in den Arterien der Schwellkörper. Anat Anz 18:79

Multidisciplinary Diagnosis of Vascular Erectile Dysfunction

W. Bähren

Department of Radiology, Federal Army Hospital Ulm, FRG

In the past 10 years extensive animal and human studies have begun to clarify the physiology of penile erection. Although there are many questions still unanswered, the evaluation of the impotent patient has reached a level of sophistication that reflects our increased understanding of the pathophysiology of chronic erectile dysfunction.

Several diagnostic methods – first being a clinical research tool – have been refined and have gained worldwide acceptance in the diagnostic workup of impotent patients.

Due to the development of new therapeutic options, the evaluation has to provide a probable etiology so that one may intelligently formulate an appropriate therapeutic plan.

Multidisciplinary Evaluation

The goal of a comprehensive diagnostic evaluation is no longer to differentiate so-called psychogenic from organic erectile dysfunction. For the patient's sake it is necessary to establish a specific etiology in regard to psychological, neurological, hormonal, arterial, corporal, venous, and end organ problems or a combination of these aspects. As Van Arsdalen pointed out, historically erectile dysfunction in a patient with no gross demonstrable neurological, vascular, hormonal, or penile abnormality has been labeled psychogenic in origin, even in the absence of positive psychogenic factors in the history (Van Arsdalen 1983). This approach undoubtedly accounts for the overestimation that as much as 90% of erectile dysfunction was thought to be psychogenic in origin.

It would be wrong, however, if the pendulum swung in the opposite direction in diminishing the problem to a mere somatic, hydraulic, or neurotransmission defect.

Even if it is not the dominant etiological factor, more than 60% of our patients show problems like changes in self-esteem and body image as well as social and partner-related conflicts mainly as a reaction to a disturbed sexual life. To make this point clear: Changes in self-esteem and body image can lead to erectile dysfunction and can easily be the consequence of it. The complex and often multifactorial pathophysiology requires a multidisciplinary approach, integrating specific knowledge of psychological, urological, neurological, andrological, and radiological disciplines.

Sexology
Eds.: W. Eicher, G. Kockott

In such a multidisciplinary center, general medical aspects, social and partner-related problems, psychosexual conditions, as well as the above-mentioned somatic factors must be considered. To manage this effectively is not easy.

History and Physical Examination

The history and physical examination have been the principal traditional means of establishing a diagnosis. This is still valid today. In addition to the classical questions related to libido, onset, course and degree of erectile dysfunction, variation with different partners or during masturbation, morning erections, ejaculatory disease, etc. it is worthwhile focussing attention toward iatrogenic causes of erectile failure.

Drug-induced or associated erectile dysfunction has been reported by Slag (1983) in up to 25% in the medical outpatient clinic. The mechanisms whereby many drugs alter erectile function are poorly understood. Antihypertensive medication, cimetidine, tricyclic antidepressive drugs, phenotiacines, and antiandrogens are common examples which have been associated in varying degrees with impotence.

An attempt has been made by Goldstein (1983) to clarify drug-induced sexual dysfunction on the basis of probable mechanism by alteration of:
- Hemodynamics of the hypogastric arterial bed
- The corporal vasomotor control system
- The endocrinology of the hypothalamic-pituitary gonadal axis
- Central and peripheral nervous systems

Surgery frequently leads to erectile dysfunction. Aortoiliac or aortofemoral bypass reduces hypogastric blood flow and or disturbs autonomic pathways of erectile and ejaculatory regulation. Renal transplantation, especially when a second renal transplant is placed on the contralateral side, is often followed by insufficient arterial inflow.

Pelvic surgery – especially radical cystectomy, radical prostatectomy, and abdominoperineal resection – are associated with high rates of impotence.

Pelvic irradiation at a higher dosage has been responsible for erectile failure in 63% as reported by Goldstein. Animal and clinical studies (Sarns 1965) show restriction of blood flow through arteries that have been exposed to radiation.

Taking the history of a patient with erectile dysfunction is usually the most time-consuming procedure in a multidisciplinary evaluation.

Nonspecific and Specific Diagnostic Measures

In the past 10 years a variety (more than 20) of nonspecific and specific, noninvasive, and invasive tests have been developed and refined objectively to demonstrate defects in the vascular, hormonal, neurological, psychological, and end organ physiology or anatomy.

Yet there is a lack of gold standards. Nocturnal penile tumescence (NTP) measurements cannot be defined a gold standard as a clinical tool for the differential diagnosis of impotence. Karacan et al. (1978) as well as Fisher et al. (1979)

have found a group of patients (15%–20% false positive) of all those tested who had abnormal NPT but no recognizable pathology. On the other hand up to 17% of patients with relatively normal circumferential changes had decreased penile rigidity, making their erection insufficient for intromission.

These false-negative responses were mainly due to sensory neuropathy, leakage of corpus cavernosum, or pelvic steal syndrome.

For arterial vascular testing there is a gold standard in regard to the morphology – unfortunately it is an invasive, time-consuming, and costly procedure which only gives diagnostic results in refined technique. I am talking about selective bilateral pharmacoarteriography of the internal iliac artery.

The arteriographic assessment of morphological changes represents the crucial step in diagnosis of *vascular* erectile dysfunction, especially prior to invasive therapeutic procedures. Michal and coworkers (1974, 1978) and somewhat later Ginestie and Romieux (1976), first described an angiographic method which regularly demonstrated pudendal and penile arteries with good contrast. Refinement of the technique by the use of intracavernous application of vasoactive substances has led to further improvement.

Arteriography as solitary investigation is worthless, since more than 50% of patients with chronic erectile dysfunction reveal more than one pathophysiological factor. Functional tests of the arterial and venous supply are necessary to evaluate the vascular nature of erectile dysfunction.

Therapeutically relevant information can be expected if the penile Doppler examination of cavernosal and dorsal arteries and pharmacological testing with vasoactive substances demonstrate a hemodynamic disturbance of arterial inflow.

In particular arteriography is indicated:

- In isolated arteriogenic erectile dysfunction if penile Doppler and vasoactive drug testing display pathological inflow to determine whether revascularization or PTA is possible.
- In primary erectile dysfunction – arterial malformation alone or combined with corporal leakage can be observed in over 60% of these patients. Even if there is no chance for promising operative procedures the positive confirmation of the organic nature gives psychological relief and prevents misleading therapeutic concepts.
- In posttraumatic erectile dysfunction, since arterial revascularization shows good results, if there is no complicating nerve injury present (Goldstein 1986).

To prepare to decide whether to use invasive diagnostic and therapeutic measures, there was a need for noninvasive, reliable, and specific tests. Functional testing of vasomotor erectile capacity by intracavernous application of a vasoactive drug combination has proven valuable in differentiating between nonvascular causes (e.g., pure neurogenic, hormonal, psychogenic), pathological diminished inflow, and pathological increased outflow.

For this purpose we use a mixture of papaverine and phentolamine individually to define the dosage required for complete erection in a standardized manner after intracavernous injection. Doses range from 0.25 to 3 ml.

Normal subjects achieve a complete erection after i.c. administration of 0.5 ml within 5–8 min, lasting at least ½ h. In the years 1985 and 1986 200 consecutive

Table 1. Multidisciplinary diagnostic approach in patients with erectile dysfunction

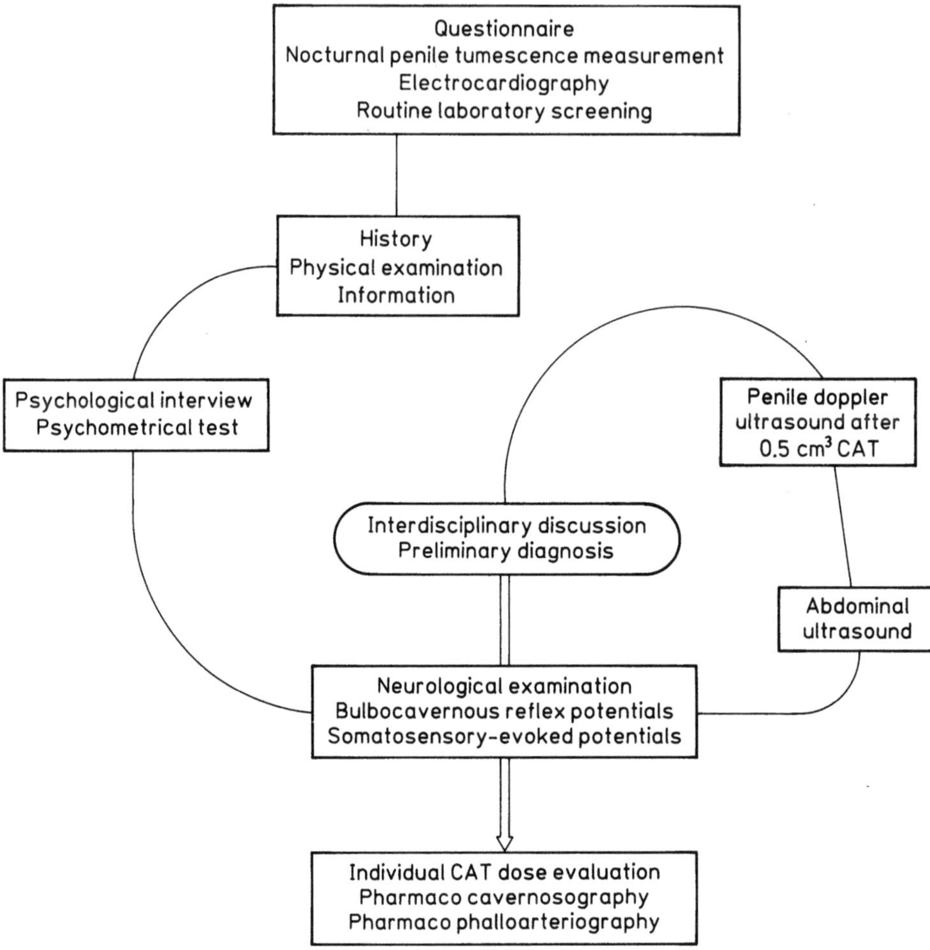

patients with erectile dysfunction of more than 1 year in duration were studied multidisciplinarily [history, physical examination, NPT measurement, laboratory evaluation, penile Doppler, Minnesota Multiphasic Personality Inventory (MMPI) and psychological interview, neurophysiological evaluation like bulbocavernous reflex (BCR) latency and somatosensory-evoked potentials (SSEP), when indicated dynamic cavernosography and pharmacoarteriography]. This study included vasoactive testing in a standardized manner (Table 1).

The multidisciplinary findings correlated well with the intracavernosal dose needed for full erection: the group without pathological hemodynamic findings ($n=36$) needed an average dose of 0.67 ml; the group with pathological inflow conditions ($n=107$) needed an average dose of 1.07 ml. In the group with pathological outflow conditions ($n=57$), 18 patients reached full erection with an average dose of 2.1 ml. Thirty-nine patients were nonresponders (19.5%) and reacted with tumescence upon 3 ml.

The combination of Visual Sexual Stimulation (VSS) and intracavernous pharmacological testing with a very small dose has been proposed by Wagner (1985) and Virag (1986) and seems to be especially effective in determining pure psychogenic etiology of the dysfunction.

Pharmacological testing cannot differentiate psychogenic from neurogenic or hormonal impotence and appropriate neurological testing, psychological consultation, and hormonal assessment are necessary to distinguish between these causes (Lue 1987).

A probable gold standard for venous and corporal insufficiency or leakage is coming up in the pharmacocavernosography and cavernosometry to assess the functional and morphological status of the venous system (Lue 1987).

If after i.c. application of a definite dosage of vasoactive drugs, intracavernous pressure increases to more than 80–100 mmHg (which is medium rigidity) after vasoactive drug administration and is sustained at that level, the venous mechanism is intact. If not – saline infusion determines the amount needed to achieve full erection. The subsequent maintenance amount indicates the venous capacity of full erection (Lue 1987).

Conclusion

The object of any test is to compartmentalize the patient's problem with respect to its etiology. After a multidisciplinary evaluation with up to ten specialized tests in difficult cases, it is necessary to communicate in an interdisciplinary council.

The use of vasoactive drugs injected into the corpus cavernosum has added a new dimension to the diagnosis of impotent patients. It serves as a functional test with high sensitivity and specificity when compared with multidisciplinary evaluation. In addition it gives a functional aspect to penile Doppler examination, selective arteriography, and dynamic cavernosography. Future research will be mandatory better to understand and hopefully measure autonomic pathways of erectile function. Furthermore we need practicable methods to evaluate the structure and pathological changes of the corpus cavernosum tissue.

In general any of the individual tests that were discussed provide only partial information, but each may be useful when considered in the context of the complete evaluation.

References

1. Fisher C, Schiavi RC, Edwards A, Davis DM, Reitman M, Fine J (1979) Evaluation of nocturnal penile tumescence in the differential diagnosis of sexual impotence. Arch Gen Psychiatry 36:431
2. Ginestie JF, Romieu A (1976) L'exploration radiologique de l'impuissance. Maloine, Paris
3. Goldstein J (1986) Arterial revascularization procedures. Sem Urol 4:252
4. Goldstein I, Krane RJ (1983) Drug-induced sexual dysfunction. World Urol 4:239
5. Goldstein I, Feldman IM, Deckers PJ, Babayan RK, Krane RJ (1984) Radiation-associated impotence, a clinical study of its mechanism. JAMA 251:903

6. Karacan I, Salis PJ, Williams RL (1978) The role of the sleep laboratory in the diagnosis and treatment of impotence. In: Williams RL, Karacan I, Frazier SH (eds) Sleep disorders, diagnosis and treatment. Wiley, New York, Chap. 14
7. Lue TF, Tanagho E (1987) Physiology of erection and pharmacological management of impotence. J Urol 137:829
8. Michal V, Pospichal J (1978) Phalloarteriography in the diagnosis of erectile impotence. World J Surg 2:239
9. Michal V, Kramar R, Bartak V (1974) Femoro-pudendal by-pass in the treatment of sexual impotence. J Cardiovasc Surg (Torino) 15:356
10. Sarns A (1965) Histological changes in the larger blood vessels of the hind limb of the mouse after x-irradiation. Int J Radiat Biol 9:165
11. Slag ME, Morley JE, Elson MK, Trence DL, Nelson CJ (1983) Impotence in medical clinical outpatients. JAMA 249:1736
12. Van Arsdalen KN, Wein AJ (1983) A critical review of diagnostic tests used in the evaluation of the impotent male. World J Urol 4:218
13. Virag R, Daniel C, Sussmann H, Bouilly P, Virag H (1986) Self intracavernous injection of vasoactive drugs for the treatment of psychogenic and neurologic impotence late results in 109 patients. 2nd world meeting on impotence, 17–20 June 1986. Prague
14. Wagner G (1986) Diagnostic methods in male impotence. 5th international symposium of operative andrology. Erection. 15 March 1986. Berlin

Intracavernous Papaverine Injections: Indications in Psychological Medicine

D. Langer

Zentrum Psychologische Medizin, Medizinische Hochschule Hannover, Konstanty-Gutschow-Str. 8, 3000 Hannover 61, FRG

As a basis for my work I conceptualize erectile dysfunctions as having multiple and interacting etiological causes. The current and widespread claim of the preponderance of somatic causes seems to me just as biased as earlier assertions of dominant psychogenetic factors. For effective therapy a precise specification of all mental as well as somatic causative factors and their interactions is essential. Until and unless it has been evidenced that a man with an erectile disorder exclusively requires either psychotherapy or somatotherapy, exploration of potential causes with their immediate therapeutic consequences should remain in one hand and be applied in cooperation with the patient.

It is essential for me to know that patients contacting the specialist in psychological medicine are different from those consulting the urologist. This is not sufficiently explained by assuming that they knew in advance what brings about their erectile disorder. It is well known that many men search for a somatic explanation and reject the thought of psychogenic causes. In this attitude they are often confirmed by physicians who would rather avoid than explore the sexual problems of their patients. On the other hand, psychopatients, too, often expect somatic diagnostics but are often frustrated by their psychotherapists on that count.

There is a considerable demand for our sexual therapeutic work by a great variety of patients applying for therapy from a large catchment area. Partly due to this factor we have been developing fairly brief, imaginative, and flexible therapeutic interventions. For us a precise diagnosis of the somatic aspects of erectile dysfunctions, including the papaverine test, has become an integral part of our psychosexual therapeutic work.

This eliminates my, as well as my patient's, fairly frequent discomfiture about a potentially hidden partial somatic factor in a picture of prevailing psychogenetic causes. These uncertainties can be quickly cleared up by measuring penile blood pressure, by Doppler sonography before and after intracavernous papaverine injections, and by the immediate effect of these injections.

The patient realizes that the somatic as well as the mental aspects of his problem are being taken equally seriously by the very same investigator. From the start the principal role of the investigator is that of the therapist. Both patient and therapist screen the process and the results of the assessment together.

If an important somatic factor is detected the patient can be directly referred, for instance, to cavernosography or he can be instructed in the technique of papaverine self-injection. This joint knowledge of the somatic factor does enable us to cooperate with the patient on a more credible basis during psychotherapy.

It is not rare that borderline conditions result or that somatic as well as mental determinants of the erectile problem can be demonstrated. This allows for additional information to be gained. In such a case papaverine in a higher dosage may force an erection by purely pharmacological means. In a lower dosage, however, papaverine is only *one* factor, i.e., a somatic one in a complex situation: not only during sexual interaction but already right away in the investigating room. Here it becomes evident how much additional sexual stimulation the patient needs – either visual or self-stimulatory – and how much privacy he requires in order to attain a rigid erection. Since even purely psychogenic erectile disorders must have a neural final pathway – such as, for instance, an excessive alpha-adrenergic innervation – it may well be that papaverine compensates for this autonomic factor.

A pharmacologically induced erection always constitutes a psychotherapeutically effective event, too, particularly for psychogenetically dysfunctional men with secondary sexual avoidance. It is different – although still comparable in principle – from the optimal situation created in sexual therapy where a patient can have a satisfying erection again, sometimes after extended periods of impotence. A common procedure is the repeated papaverine induction of erections by the physician. However, the actual period of the pharmacologically induced erection can also be used to impart cognitive and emotional experiences, i.e., for psychotherapy.

Hereby I am aware of the fact that this is psychotherapy under threat from a pat solution, which readily lends itself to abuse by uniting physicians and patients with erectile dysfunctions in a collusion of exclusive and hasty somatic orientation. As far as I am concerned I feel that patients with predominantly either somatic or psychogenic erectile dysfunctions always require psychosomatic sexual counseling if not sexual therapy. Specific somatodiagnostics, including the papaverine test as well as instruction in self-injection, if indicated, should always be seen in a sexual psychotherapeutic context. Somatodiagnosis clearly delineates the somatic factors, thus enabling a clearer identification of any psychogenic components. This is why I consider somatodiagnostics for erectile dysfunctions to be an integral part of sexual therapy along the guideline of utmost flexibility in order adequately to meet each patient's individuality.

Male Impotence – No Further Diagnostic and Therapeutic Dilemma

T. Block, W. Sturm, and G. Ernst

Department of Urology, University of Munich, Marchionistr. 15, 8000-Munich, FRG

For a long time male impotence was mainly classified – more or less unsatisfactorily – as psychologically caused. However, an analysis of patients afflicted with male impotence demonstrated that more than 50% of erectile disorders were of organic origin (Porst et al. 1983).

Recent advances in erection research have enabled us to classify the etiology of male impotence – or in the newer term: erectile dysfunction – closer.

Organic causes of erectile disorders are arterial reduction of penile perfusion, increase of penile venous outflow, and neurogenic failure. Other causes are hormonal and neurogenic imbalances as well as local penile disorders, i.e., Peyronie's disease.

Subtile diagnostic methods are able to evaluate these causes of male impotence: obligate diagnostics (Table 1) begins with sexual history-taking, for instance beginning and course of erectile dysfunction, associated diseases, arterial risk factors, psychosexual development, actual sexual behavior etc. A physical examination, particularly of the genital region and the cardiovascular system, follows. In laboratory tests testosterone, prolactin, creatinine, GPT, γGTP, triglyceride, cholesterol, glucose, parameters of blood coagulation and leukocytes are determined. A very important diagnostic tool is the Doppler sonography of penile dorsal and cavernosal arteries before and after intracavernous application of 25 mg papaverine (Porst et al. 1983; Virag et al. 1986). In healthy men amplitudes of wave forms of penile dorsal arteries are increased two to three times and pulse sounds of both cavernosal arteries are heard after papaverine injection.

Facultative diagnostic investigations (Table 2) consist of special laboratory tests when indicated, i.e., follicle stimulating hormone, luteinizing hormone, thy-

Table 1. Obligate diagnostics of erectile dysfunction

1. *Sexual History*
   (Beginning and course of e.d., associated diseases, arterial risk factors, psychosexual development, actual sexual behavior)
2. *Physical examination*
   (Particularly of genital region and cardiovascular system)
3. *Laboratory tests*
   (Testosterone, prolactin, creatinine, glutamic-pyruvic transaminase, γ-glutamyl transpeptidase, triglyceride, cholesterol, glucose, blood coagulation, leukocytes)
4. *Doppler sonography* of penile dorsal and cavernosal arteries before and after i.c. application of 25 mg papaverine

Sexology
Eds.: W. Eicher, G. Kockott

Table 2. Facultative diagnostics of erectile dysfunction

Special indicated laboratory tests (FSH, LH, t_3, T_4, etc.)
2. *Dynamic Cavernosogram with artificial erection*
3. *Psychological assessment*
4. *Neurological evaluation* (Bulbocavernous reflex latency time)
5. *Selective angiography* of internal pudendal arteries

roid hormones etc. Dynamic cavernosography with artificial erection is able to determine an increase of penile venous outflow with consecutive erectile dysfunction (Buvat et al. 1986; Wespes et al. 1984). Psychological examination of patients is indicated when no organic disorder can be evaluated. Determination of bulbocavernous reflex latency time (Lue et al. 1985; Tackmann and Porst 1986) allows the identification of neurogenic causes of erectile disorders. Up to now the neurological assessment has been without therapeutic consequence but serves as an evaluation of underlying disease. Because of the high correlation of the results of angiography and Doppler sonography of penile arteries, selective angiography of pudendal arteries is only indicated prior to penile revascularization procedures.

Patients

In a special out-patient clinic at our hospital 160 patients between the ages of 19 and 75 (median age: 48.0±12.7) years were examined concerning erectile dysfunction between April 1986 and April 1987. Organic disorders were found in 98 patients (61.3%) with a median age of 53.7±10.8 years: reduction of arterial penile supply was diagnosed in 82 men, an increase of venous drainage was identified in ten patients, and in six patients there was neurogenic failure. Psychogenic-linked erectile dysfunction was diagnosed in 57 patients (35.6%). The median age of patients with psychogenic-linked erectile dysfunction was lower (39.4±11.1 years) than that of patients with impotence due to organic causes.

Hormonal imbalances were stated in three patients (1.9%) with a median age of 36.3±10.7 years. In two patients no erectile dysfunction could be diagnosed.

Therapy

An intracavernous injection of papaverine or a mixture of papaverine and phentolamine was offered to 88 patients with arterial or neurogenic-linked erectile dysfunction. The dosages of these vasoactive drugs were adjusted individually. Of these 88 patients, 70 (79.5%) accepted this therapeutic approach (Table 3): 36 patients received their injections in the hospital temporarily, 34 patients were given detailed training in the technique of self-injection and performed intracavernous administration of vasoactive drugs by themselves or their partners did this. Both groups were thus once again capable of – weekly – sexual intercourse with suitable

Table 3. Therapy of arterial or neurogenic-linked erectile dysfunction

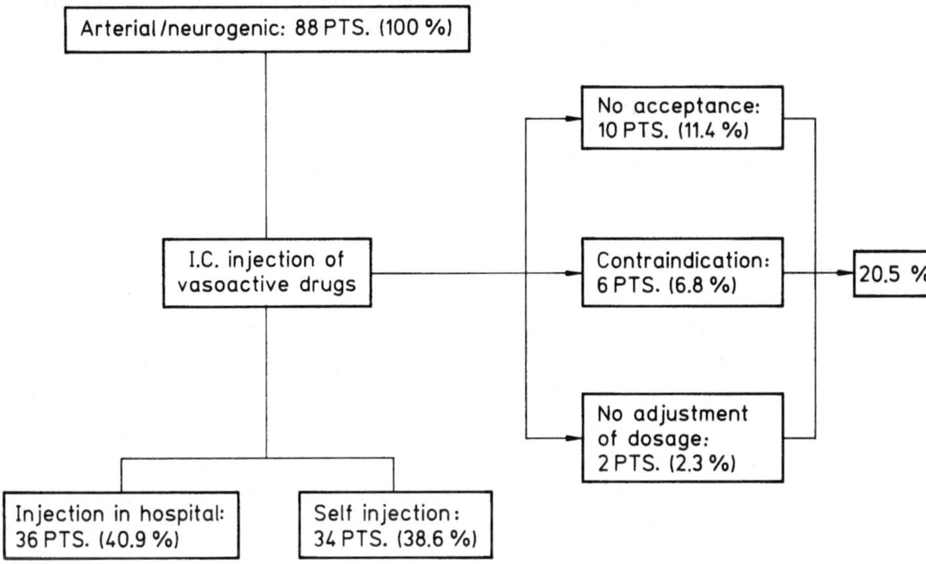

Table 4. Contraindications of intracavernous injection in treatment of erectile dysfunction

- Cardiac dysrhythmia
- Glaucoma
- Hepatic disease
- Adenoma of the prostate
- Increase of penile venous outflow
- Low patient compliance

quality and duration of erections. In 20.5% this therapeutic modality did not work: ten patients (11.4%) refused intracavernous administration of drugs, a contraindication of therapy (Table 4) had to be stated in six patients (6.8%), in two patients (2.3%) penile perfusion was too poor to determine a dosage of vasoactive drugs without systemic side effects for complete erection and suitable intercourse.

Results of surgical treatment of increased venous outflow (Buvat et al. 1986; Wespes and Schulman) remain controversial. In one out of ten patients a ligation of the deep and superficial dorsal vein was performed in order to decrease penile outflow via these veins; in three patients with diffuse venous drainage penile prostheses were implanted; six of these patients with erectile dysfunction due to venous leakages refused further therapy. Patients with mainly psychogenically induced impotence were transferred to a very experienced sexologist; hormonal imbalances were treated with bromocriptine and substitution of testosterone respectively.

The overall complication rate was 9.8%: In six patients a pharmacologically induced prolonged erection occurred which was treated by intracavernous administration of the alpha-adrenergic drug metaraminol. Eight patients developed a penile hematoma which was reversible spontaneously. In a 72-year-old patient small plaques around the proximal cavernous bodies with slight penile deviation were diagnosed after 1 year of intracavernous injection of papaverine. No infection of cavernous bodies was observed in any patient.

Discussion

In 158 out of 160 patients the main cause of erectile dysfunction could be evaluated in more detail; 140 (87.5%) were transferred to a suitable therapy.

Seventy patients with arterial or neurogenic-linked erectile dysfunctions received injections into cavernous bodies in order to induce penile erection of suitable duration and quality. One injection weekly is recommended in order to reduce local penile side effects like fibrosis. Intracavernous injections of papaverine or simultaneous administration of papaverine and phentolamine were first published by Virag (1982) and Brindley (1983).

Papaverine induces relaxation of the smooth muscle cells of the cavernous bodies with consecutive arteriolar dilatation and sinusoidal relaxation. Due to a decrease of intracavernous resistance the arterial influx increases (Juenemann et al. 1986). Dilated sinusoidal spaces cause a compression of intracavernous veins resulting in reduced venous penile drainage. In contrast, phentolamine has a direct effect on the increase of arterial perfusion. The attempt should be made to induce full erection without phentolamine because this drug seems to increase the incidence of pharmacologically induced prolonged erections. However, in some patients a combination therapy of papaverine and phentolamine is necessary in order to achieve a suitable quality and duration of erection (Sidi et al. 1986). The treatment of pharmacologically induced prolonged erection is indicated 3–5 h after the onset of erection because at this time gas checks of intracavernous blood demonstrate the beginning of the deterioration of the intracavernous metabolism. Therapy consists of the unilateral puncture of cavernous bodies in the area of the coronal sulcus, aspiration of intracavernous blood, and consecutive administration of metaraminol. Because of systemic hemodynamic side effects this therapy has to be performed with close supervision of the patient's circulatory system. Conservative treatment of persistent erection by alpha-adrenergic drugs causes pharmacologically induced prolonged erection to recede; this therapy should avoid the necessity to perform surgical shunt procedures.

Intracavernous injection of vasodilating drugs is a sufficient modality of treatment of erectile impotence. Patients treated with intracavernous injections have to be followed up carefully in order to recognize and to treat therapy-related-complications as soon as possible. At present the long-term complication rate of intracavernous application in the treatment of erectile dysfunction cannot be finally evaluated.

References

Brindley GS (1983) Cavernosal alpha blockade: a new technique for investigating and treating erectile dysfunction. Br J Psychiatry 43:332–337

Buvat J, Lemaire A, Dehaene JL, Buvat-Herbaut M, Guieu JD (1986) Venous incompetence: critical study of organic basis of high maintenance-flow rates during artificial erection test. J Urol 135:926–928

Juenemann KP, Lue TF, Fournier GM Jr, Tanagho EA (1986) Hemodynamics of papaverine- and phentolamine-induced penile erection. J Urol 136:158–161

Lue TF, Schmidt RA, Tanagho EA (1985) Electrostimulation and penile erection. Urol Int 40:60–64

Porst H, Bähren W, Altwein JE (1983) Diagnostic and therapeutic possibilities in vascular erectile dysfunction. Urol Int 38:5–11

Sidi AA, Cameron JS, Duffy LM, Lange NH (1986) Intracavernous drug-induced erections in the management of male erectile dysfunction: experience with 100 patients. J Urol 135:704–706

Tackmann W, Porst H (1986) Der Bulbus-Kavernosusreflex bei Kontrollen und Patienten mit Potenzstörungen. Z EEG-EMG 17:1 147–152

Virag R (1982) Intracavernous injection of papaverine for erectile failure. Lancet II:938

Virag R, Bouilly P, Daniel C, Virag H (1986) Intracavernous injection of papaverine and other vasoactive drugs: a new era in the diagnosis and treatment of impotence. In: Virag R, Virag H (eds) Proceedings of the first world meeting on impotence, Editions du Ceri, Paris, p 187

Wespes E, Delcour C, Struyen J, Schulman CC (1984) Cavernosometry – cavernosography: its role in male impotence. Eur Urol 10:229–232

Wespes E, Schulman CC (1985) Venous leakage: surgical treatment of a curable cause of impotence. J Urol 133:796–798

Priapism: An Improved Strategy in Treatment

T. Block, W. Sturm, and G. Ernst

Department of Urology, University of Munich, Marchionistr. 15, 8000-Munich, FRG

Priapism is a state of persistent erection without sexual desire. Primary priapisms are of unknown etiopathogenesis. Secondary forms might be induced by refuded or no venous drainage either of the cavernous bodies of the penis or of the pelvic veniplex as well as by neurofunctional disorders affecting the CNS or the urogenital tract. Drugs are also able to cause persistent erection: antihypertensives (prazosin, dihydralazine, guanethidine), chlorpromazine, trazodone, fluphenazine, heparin, but also intracavernous administration of vasodilating drugs in the treatment of erectile dysfunction. Rare causes of secondary priapisms might be Fabry's disease, hemodialysis, and penile vascular anastomosis and direct revascularisation of the cavernous body. Up to now the main therapy for primary and secondary forms of priapisms has consisted in various surgical shunt procedures (Ebbehoj 1974; Al Ghorab 1981; Grayhack et al. 1964; Quackles 1964; Winter 1976). A frequent complication of the surgical shunt procedure in the treatment of priapism is irreversible erectile impotence (Marx 1981). The recession of priapism after intracavernous application of the alpha-adrenergic drug metaraminol was first described by Brindley in 1984. This pharmacological therapy might render unnecessary the surgical treatment of priapism and – in consequence – the postoperative complication of male impotence. Preliminary data of intracavernous administration of metaraminol in the treatment of persistent erection are presented.

Patients

Twelve patients between the ages of 17 and 66 (median age: 43.8 ± 16.5) years have been treated for priapism and pharmacologically induced prolonged erection (PIPE) between April 1986 and May 1987 (Table 1): Pharmacologically induced persistent erection occurred in six patients after intracavernous injection of papaverine and in four patients after simultaneous intracavernous administration of papaverine and phentolamine. In a 65-year-old-patient there was sustained priapism for 6 weeks, resulting from an infiltration of a rectal carcinoma into cavernous bodies. In one 17-year-old patient priapism appeared in conjunction with Fabry's disease (Funderburk et al. 1974; Wilson et al. 1973).

Sexology
Eds.: W. Eicher, G. Kockott

Table 1. Etiology of treated priapisms and PIPE

Patients	Age (years)	Duration	Etiology
1	25	19,00 h	20 mg papaverine/1 mg phentolamine
2	65	6 weeks	Intracavernous infiltrating rectumcarcinoma
3	59	13.50 h	40 mg papaverine/0.5 mg phentolamine
4	17	24.00 h	Fabry's disease
5	36	10.25 h	40 mg papaverine/0.5 mg phentolamine
6	66	19.50 h	50 mg papaverine
7	45	12.75 h	25 mg papaverine
8	48	4.00 h	25 mg papaverine
9	48	4.00 h	25 mg papaverine/1 mg phentolamine
10	33	4.75 h	40 mg papaverine
11	34	15.00 h	50 mg papaverine
12	49	20.25 h	60 mg papaverine

Treatment

After histologically proven infiltration of cavernous bodies by an adenocarcinoma of the rectum patient 2 was surgically treated in order to reduce intracavernous tumor volume. As this attempt failed a cavernosoglandular shunt was applied as described by Al Ghorab (1981) and the patient subsequently subjected to palliative radiation.

The remaining patients were primary treated by unilateral puncture of cavernous bodies in the region of the coronal sulcus. After aspiration of intracavernous blood the alpha-adrenergic drug metaraminol (2 mg/4 cc NaCl) was injected into one cavernous body with close surveillance of patients' circulation. Repitition of metaraminol injection was indicated when no or only little penile

Table 2. Blood-gas analysis of priapisms and PIPE induced by intracavernous application of vasodilating drugs

Pts	Duration of erection (h)	Intra-cavernous blood aspiration (cc)	Blood gas analysis of cavernous blood (before and after aspiration) pH		pO_2 (mmHg)		pCO_2 (mmHg)		O_2-saturation (%)	
1	19.00	260	–	7.37	–	58.1	–	41.2	–	88.8
3	13.50	80	7.07	7.33	41.7	51.3	86.9	44.6	56.3	83.3
5	10.25	80	7.02	7.24	56.8	67.4	94.0	56.2	79.6	83.8
6	19.50	100	6.83	7.21	12.0	37.1	102.4	53.1	10.2	57.9
7	12.75	100	6.88	7.14	17.5	34.8	109.4	68.2	8.7	46.5
8	4.00	80	7.07	7.25	56.6	54.3	80.4	60.2	75.6	82.2
9	4.00	80	7.07	7.20	59.7	57.3	74.5	59.8	76.9	81.7
10	4.75	65	7.08	7.22	70.2	62.7	71.1	57.9	84.7	86.1
11	15.00	80	6.89	7.15	31.8	41.0	107.7	67.7	27.1	60.2
12	20.25	80	6.93	7.29	25.9	48.1	96.8	52.8	20.2	78.2

Table 3. Blood-gas analysis of intracavernous blood in a patient with priapism associated with Fabry's disease

H	0		2		12	
Blood aspiration (cc)	100		100		160	
pH	7.02	7.37	7.32	7.36	7.00	7.39
pO_2 (mmHg)	34.1	67.1	75.3	82.6	30.8	76.4
pCO_2 (mmHg)	59.8	37.6	28.1	26.3	60.2	25.0
O_2-saturation (%)	41.1	92.5	94.9	96.8	31.5	94.7

detumescence occurred 10 min after the first intracavernous administration. At the beginning and the end of aspiration blood-gas analysis was performed. After this puncture digital compression was applied for a 5-min period in order to avoid penile hematoma. Pharmacologically induced prolonged erections by vasodilating drugs were treated by metaraminol injections (Table 2) after 4.0–20.25 (median duration: 12.3 ± 6.5) h. Prior to the administration of metaraminol 65–260 ml (median volume of aspiration: 100.4 ± 75.0 ml) of intracavernous blood was aspirated. In patients 3 and 5–12 complete penile detumescence occurred 2–3 min after intracavernous administration of 2 mg metaraminol. In the case of the first 25-year-old patient who, out of mere curiosity, had administered a papaverine-phentolamine mixture to himself, complete penile detumescence did not occur until 2.5 h after administration. After completion of treatment this patient has a normal degree of potency; the remaining patients perform complete and painless erections after intracavernous injections of vasodilating drugs. Hemodynamic side effects were not observed, but in three patients a penile hematoma developed due to the puncture of the cavernous body which receded spontaneously.

Gas checks from the aspirated cavernous blood (Table 2) demonstrated a development of intracavernous acidosis with pH values between 7.0 and 7.1, 4–5 h after the onset of erection. Acidosis was accompanied by marked hypercapnia. In the subsequent hours pH and carbon dioxide changed only slightly. However, during this period a marked hypoxia with consecutive reduction of oxygen saturation level became more apparrent.

Priapism caused by Fabry's disease could not be treated by metaraminol successfully (Table 3): Aspiration of 100 ml of intracavernous blood and intracavernous administration of 2 mg metaraminol led only to a moderate penile detumescence. However, after 2 h priapism had recurred, necessating aspiration of 100 ml intracavernous blood. At this time blood-gas analysis showed only minor deterioration of intracavernous metabolism. Injection of 2×2 mg metaraminol at short intervals under close surveillance of hemodynamic parameters led again only to a slight decrease of penile tumescence. Ten h after this second treatment priapism had recurred completely. Again blood-gas analysis demonstrated marked hypoxia, hypercapnia, and extensive acidosis. With close surveillance of the patient's circulation in an intensive care unit 11 mg metaraminol was administered intermittently into both cavernous bodies within a period of 20 min. Although this high dose initially led to penile detumescence, priapism recurred shortly afterwards. As the priapism did not recede after such a large dose of metaraminol into both cavernous bodies, a cavernosoglandular shunt was performed according to Al Ghorab (1981). One year after treatment the patient complained about impotence.

Discussion

Despite the availability of various surgical shunt procedures as well as conservative methods of treatment only 50% of patients suffering from primary priapism remained potent; in those patients with secondary priapism prognosis remained poor for restoring potency (Marx 1981). Consequently the primary aim of priapism therapy has to be to preserve erectile potency. Therefore in every patient afflicted with priapism the attempt should be made to treat persistent erection by intracavernous injection of alpha-adrenergic drugs such as metaraminol, norepinephrine, and epinephrine. In order to understand the mode of action of alpha-adrenergic drugs in the treatment of priapism one has to consider the hemodynamics of penile erection. First: the relaxation of cavernous and arteriolar smooth muscle cells occurs after sexual stimulation. In consequence the increase of compliance of sinusoidal spaces with an accompanying reduction of penile venous outflow then follows (Lue et al. 1983). Metaraminol, norepinephrine, and epinephrine lead to the contraction of unstriated cavernous arteriolar smooth muscle cells resulting in a lowered arterial inflow as well as increased venous drainage with consecutive penile detumescence. Because of systemic vasoconstructive side effects the administration of alpha-adrenergic drugs into the cavernous bodies has to be carried out with strict surveillance of the patient's circulatory system.

Results of blood-gas analyses obtained from the cavernous body demonstrate the beginning of a marked deterioration of the intracavernous metabolism 4–5 h after the onset of prolonged erection. Early deterioration of the intracavernous metabolism is characterized by marked hypercapnia and severe acidosis.

During the subsequent hours a decrease of O_2 saturation level and oxygen pressure appears. Progressive intracavernous ischemia leads to the damage of erectile tissue and to pain inside the penis. Consequently, treatment of prolonged erection or priapism is indicated 3–5 h after the onset of erection.

When repeated injections of alpha-adrenergic drugs remain ineffective, it is mainly attributable to the fact that treatment has begun too late. In these cases temporary penile detumescence is the result of paralyses of the unstriated muscle cells in cavernous bodies (Lue et al. 1986). It seems possible to treat priapisms and pharmacologically induced prolonged erections conservatively with alpha-adrenergic drugs successfully, but therapy of persistent erection has to begin as soon as possible.

With regard to the data presented, the following strategy in the treatment of priapism – analogous to the therapeutic concept published by Lue et al. (1986) – seems appropriate (Fig. 1): If remission of priapism is induced by aspiration of intracavernous blood no further therapy should be applied. However, in cases of severe ischemia (O_2 saturation $<60\%$) aspiration of blood must be continued in order to improve the intracavernous metabolism. After improving the intracavernous metabolism 2 mg metaraminol/4 cc NaCl should be injected into one of

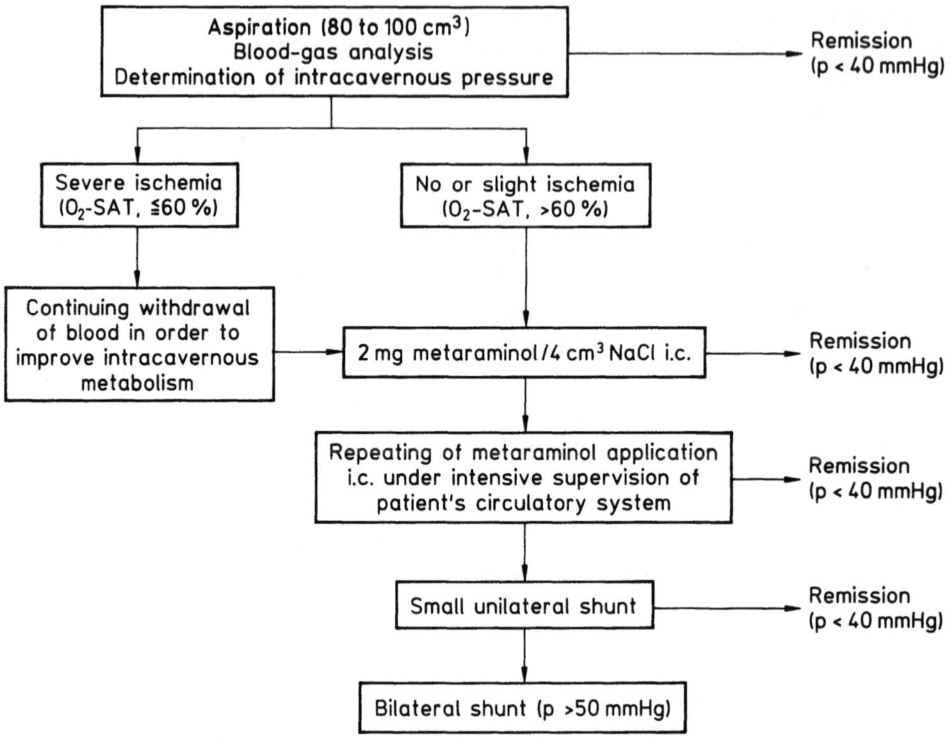

Fig. 1. Blood gas → blood-gas, metaraminol-application → metaraminol application p→*p*

the cavernous bodies. If no or only slight ischemia is present intracavernous injection of the alpha-adrenergic drug should be performed immediately. If the prolonged erection does not recede (intracavernous pressure >40 mmHg) the application of alpha-adrenergic drugs should be continued. This treatment must, by all means, be performed under intensive surveillance of the patient's circulatory system. Step-by-step shunt procedures are ultimate therapeutic approaches if penile detumescence still does not occur after this pharmacological therapy: In these cases the attempt should be made to recede priapism first by a small unilateral shunt in order to increase the chance of spontaneous shunt occlusion postoperatively. Only in cases when intracavernous pressure is >50 mmHg is a bilateral shunt procedure indicated. Further investigations are required to determine whether or not this pharmacological mode of treatment could be applied successfully in all cases of priapism.

References

Al Ghorab MM (1981) Personal communication in: Ercole CJJ, Pontes JE, Pierce JM Jr (1981) Changing surgical concepts in the treatment of priapism. J Urol 125:210
Brindley GS (1984) New treatment for priapism. Lancet 2:220
Ebbehoj J (1974) A new operation for priapism. Scand J Plast Reconstr Surg 8:241
Funderburk SJ, Philipart M, Dale G, Cederbaum SD, Vyden JK (1974) Priapism after phenoxybenzamine in a patient with Fabry's disease. N Engl J Med 290:630

Grayhack JT, McCullough W, O'Conor VJ, Trippel O (1964) Venous bypass to control priapism. Invest Urol 1:509
Lue TF, Takamura T, Schmidt RA, Palubinsuas AJ, Tanagho EA (1983) Hemodynamics of erection in the monkey. J Urol 130:1237
Lue TF, Wayne J, Hellstrom G, McAninch JW, Tanagho EA (1986) Priapism: a refined approach to diagnosis and treatment. J Urol 136:104
Marx FJ (1981) Zur Therapie des Priapismus. Urologe [A] 20:353
Quackles R (1964) Cure of a patient from priapism by cavernospongiosa anastomosis. Acta Urol Belg 32:5
Wilson SK, Klionsky BL, Rhamy RK (1973) A new etiology of priapism: Fabry's disease. J Urol 109:646
Winter CC (1976) Cure of idiopathic priapism: new procedure for creating fistula between glans penis and corpora cavernosa. Urology 8:389

Group Therapy with Single Males with Erectile Difficulties

B. Møhl and G. Winther

Department of Clinical Sexology, Rigshospitalet, University of Copenhagen, Copenhagen, Denmark

Until recently the psychotherapeutic treatment of psychogenic sexual dysfunction has been based on couples. According to the classical Masters and Johnson technique (Masters and Johnson 1970), the patient had to have a partner – either a real partner or a surrogate one. This approach is problematic for patients living alone or for those who could not benefit from a surrogate partner. (In Denmark we have never used surrogate partners for many reasons.)

Many patients with sexual dysfunctions are single and they suffer from loneliness. They have a partner problem and so has the therapy as long as it is couple-based.

But now individual treatment for this category of patients have been tried out with a modified Masters and Johnson model. These techniques have also been applied to group therapy, which is the subject of this paper.

Inspired by people like Zilbergeld (1978) and Lobitz and Baker (1979), the Sexological Clinic at Rigshospitalet, Copenhagen, has established group treatment of single men with premature ejaculation and single men with erectile difficulties. I want to describe a group treatment of erectile dysfunctioning men in order to point out the principles and techniques of the treatment that we are using.

The group consisted of seven single men with primary or secondary psychogenic erectile dysfunction. (Excluded were patients where the dysfunctions had organic reasons.) The group was conducted by one male and one female psychotherapist. This was to allow the parental transference to develop, and in order to have a feminine aspect present in the group.

The group met once a week for 2 h during 12 sessions. Then we had three more sessions every 2 weeks. This was a short-term, focused therapy based on psychodynamic principles. But it also had elements of social skill training. The goals in the group were:

1. Enhancement of a feeling of adequacy and comfort in sexual relations
2. Development of skills to facilitate the acquisition and maintenance of an erection which is sufficient to complete intercourse.

Between the group sessions the group members had homework assignments which were discussed during the following session. The homework assignments were:

1. Nongenital sensate focus with soap in shower. Ban on intercourse/masturbation
2. Nongenital sensate focus with body lotion – tactile exploration of the body
3. Genital sensate focus
4. Genital sensate focus with masturbation

Sexology
Eds.: W. Eicher, G. Kockott

5. Masturbation with "tease technique"
6. Fantasy: nongenital sensate focus with partner
7. Fantasy: genital focus with partner
8. Fantasy: intercourse with partner
9. Fantasy: intercourse with partner including fantasy about sexual difficulties
   – plus individual assignments

During the sessions *role playing* was used (how to date, telling partner about nervousness or erection problems) and *didactic material* like pictures and videotapes (e.g., with masturbation techniques or nondemanding intercourse). For one session we had a female guest therapist – a doctor from the Clinic – again to represent the female sex. We used her for role playing.

So much about the setting of the group.

Common to the men was lack of self-confidence and dependency, unrealistic views of women, performance anxiety, and "spectatoring" in sexual situations. Therefore the sessions concentrated on themes like performance anxiety and lack of self-confidence, especially in sexual situations, latent homosexuality, contact problems. (All the men were so afraid of women that they did not dare even talk to them. They stopped before they started.) Furthermore members of the group were occupied with jealousy, envy, myths about male and female sexuality (the men thought of women as unobtainable and as extremely occupied with sex). It was extremely useful for the group members to discuss these topics and during the sessions a lot of "aha" experiences were noticed.

The outcome of this group therapy seems to document the effectiveness of this approach to erectile difficulties. After the terminations of the group sessions all members reported satisfaction with the treatment. All of them felt a higher degree of self-confidence in relation to women. In regard to the sexual problems three out of seven men had improved considerably. The rest – with the exception of one – reported a better understanding of their problem leading to another perspective, "this is not the overwhelming problem in my life any longer" as one group member said. This made the performance anxiety decrease.

Before the group started, after the fifth session, and after the termination of the group, the members took the DAP test.

Group treatment of erectile dysfunctions differs primarily from individual and couple treatment by the *mirror effect*. The group members can identify with each other; they have the feeling of "we are all in the same boat." They can help and support each other and learn from each other's experiences. By *sharing* the problems with others in the same situation, the problems are easier to handle and to overcome.

It is our experience that short-term, focused group treatment of sexual dysfunctioning men or women without regular sex partners is now an attractive alternative to individual treatment.

The cost is lower and there seem to be psychodynamic advantages.

References

Lobitz W, Baker EL, (1979) Group treatment of single males with erectile dysfunction. Arch Sex Behav 8:2
Masters WS, Johnson VE (1970) Human sexual inadequacy. Little, Brown, Boston
Zilbergeld B (1978) Men and sex. Fontana/Collins, New York

Impotence as Seen in an Australian Sex Therapy Practice

J. D. Richardson

G.P.O. Box 3712, Aus 2001 Sidney, N.S.W., Australia

This paper reviews 215 consecutive male patients seen over a period of 7 months, from July 1986 to February 1987, by a medically qualified sex therapist, working in solo private practice in Sydney, New South Wales, Australia. Those presenting with erectile incompetence (impotence) are compared with patients presenting with other problems. The age distribution between the two groups is compared, as are religious affiliation, country of birth, marital status, referral source, and diagnosis, together with alcohol and smoking habits, and the results of pathology and blood flow investigations performed.

All patients making appointments with the practice were seen, and any selection that occurred was made by the referring source, presumably on the grounds that this was an appropriate referral.

When the review was set up it was expected that the time period chosen would be based on the period needed to have seen 100 patients with impotence, but in fact the potent patients proved to be the governing factor. The final sample contained 113 impotent and 102 potent patients.

Table 1 shows that the bulk of those seen were referred from medical sources.

In addition referrals were received from psychologists (five), social workers (five), marriage guidance counselors (four), Family Planning Association (four), solicitors for legal opinions (three), university counselors (three), hypnotherapists (three), and specialist physicians (one).

The high figure for media referrals reflects the fact that there is no Sexual Difficulties Clinic attached to a Hospital or other institution in NSW, and it is there-

Table 1. Referral source

Referral sources	Total number seen	Impotent	Non-impotent
General practitioner	104	68	36
Telephone counseling service	18	6	12
Media	18	9	9
Psychiatrist	12	6	6
Friends	9	4	5
Endocrinologist	7	6	2
Obstetrician and gynecologist	6	4	2
Urologist	6	4	2
STD clinic	6	2	4

Sexology
Eds.: W. Eicher, G. Kockott

Table 2. Age distribution

Age (years)	15–19	20–29	30–39	40–49	50–59	60–69	70–79
Total numbers	4	36	66	43	38	23	5
Impotent	2	5	25	27	30	21	4
Nonimpotent	2	31	41	16	8	2	1

Table 3. Country of birth

Country of birth	Total	Impotent	Potent
Australia	133	67	66
United Kingdom	11	6	5
Egypt	6	3	3
New Zealand	5	3	2
Lebanon	5	2	3
Hungary	5	3	2
Italy	5	2	3
Other	45	27	18

Table 4. Religious affiliations

Religion	Impotent	Potent
Church of England	44	28
Catholic	32	45
Presbyterian	14	7
Jewish	7	6
Greek Orthodox	5	4
Armenian Orthodox	2	0
Russian Orthodox	4	1
Ukranian	0	1
Muslim	4	5
Miscellaneous	0	5

fore common for people to approach those conducting radio talkback shows, writing for newspapers and magazines, or telephone counseling services, for information as to where help can be found.

The age distribution of patients presenting with problems of erectile incompetence showed, as might be expected, more patients in the older age groups, which was not mirrored in the potent group.

In a study by Lane (1987) the relationship between vascular disease in the pelvis and age showed a linear pattern on regression analysis.

As might be expected the majority of those presenting were born within Australia.

The countries represented among others were drawn from Asia, Europe, Africa, and North and South America, but in no case were there more than five representatives of any country.

Table 5. Marital status

Marital status	Married	Single	Divorced	Separated	Widowed
Impotent	60	31	11	5	8
Potent	58	38	3	2	1

Table 6. Smoking habits

Amount smoked/day	Nil	1–10	11–20	21–30	31–40	41+
Impotent	84	9	12	4	0	2
Potent	69	11	9	5	2	2

Enquiries were made about the primary religious affiliation of the parents, with it being the norm to find mother and father embracing the same religion. The Table 4 shows the religions most commonly seen, and their numbers, in both the impotent and potent groups.

The marital status did show a definite shift toward the problem being more common in those divorced, separated, or widowed. Table 5 shows these results.

In Table 6 it can be seen that whereas 73% of those who were impotent were nonsmokers only 67% of the potent did not smoke cigarettes.

In addition to these cigarette smokers there were two pipe smokers who reported impotence, and one pipe smoker who had no problems.

Lane (1987, personal communication) reported that regression analysis of over 1000 patients who attended for infrared photoplethysmography showed that there was an increase by a factor of 2.5 in the incidence of vasculogenic impotence comparing smokers of 45 years or less with nonsmokers of over 65 years. These findings were confirmed by angiography, to a probability of $P<0.001$.

It is notoriously difficult to get accurate and reliable statistics on the amount of alcohol consumed, that the patients' statements were collated. A standard drink was taken as the equivalent of 10 g alcohol, and the consumption levels were graded as:

Nil – No alcohol consumed at any time
Low – One to three drinks weekly
Moderate – One to two drinks daily
Medium – Three or more drinks daily
Heavy – Five or more drinks daily

The patterns of drinking are shown in Table 7.

Table 7. Drinking patterns

Amount drunk	Nil	Low	Moderate	Medium	Heavy
Impotent	8	42	23	20	10
Potent	14	36	20	20	12

Where there were any doubts about the patient's truthfulness, liver function tests were performed, with the gamma-glutamyl transferase being regarded as a significant indicator of current high alcohol consumption, and the whole pattern of the tests gave an indication of past habits (although it is accepted that hepatitis and certain other conditions can also affect the results of the liver function tests).

Increased awareness that organic causes may underlie erectile incompetence has led to major changes in the way in which this condition is investigated and treated. There is now a general acceptance amongst sexologists that up to 50% of patients presenting may have medical causes for their symptoms.

Unfortunately in countries like Australia, where human sexuality does not form a major part of the undergraduate medical curriculum, there is little appreciation of the wide range of tests needed to eliminate medical causes. Clinically 40%–50% of cases can be seen to be probably psychologically based, on the history and clinical examination, and they should be treated with counseling, education, and psychotherapy before further investigations are instigated, but recent advances, particularly in penile vascular surgery, and the development of more acceptable prostheses such as the Hydraflex, Mentor, or Flexiflate have made full investigation imperative. As a result all cases where there were clinical grounds for doing so were investigated further. Of the 113 patients in the impotent sample 46 had no pathology testing done, but of the 102 potent patients, who presented with other symptoms, only 2 had had any hormone studies or other pathology tests performed. The basic tests undertaken were serum testosterone levels, luteinizing hormone, follicle-stimulating hormone, sex hormone binding globulin, serum prolactin, liver function tests, thyroid function tests, serum acid phosphatase, random blood sugar, fasting cholesterol and triglycerides, and penile artery blood flows using the infrared photoplethysmograph, followed by angiograms or cavernosograms where appropriate. It was *not* the practise to repeat estimations carried out previously by other doctors, nor ones that were not clinically indicated.

The cases presented in this paper are those seen clinically, and the patients pay the cost of all investigations, so extensive investigation for research purposes could not be justified. In Australia all residents are covered by "Medicare," which pays 85% of a standard or scheduled fee; if it was believed by the Government-appointed Health Insurance Commission that the testing was done for screening purposes, or without good clinical grounds, then the patient would not be reimbursed for the fees charged.

The first of the tests undertaken was an assessment of the serum testosterone level, and where this was done it was usual to measure two values, at least 1 h apart, because there can be a very wide variation between samples and the actual figures obtained are listed in Table 8.

It can be seen that serum testosterone levels were measured in 66 out of 113 impotent patients, while these tests were only done on two of the 102 patients who were potent. In Table 8 two patients are reported to have normal values, which is all the information which could be obtained from the referring source.

Testosterone levels are believed to vary with age, so the age distribution curve is shown in Table 9.

Table 8. Serum testosterone values (nmol/liter)

0–12	12–19	20–25	26–30	30–40
(7.0, 5.0) (13.5, 10.1)	(18.2, 16.3) (19.1, 16.7)	(19.6, 25.8)	(28, 35)	(33.2, 38.0)
(7.9, 7.4) [6.1]	(13.0, 14.0) (17, 35)	(25, 25)	[26]	(37.7, 35.5)
(11.7, 13.4) (11, 16)	(13.7, 18.2) [13]	[22.4]		
(9.2, 12) (18.4, 6.2)	(15, 15) (13.8, 17.4)	(19.5, 28.1)		
(12.5, 10.0) (6.9, 0.9)	(13, 13) (16.0, 23.8)	"Normal"		
(1.7, 9.7) (11, 9.7)	(16.7, 15.9) (18.0, 32.0)	"Normal"		
(0.6, 0.6) (14, 9.5)	(18.0, 18.5, 16.0)	(20.9, 24.0)		
(13.3, 11.7) [9.6]	(15.6, 25.9) (15.3, 15.1)	(27.1, 20.5)		
	(16.6, 15.3) (13.6, 16.0)	(23.6, 25.5)		
	(24.3, 16.9) (16, 13)	(21, 20)		
	(22.0, 26.0) (27.5, 13.0)	(23, 22) [23]		
	[15] (16.9, 18.5)			
	(12.1, 12.6) (19.7, 13.5)			
	[14] (15.0, 14.0) (16, 17)			
	(14, 15) (15, 12)			
	(13.1, 17.2) (19.1, 21.5)			
	(19.3, 28.4) (16.4, 15.1)			
	(20.0, 13.9) (17.4, 18.3)			
	(21.4, 15.4)			

Table 9. Age distribution

Age	15–20	21–30	31–40	41–50	51–60	61–70	70+
Numbers	0	1	16	14	20	12	4
Testosterone (nmol/liter)		25	18.53	15.62	17.94	16.88	14.64

Table 10. Sex hormone binding globulin (nmol/liter)

0–10	10–40	40–60	80+
1	43	4	5

As free testosterone, not the bound form, appears to be the relevant factor, hormone-binding globulins were measured, and essentially these were found to be well within the normal range in the majority of cases, with the laboratory reference range being 10–40 nmol/liter. The vast majority of patients fell into this range when the test was carried out. Table 10 shows the values obtained.

However, it was felt worthwhile to check the testosterone levels where high levels of sex hormone binding globulin were found and these are shown in Table 11.

It is interesting to note the increased numbers of abnormal values in the 31- to 40-year-old age group.

Table 11. Testosterone levels of patients with high levels of sex hormone binding globulin

Sex hormone binding globulin	Testosterone
39	(24.3, 16.9) (15) (19.1, 21.5)
39.6	(19.7, 13.5)
40	(7.0, 5.0)
41	(16, 17)
45	(23)
53	(–)
54	(33.2, 38.0)
57	(0.6, 0.6)
58	(35, 28)
64	(16.4, 15.1)
66	(17.4, 18.3)
82	(21, 20)
118	(1.7, 9.7)

Table 12. Follicle-stimulating and luteinizing hormones

	0–5	6–10	11–15	16–20	20+
Follicle-stimulating hormone (mU/ml)	21	24	7	5	11
Luteinizing hormone (mU/ml)	21	26	13	1	8

Table 13. Infrared photoplethysmography

Index	0.72	0.72–0.80	0.81–0.85	0.85
Number	31	30	17	32
Right	6	11	8	8
Left	13	8	4	7
Both	12	11	5	16

The follicle-stimulating hormone and luteinizing hormone estimations showed a relationship with testosterone levels but these details are not listed. The distribution of follicle-stimulating hormone and luteinizing hormone was as shown in Table 12.

Penile blood flow studies were assessed using the infrared photoplethysmograph, the majority of tests being performed by Dr. Rodney Lane, the vascular surgeon from the Royal North Shore Hospital in Sydney. His work during the early days of the investigation of vasculogenic impotence has been invaluable to sex therapists in Sydney. He expresses the results of the infrared photoplethysmography as an index, which is the ratio of penile artery pressure to brachial artery pressure, and where this is above 0.86 there is no vascular problem, while below 0.72 the penile vessel is completely blocked. The results of the tests performed are summarized in Table 13.

Dr. Lane analyzed his figures and found that the lower the index the more proximal was the lesion in the penile arteries. Other correlations found were that

Table 14. Levels of fasting cholesterol and triglycerides

Fasting cholesterol (mmol/liter)	0–5.5 30	5.5–6.5 20	6.5–7.5 10	7.5+ 7
Triglycerides (mmol/liter)	0–1.7 41	1.8–2.0 8	2.0–2.5 4	2.5+ 14

Table 15. Problems seen

	Impotent	Potent
Performance anxiety	45	25
Rapid ejaculation	17	30
Communication difficulties	3	30
No difficulty except impotence	27	0
Marital problems	2	16
Relationship problems	0	14
Loss of libido	9	10
Inhibited sexual desire	2	6
Retarded ejaculation	6	3
Orientation	0	4
Other	20	37

Table 16. Main types of therapy used

	Impotent	Potent
Education	21	49
Psychotherapy or counseling	22	30
Discussion of options	46	–
None	15	19
Diet	6	0
Surrogate therapy	5	2
Life style change	5	2
Other	45	4

approximately 83% of patients with peripheral vascular disease would have one or both penile vessels blocked, while the percentage was 68 in long-term diabetics, 60 in those with coronary artery disease and hypertension, but only 25 in men with no vascular disease.

Apart from smoking, another factor of significance was the level of fasting cholesterol and triglycerides.

It was felt appropriate to assess the problems being seen, and Table 14 shows those commonly seen in both the impotent and potent groups.

Therapy was directed to discussion of the options for the impotent patient; counseling, psychotherapy, education, vaginal containment with penile stuffing, papaverine or papaverine with regitine injections intracorporally (Table 15), angioplasty, bypass surgery, or penile prosthesis. The main types of therapy used are shown in Table 16.

Discussion

Age distribution, marital status, religious affiliations of parents, and smoking and drinking habits were all reviewed. The myth that Catholicism was related to sexual disfunction was not confirmed, nor that smoking had a major effect on impotence, but the figures relating to smoking must be viewed with caution because they referred to current smoking habits, not those of the past. Similarly no direct relationship with alcohol intake could be established in this study.

The conclusion reached was that in the absence of a clear clinical history of psychological factors it was necessary to undertake extensive investigation of the patients presenting if organic causes for the symptoms were not to be missed. A careful history was always necessary to separate these two groups, but clinical examination was often unrewarding. An appreciable number of men did have obvious marital, relationship, stress-related, or similar problems which were sufficient to explain their erectile incompetence, but most of the clinical abnormalities found were only shown up after blood testing or the penile blood flow studies.

IV. Sexuality in the Elderly and Marriage

Endocrine Aspects of Sexuality in the Elderly

A. K. Slob

Department of Endocrinology, Growth and Reproduction, Faculty of Medicine, Erasmus University, P.O. Box 1738, 3000 DR Rotterdam, The Netherlands

Introduction

The interaction of categories and components of human sexual behavior is depicted in Fig. 1. This scheme originated with Davidson et al. (1983). A few of his own words will elucidate. "Libido" comprises those aspects of sexuality which concern conscious experience. "Potency" encompasses those aspects which can be measured in the laboratory. The various components of sexual behavior/experience listed below the libido category are assessed through verbal report; those listed below the potency category via physical measurements.

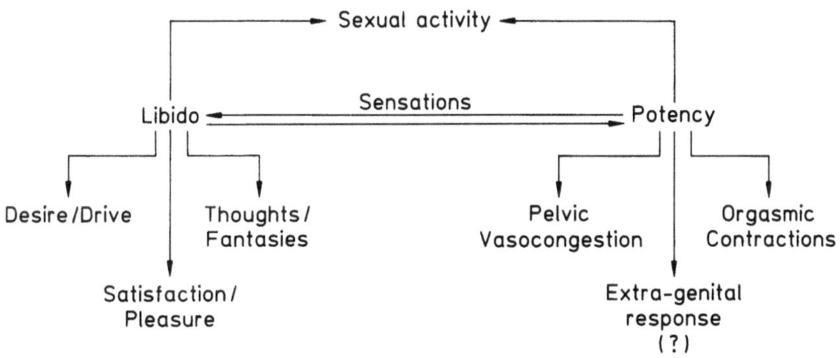

Fig. 1. Interaction of categories and components of human sexual behavior

Sexual Response

Part of human sexuality is the so-called sexual response (Fig. 2). This physiological response comprises four stages or phases: excitement, plateau, orgasm, and resolution or refractory phase. Another phase was added by Kaplan: the phase of sexual desire. In her concept of the sexual response it is a three-phase model: desire – excitement – orgasm (Kaplan 1974). An important psychological addition to this concept comes from Everaerd and Dekker (1981). They added the conceptions "solo phase" and "interaction phase." With this idea they emphasize that during excitement and the first part of plateau phase people that make love can or will be focussed on each other: interaction. When the sexual arousal further increases and people want to make an orgasm, it is of great significance to turn inwards and concentrate on their own feelings: solo phase. In the practice of sex therapy, especially with orgasmic dysfunction, the concept appeared to be valuable.

Sexology
Eds.: W. Eicher, G. Kockott

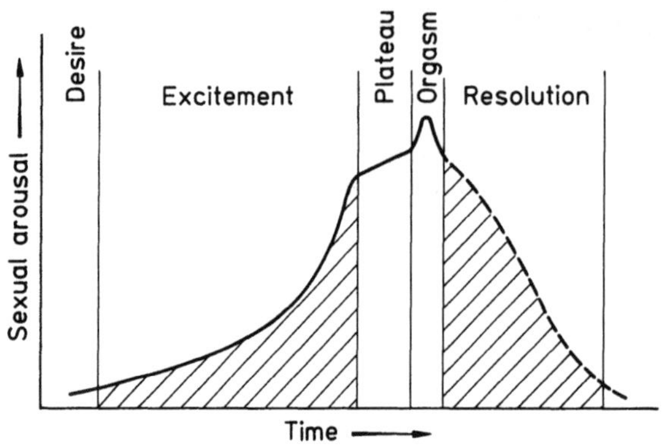

Fig. 2. The so-called sexual response

Sexual Behavior of Elderly Men and Women

In modern books and papers dealing with sexuality and elderly people it is stated that sexual behavior is optional. Sometimes, however, it seems as if sex is obligatory. But what is normal for elderly men and women with regard to making love, frequency of intercourse, frequency of masturbation, frequency of orgasm, etc.? To find out I reviewed the literature (Slob 1987).

In this review an age of 50 years and older was chosen. For women it is perhaps a logical line because at that age most women are in a biological/psychological transition. For men there is no such biological climacteric phase, but the age of 50 is experienced as a turning-point by many males. Masters and Johnson (1966) stated: "The incidence of sexual inadequacy in the human male takes a sharp upturn after 50 years of age."

Reviewing the literature on sexuality and the elderly revealed the following striking factors: (1) There were relatively few studies, especially with regard to women. (2) There was a lack of studies that could be considered representative for the older population as a whole. (3) There was quite often limited data on sexuality and sexual behavior. (4) Too many studies dealt with geriatric patients and were thus medically oriented. With these points in mind the following global overview of sexually active elderly men and women can be seen in Fig. 3.

In summary, about 75% of men between 50 and 70 years of age are sexually active. These men are healthy and usually have a partner. Above 80 the number of sexually active men is relatively small. For women the picture is different. Up till 60 years about 75% are sexually active, between 60 and 70 a little more than one-third, and between 70 and 80 only 7% are sexually active. This sex difference is conspicuous. It can be partially explained by the difference in marital status between elderly men and women. Many elderly men live with a partner, whereas many women live single because there is no partner available. Or, to cite Freeman (1961), "Old men tend to get married, while old women tend to get lonesome." It is obvious that research into sexual activity, especially coital activity, is affected by the marital status of the people investigated. But it is not the only explanation for the sex difference in sexual activity of elderly people. The studies of Verwoerdt and coworkers (Verwoerdt et al. 1969 a, b) are relevant in this respect, as can be illustrated by the following citation: "In men, the factor of marital status has little

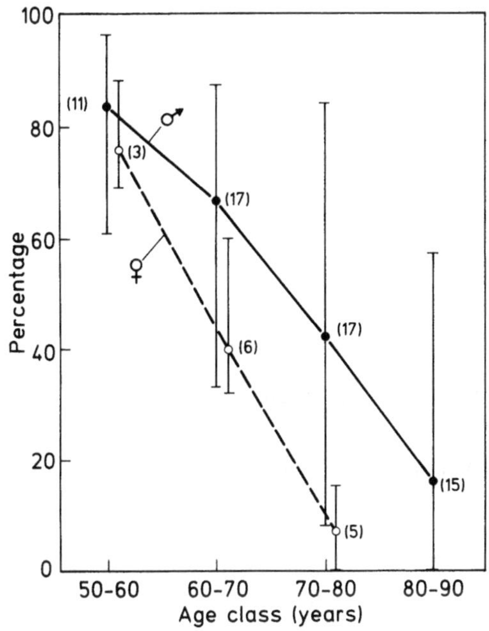

Fig. 3. Percentage sexually active (mean + range) older males (●) and females (○) in a literature survey (number of studies in parentheses)

or no effect on sexual activity and interest; in women marital status has considerable effect on activity but relatively little effect on interest. Generally, the sexual activity and interest of men is greater than that of women, regardless of marital status, but with advancing age, marital status becomes less important in its effect on activity."

Sexuality and Endogenous Hormones

Males

As depicted in Fig. 4 the total plasma levels of testosterone show a decline with advancing age (Vermeulen et al. 1971 a). From the age of 60 years onwards the mean levels are significantly lower than the levels between 20 and 30 years of age. From Fig. 5 it is obvious that a similar decline has been shown to occur for the free plasma testosterone levels (Vermeulen et al. 1971 b). The free testosterone fraction is supposed to be the biologically active component. From the work of Davidson et al. (1982, 1983), it is clear that there is also a significant decline with age of various behavioral/affective measures. In Fig. 6 mean scores on measures of sexual function by decade of life are presented: sexual activity with orgasm, morning erections, sexual thoughts, and enjoyment of sex. As shown in Table 1, all four behavioral/affective measures were highly significantly correlated with age. Frequency of masturbation (not depicted) showed the least decline with age. This was largely due to the high percentage of men reporting a frequency of zero to once per year throughout the age span, particularly within the last three age groups. Total testosterone, estradiol, and prolactin levels were not significantly

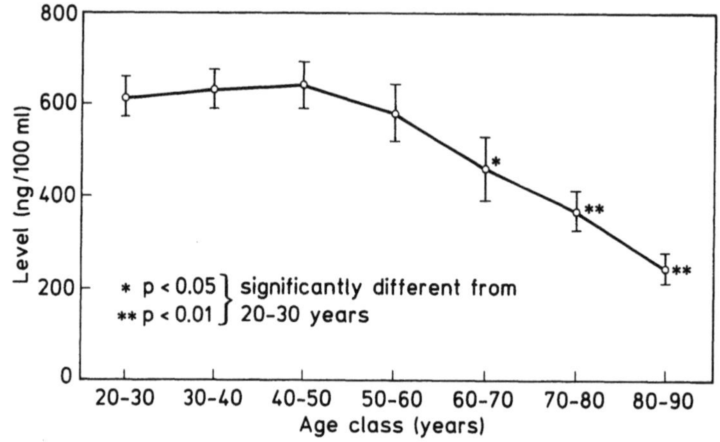

Fig. 4. Plasma testosterone levels (mean ± SE) in males from young to old age (Vermeulen et al. 1971 a, b)

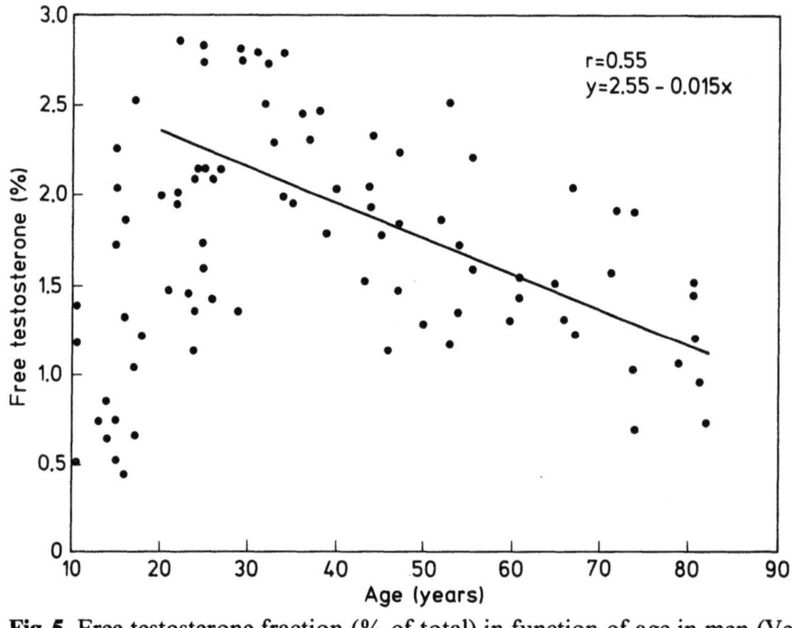

Fig. 5. Free testosterone fraction (% of total) in function of age in men (Vermeulen et al. 1971 a, b)

related to any measure of sexual function. Masturbation did not correlate with any hormonal variable.

Besides plasma testosterone levels, testosterone concentration in target and nontarget tissues in men and women decline in old age (Fig. 7). There are obvious age-related differences in testosterone content in genital tissues: scrotal skin and pubic skin in men; labia majora, clitoris and pubic skin in women. No age-related differences were found in thigh skin and striated muscle, neither in men nor in women. However, there still seems to be a sex difference: males having somewhat higher concentrations than females (Deslyperre and Vermeulen 1985).

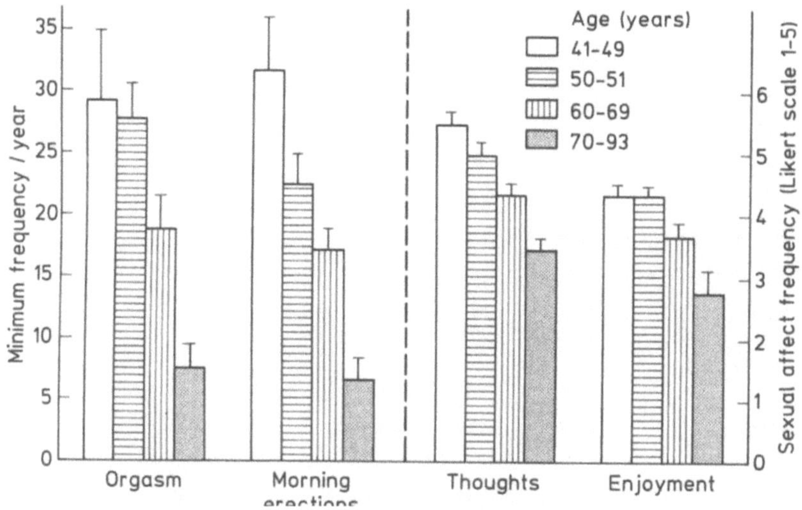

Fig. 6. Age and frequency of sexual events in men (Davidson et al. 1983). *Left*, sex activity with orgasm and nocturnal erections (minimum frequencies); *right*, sex thoughts/fantasies and enjoyment

Table 1. Significant Pearson correlations among hormone levels, age, and behavioral/affective measures. (Davidson et al. 1983)

Hormones	Activity with orgasm	Morning erections	Sexual thoughts	Sexual enjoyment	Age (years)
Total T	–	–	–	–	−0.18
Free T	0.20	0.12	0.18	–	−0.34
LH	−0.21	−0.27	−0.15	−0.19	0.25
FSH	–	−0.18	–	−0.14	0.22
PRL	–	–	–	–	–
Estradiol	–	–	–	–	–
Free T/Estradiol	0.20	0.16	0.17	–	−0.33
Free T/LH	0.30	0.27	0.18	0.16	−0.27
Age	−0.34	−0.39	−0.40	−0.39	

Back to the elaborate studies of Davidson and coworkers (Davidson et al. 1982, 1983). They found that with increasing age both potency and libido factors were affected. Declining androgen levels, reduced sexual activity, and decreased sexual interest thus appear to be related sequelae of the aging process in men. Hormonal factors do not completely account for age-related changes in sexuality, although the full explanation of these changes must include a consideration of hormonal factors. Therefore, they concluded that the changing hormone levels of total and of free testosterone could account for a definite, though small, portion of the age-related changes observed in sexual activity, capacity, and experience. Hormonal change is not the major determining factor in the decline in male sexuality.

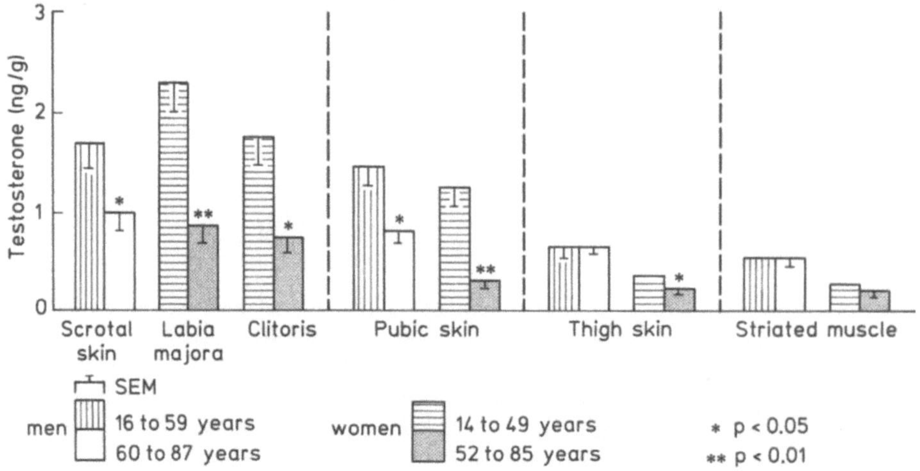

Fig. 7. Age and testosterone levels in target and nontarget tissues in men and women (Deslijpere and Vermeulen 1985)

It has been suggested that administration of androgen may be indicated for a subgroup of elderly men who have low endogenous testosterone levels, sexual dysfunction, and the desire to correct it. Target tissue insensitivity for testosterone, produced by aging, has also been suggested (Tsitouras et al. 1983).

Females

After menopause the ovaries virtually cease to produce physiologically active sex steroids. The persistence of sexual behavior with a completely normal sexual response illustrates the relative independence of such behavior from ovarian hormones.

The most significant postmenopausal change is a drastic decrease in plasma estradiol levels. The concentration of estradiol, derived mainly from estrone in peripheral tissues, is about 10% of the premenopausal levels. Up till old age (83 years) this remains constant (Meldrum et al. 1981). The plasma estrone concentration decreases to about 30% of the premenopausal value. This means that postmenopausally the estrone concentration (about 40 pg/ml) is higher than the estradiol concentration [about 15 pg/ml; Meldrum et al. (1981)]. Estrone is derived from peripheral conversion of androstenedione.

In elderly women there is also a decrease in androgens from adrenal origin: dehydroepiandrosterone, androstenedione, testosterone, and dihydrotestosterone, as can be seen in Fig. 8 (Roger et al. 1980; Persky et al. 1982).

The significance of androgenic steroids for "libido" and for sexual activity was suggested about 30 years ago and is still being investigated. In a critical review of the nonhuman primate and the human literature, Baum stated that more research was needed to determine whether circulating androgens promote the expression of certain types of sexual behavior in different primate species (Baum 1983).

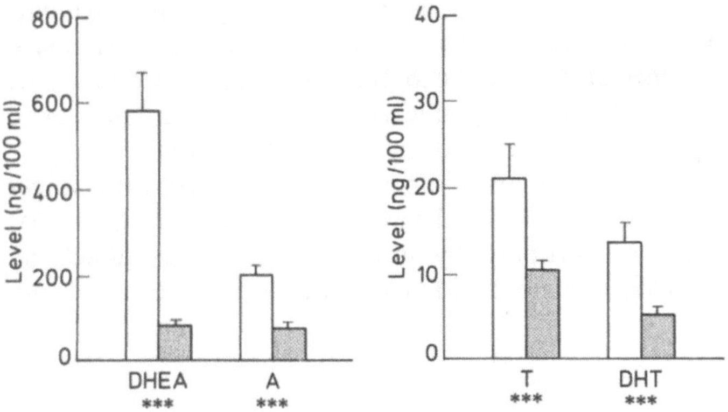

Fig. 8. Plasma androgen levels (means ± SE): young (□, x̄: 24 years; $n = 11$) and postmenopausal (■, x̄: 54 years; $n = 19$) women. (Persky et al. 1982)

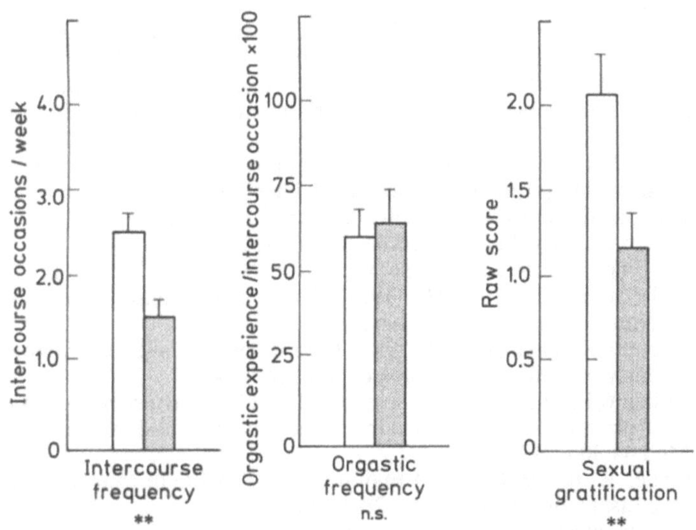

Fig. 9. Intercourse and orgastic frequency and sexual gratification scores (means ± SE) for young (□ 24 years) and postmenopausal (■ 54 years) women. (Persky et al. 1982)

In a study using vaginal photoplethysmography, it was found that postmenopausal women (mean age 57 years) had significantly lower responses to erotic film than premenopausal (51 years) women (Morrell et al. 1984). The subjective ratings of arousal, however, did not differ between the groups. Also the reported sexual arousability and sexual behavior outside the laboratory were similar in the two groups: apparently the physiological changes did not cause any sexual dysfunction. The low endogenous estrogen levels may cause problems with coital activity such as dyspareunia.

In the study by Persky et al. (1982) (Fig. 9) the older women reported the same level of sexual desire and sexual arousal as the younger women (an age difference of 3 decades). Their intercourse frequencies and self-rated gratification scores were significantly lower than the values obtained for the younger wives. All participants were in good physical and emotional health. Whether the lower sexual gratification was a consequence of the higher expectations of intimacy on the part of the older women as reflected in their equal levels of desire and arousal, or to some deficiencies on the part of their husbands, was not yet apparent.

In conclusion: both in elderly men and women there are significant changes in plasma sex steroid hormone levels. From the available literature it seems that these changes do play a role, at least partially, in the decrease of sexual activity and sexual gratification in elderly males and females. But other factors are very likely also to be involved.

References

Baum MJ (1983) Hormonal modulation of sexuality in female primates. Bisc 33:578–582

Davidson JM, Kwan M, Greenleaf WJ (1982) Hormonal replacement and sexuality in men. Clin Endocrin Metabol 11:599–623

Davidson JM, Chen JJ, Crapo L, Gray GD, Greenleaf WJ, Catania A (1983) Hormonal changes and sexual function in aging men. J Clin Endocrin Metab 34:71–77

Deslyperre JP, Vermeulen A (1985) Influence of age on steroid concentrations in skin and striated muscle in women and cardiac muscle and lung tissue in men. J Clin Endocrin Metab 61:648–653

Everaerd W, Dekker J (1981) A comparison of sex therapy and communicative therapy: couples complaining of organic dysfunction. J Sex Marit Ther 7:278–285

Freeman JT (1961) Sexual capacities in the aging male. Geriatrics 16:37–43

Kaplan HS (1974) The new sex therapy. Penguin Books, Middlesex

Masters WH, Johnson VE (1966) Human sexual response. Little, Brown & Co, Boston

Meldrum DR, Davidson BJ, Tataryn IV, Judd HL (1981) Changes in circulating steroids with aging in postmenopausal women. Obstet Gynecol 57:624–628

Morrell MJ, Dixen JM, Carter CS, Davidson JM (1984) The influence of age and cycling status on sexual arousability in women. Am J Obstet Gynaec 48:66–71

Persky H, Dreisbach L, Miller WR, O'Brien CP, Khan MA, Lief HI, Charney N, Strauss D (1982) The relation of plasma androgen levels to sexual behaviors and attitudes of women. Psychosom Med 44:305–319

Roger M, Nahoul K, Scholler R, Bagrel D (1980) Evolution with ageing of four plasma androgens in postmenopausal women. Maturitas 2:171–177

Slob AK (1987) Seksuele aktiviteit van vrouwen en mannen boven 50 jaar (sexual activity of men and women over 50 years). In: Goedhard WJA, Knook DL (eds) Geriatrie Informatorium. Stafleu/Samsom, Alphen aan den Rijn

Tsitouras PD, Martin CE, Harman SM (1983) Relationship of serum testosterone to sexual activity in healthy elderly men. J Gerontol 37:288–293

Vermeulen A, Rubens R, Verdonck L (1971 a) Testosterone secretion and metabolism in male senescence. J Clin Endocrin 34:71–77

Vermeulen A, Stoica T, Verdonck L (1971 b) The apparent free testosterone concentration, an index of androgenicity. J Clin Endocrin 33:759–767

Verwoerdt A, Pfeiffer E, Wang HS (1969 a) Sexual behavior in senescence; changes in sexual activity and interest of aging men and women. J Geriatr Psychol 2:163–180

Verwoerdt A, Pfeiffer E, Wang HS (1969 b) Sexual behavior in senescence. II Patterns of sexual activity and interest. Geriatrics 24:137–154

Age-Related Subjective Importance of Sexuality in the Elderly

W. Zwanikken

Oudegracht 333, 3511 PC Utrecht, Niederlande

In publications on the sexuality of elderly people we come across a limited number of frequently used concepts: drive level, sexual capacity, sexual interest, sexual motivation, taboo, negative attitude, social desirability. These are useful concepts. As people grow older, however, they grow more complicated. Inter- and intrapersonal variability seem to increase, making gerontology the science of exceptions. That is why I have tried to construct a more or less new concept at the psychological level. This concept implies that the continuity or the stopping of any sexual activity in elderly people is based on a cost-benefit consideration.

In this paper I will deal with three questions:

1. What do I mean by the concept of "subjective importance of sexuality"?
2. From which point in the life history can we use this concept successfully to explain or describe sexual patterns of elderly people? Can we use the concept as well for the sexual life histories of men as for those of women?
3. In which field of research has the concept any use as a supplementary or alternative explanation for sexual patterns in elderly people?

Now let me tell you about two recent experiences with elderly people's sex life. One of the family doctors I used to work with told me about an older couple. He is 83 years old, she is 80 years old. They had been his patients for years. One day she came to his office and asked for treatment of fluor vaginalis. She explained to the doctor: "I had intercourse with my husband on the occasion of my eightieth birthday, the first time for years." Soon afterwards they left his practice for good. The doctor was very disappointed because he thought of himself as a confidant of these people. He decided to write them a letter and ask them why they had left his practice. Their answer was: "because you should not have known about our latest lovemaking."

A second situation: Mr. L. is a newspaper man about 50 years old. He is a young old man. He had overworked himself. He now suffers from depressions, hypertension, headaches, alcohol abuse, and sleeplessness. After 1 year of therapeutic treatment he told me, pretty embarrassed, that he wanted to talk about sex, because for some time he had had a morning erection. During the past 5 years he had had no intercourse with his wife, he had not masturbated, nor had he had any sexual fantasies or dreams. His partial sexual revival made him unhappy. He tried to hide his erections from his partner for fear of possible overtures on her part.

These examples demonstrate two things:

– Sex in elderly people can be absent for a long time.
– Sex can return after a long time.

Sexology
Eds.: W. Eicher, G. Kockott

The question of whether sex will be missed and whether the comeback of sex will be a welcome event is subject to a cost-benefit consideration.

What Do I Mean by the Concept of "Subjective Importance" of Sexuality?

By "subjective importance" I mean:

– The relative weight that a person more or less habitually attributes to sexuality as compared with other aspects of life, and as a means to acquire specific, highly valued emotional and/or social goods or to prevent the loss of these goods. These goods are pleasure, excitement and satisfaction, warmth, tenderness, power, friendship, company, partnership, reinforcement, help, emotional, social, even economic security, etc. A more or less close, personal tie with one or more of these goods and sexuality is been formed in early youth, is reinforced by life experiences, and is transported to old age. A study by Christenson and Johnson (1973) demonstrated that women who are not reared – as the most of us are – on the belief that sex is very important, for the greater part live without any overt sexual behavior without missing it.

The subjective importance of sexuality may be consistent during the life course, it may increase, or it may decrease. Decreasing subjective importance will be reflected by:

- lower levels of sexual thought, sexual interest, and sexual behavior, and at the same time:
- higher levels of thought, interest, and behavior around a current nonsexual concern that successfully competes with sexuality.

Such concerns may be: important encounters, new jobs, the resolution of a conflict, pain, housing problems, health problems, worrying about relatives; decisions to be taken with respect to one's place in the family or neighborhood, with respect to maintaining one's independence, with respect to one's financial position, with respect to one's religious commitment, etc. People who are brought up with the idea that sex is not very important or even a bad, tricky thing, who in their life history had little profit from their sexuality, will – according to the concept of subjective importance – be the first to leave their sexuality "at the side of the road" like you do with a superfluous piece of luggage.

From Which Point in the Life History Could the Concept of "Subjective Importance" Become Significant?

From the moment that any sexual habit, any habitual level of sexual functioning, any lasting sexual relationship is no longer taken for granted by the person involved. The choice of a fixed chronological age is arbitrary. Choosing the age of 50 years has some advantages: at this age for many men and women a time of many transitions has come: for the women menopause, for many men according to Masters and Johnson (1970) "a sharp upturn of sexual dysfunctions," children leaving the parental home, many men and women taking care of their own aged parents. Actually at any point in the life history such transitions may occur: either a period of disease, a prolonged absence from home, or the end of a significant intimate relationship by death or divorce can have the same effects.

Is the concept of "subjective importance" as useful to describe or explain the sexual life histories of men as of women?

As far as I can see, it is not, because until now in our culture in every stage of life the sexuality of men and the expression of it is socially more accepted than that of women. In every age group men report a higher level of sexual activity, sexual thought, and sexual interest than women in the corresponding age group. Men's sexuality is a low-cost and high-benefit good. Women's sexuality is not. Besides, as far as married women are concerned, their sexual (coital) behavior in many cases seems to be a function of their husband's sexual wishes.

In Which Field of Research Has the Concept of "Subjective Importance" Any Use as a Supplementary or Alternative Explanation of Sexual Patterns in Old Age?

I will try to demonstrate that the concept of "subjective importance" is a good supplement to the hypothesis that elderly people will abstain from sexual behavior on account of social pressure from the environment. From the point of view of social desirability, the sexuality of elderly people is evolving from a DON'T to a MUST. Advocates of the social desirability theory state that society at large wants the elderly to live asexually. The supposed basis of this attitude is the children's fearful denial of their parents' sexuality or – according to others – it is their revenge for the sexual restriction with which they were brought up by these parents. For instance, Gochross (1972) considers the aged a "sexually oppressed" group, like the inmates of prisons and mental hospitals and homosexuals. And so does Kaas (1978). Advocates of this theory want to protect elderly people from the negative social influences. Comfort (1976) writes: "We have to make society understand that all humans are sexual beings, retaining the same needs until they die." and: "We need to support and encourage their sexuality. It is a mental, social, and probably a physical preservative of their status as persons, which our society already attacks in so many cruel ways."

One of the most complete descriptions of how such a process of disapproval and social pressure could take place has been published by Merrie-Jean Kaas. She called it the "geriatric sexuality breakdown syndrome." One assumption of this theory is that people in general will obey sexual prohibitions. Now, as Abraham (1973) states in the context of sexuality in old age, a sexual prohibition can also act as a stimulus. In that case the sexual prohibition would give rise to the formation of a sexual "underground movement" and a heightened level of sexual thought, especially in communities of elderly people. The concept of "subjective importance" is in my opinion completely compatible with the "geriatric sexuality breakdown syndrome" (GSBS) of Merrie-Jean Kaas, but it could explain why some people do not give up their sexuality, even in the nursing home. Kaas suggests that the GSBS is the typical reaction of old people to the social taboos on sexuality in old age. I think that the GSBS is typical for these elderly people who use to react to environmental demands with submissive and subassertive behavior: people who consider themselves unimportant in every respect, sexuality included. For them being accepted and respected by the caring environment is a highly valued and scarce social good. This reaction is not typical for men, nor for women with some formal education. (Take for instance: Szasz 1983.)

The most convincing proof that in the field of social desirability the concept of "subjective importance" has a supplementary function consists of the findings of Cameron and Biber (1973), Giambra and Martin (1977), and Giambra (1983).

Sexual Thought and Daydreaming

Cameron and Biber (1973) asked 4420 people between 9 and 99 years of age, in a representative time-sampling study, what they had thought about for the past 5 min. They found that the frequency of reported sexual thought reaches a highpoint in the teenage and young adult years and then decreases in every subsequent age group. If elderly people as a group were sexually oppressed, this would in my opinion manifest itself as an increase in sexual thought as an expression of current concern. They do not, not even elderly men, who in every stage of life think more about sex than women, and are less inclined to underreporting of sexual matters than women. The findings of Giambra and Martin and Giambra concerning age-related frequencies of sexual daydreaming reflect the same tendency.

My conclusion is that for elderly people nonsexual aspects of their daily life gain in relative importance. At the end of this paper I will summarize what advantages I see in the concept of "subjective importance."

- I consider it a good common sense concept in the psychotherapeutic contacts with elderly clients. By using the concept they can make clear what sexuality in a given situation or relation brings and what it costs.
- I consider the concept a good instrument to connect a series of life stages in one comprehensive research design.
- The concept is in my opinion a source of new – until now mostly unanswered – questions. I will give some examples:
- Can we define different styles of early sexual socialization (one source of subjective importance)? Can we define different ways in which people use their sexuality instrumentally in their life history (another source of subjective importance)? Can we relate these two sources of subjective importance in the context of individual life histories?
- What is the role of an early parental loss on the subjective importance of sexuality in later years?
- What is the quality of life of elderly people with and without sex? There are four possible combinations of sexual activity and satisfaction:
  Sexually active and satisfied
  Sexually inactive and satisfied
  Sexually inactive and dissatisfied
  Sexually active and dissatisfied

How many elderly people in a given time and place belong to each of these categories? I am impressed by the large numbers of widowed women, who miss their husbands, but who declare themselves to be relieved from their sexual "duties."

I am curious to know what a so-called asexual old age is like. Do elderly people have a restricted life space and a poor environment? Do they feel sad, guilty, disappointed, relieved? Do these people have sexual reminiscences, desires? Do they avoid sex in their conversation? Will they try to prevent other elderly people engaging in sexual relations? Will an asexual life facilitate noncompetitive relations with age mates? Under what kind of emotional and social circumstances can sexuality revive? What kind of encounters will be needed for that?

In this paper I have tried to demonstrate some possibilities of a common sense concept in the study of sexuality in elderly people. The preparation of this paper made me aware of the many gaps in our knowledge of the subject and of my desire to answer some of the questions I asked myself.

References

Abraham G (1973) Lebensalter und Sexualität. Sexualmedizin 2:450–452

Cameron P, Biber H (1973) Sexual thought throughout the life span. Gerontologist 13:144–147

Christenson CV, Johnson AB (1973) Sexual patterns in a group of older never-married women. J Ger Psychiatr 6:80–98

Comfort A (1976) Sexuality and aging. Siecus Report 4(6):9

Gochross HL (1972) The sexually oppressed. Soc Work 17:16–23

Giambra LM (1983) Daydreaming in 40–60-year-old women: menopause, health, values, and sexuality. J Clin Psychol 39:11–21

Giambra LM, Martin CIE (1977) Sexual daydreams and quantitative aspects of sexual activity: some relations for males across adulthood. Arch Sex Behav 6(6):497–505

Kaas M-J (1978) Sexual expressions of the elderly in nursing homes. Gerontologist 18:372–378

Kaas M-J (1981) Geriatric sexuality breakdown syndrome. Intern J Aging Hum Develop 13:71–77

Masters WH, Johnson VE (1970) Human sexual inadequacy. Little Brown, Boston

Szasz G (1983) Sexual incidents in an extended care unit for aged men. J Am Geriatr Soc 31:407–411

Does Marriage Inhibit Sexual Desire?

C. Buddeberg

Abteilung für Psychosoziale Medizin, Universitätsspital Zürich,
CH-8091 Zürich, Switzerland

Until a few decades ago, marriage was the only place where sexual desire could be shown and lived without scruples. The limitations of personal freedom through marriage were compensated for by the attainment of sexual possibilities and rights. Today, premarital sex is accepted quite widely and is practiced by a large part of the population. As a rule, conclusion of marriage does not mean any longer a gain today, but rather a limitation of sexual freedom to the relation with the marital partner. Is it a consequence of this limitation that ever more men and women have come in recent years to consult physicians, psychotherapists, and sexologists because of lack of libido? It would be too simple to attribute the increase of disturbances of libido to this aspect alone. Sexual appetence is the expression of a complex occurrence, in which biological, psychological, and social factors have their parts. I limit myself in the following to three aspects that make understandable in part why disorders of sexual desire are so frequent today: They are *the change in the social meaning of marriage, the discrepancy between the ideal of marriage and its reality, and the value of sex within marriage today*.

What Is Sexual Desire?

Levine (1987, p. 44) described the essential characteristics of sexual desire as follows: "Sexual desire is the psychobiologic energy that precedes and accompanies sexual arousal and tends to produce sexual behavior. It is the product of the interaction of the neuroendocrine system that produces drive, the cognitive processes that generate wish, and the motivational processes that result in willingness to behave sexually." This conceptual determination shows that libido is a psychosomatic phenomenon, and inhibition of sexual desire mostly a multifactorially caused symptom. Therefore, the diagnosis and treatment of disorders of sexual desire requires the consideration and evaluation of various factors such as, for example, age, hormonal status, and sexual attitudes, as well as life cycle and the quality of the current relationship of the marital partners. I should like to refer to three studies indicating that deficiency of libido is today a frequent problem with which we as sexual therapists are confronted in the treatment of patients and perhaps ever again in our private life.

Clement (1986) found in an empirical comparative study of German students that in the years between 1966 and 1981 the attitude toward sexuality and sexual behavior had changed in some kind foremost among the women. Whereas no

Sexology
Eds.: W. Eicher, G. Kockott

changes were found in the masturbatory behavior of the male students, there was a clear increase of experience of masturbation in the female students. In 1981 three-fourths of the women reported masturbating from time to time, while in 1966 42% had stated so, whereby the frequency of masturbation was independent of whether heterosexual contacts existed at the same time or not. Married students answered in the inquiry of 1966 that after marriage their sexual activity and satisfaction had increased; in 1982 the married one stated that since marrying they were less active sexually and less satisfied. Thus while in 1966 conclusion of marriage was attended by an intensification and improvement of sexual life, in 1981 an opposite trend was found; marriage led to lessening and worsening of partnership sex.

Elliott and Watson (1985) in a prospective study of young married couples examined changes in sexuality during pregnancy and after the birth of a child; 50% of the women and 20% of the men judged their ability for sexual response 1 year after the birth of a child, mainly of the first child, to be worse than before the pregnancy. Also, a third of the women were less content with their sex lives than before pregnancies.

An evaluation of the patients treated for sexual disorders in our outpatient service at the University Hospital of Zurich between 1976 and 1985 yielded an increase of disorders of sexual desire in both sexes (Buddeberg 1987; C. Buddeberg, H.J. Furrer, M. Sieber, 1987, 10 Jahre sexualmedizinische Sprechstunde am Universitätsspital Zurich, Switzerland, unpublished paper). The age of the women was between 20 and 35 years, while the men with libido problems were almost all over 35 years old. The trends that these three studies showed may be summarized as follows: Among young adults with a liberal attitude to sex, marriage marks a change toward a quantitative and qualitative worsening of their sexual life. The phase of founding a family, that is the change from the marital relationship of two people to the familial relationship of three, is accompanied in both sexes by a worsening of sexual life, whereby the changes are more obvious among the women than among the men. Whereas the women suffer from deficiency of libido rather in that phase of life in which they have young children, men are afflicted rather more during middle age. How are these fluctuations of sexual desire to be explained?

Change of the Social Meaning of Marriage

The social change in marriage is to be attributed foremost to three causes, namely to the increase of the average expectancy of life, to changes in the relation of the sexes to one another, and to a fundamental change in the meaning of marriage.

In the course of the past hundred years the *average expectancy of life* has lengthened from about 40 years to more than 70. This lengthening of life has led to profound changes of ordinary daily life, but also of life in marriage (Imhof 1981). The duration of marriages that are not divorced has increased from an average of about 31 to an average of about 45 years and so now exceeds 60% of the full length of life. Even more obvious are the changes of the proportions of the single phases of life. For women that married, childhood, measured as the time from birth to menarche, was previously more than a fourth of the full span of life; its proportion is now reduced to 15%, thus less than a sixth. In contrast thereto the length of the period of the so-called "unused fruitful years," that is after the birth of the last child until menopause, has increased most markedly to become the longest single period of life, 31% or nearly a third, whereas it was once only 8%, about a twelfth in the life of a woman who married.

The *change in the relation of the sexes to one another* is shown in, among other matters, the fact that with the exception of the biologically determined functions, such as procreation, pregnancy, and bearing children, today all the tasks of a marital partnership can be undertaken by the woman as well as the man. It is true that the traditional division of functions which gives to the woman tasks inside the home and to the man tasks outside the home, is still the dominant one; but marriages between housemen and professionally employed women show that the sharing of roles and tasks need not be as it was for hundreds of years and as many men still wish it to be today. With this is indicated that the tasks that must be done by a family, such as earning money, raising children, support during illness and disability, nutrition, care of the home and planning of leisure, need not be distributed a priori in a sex-specific way between man and woman, but may be discussed and distributed anew repeatedly.

The *change in the ideal of marriage* may be characterized in brief: In past centuries the selection of partners and marriage were subject to a large degree to the control or regulation by the environment and to strict social norms; marriages were arranged often by the partners and concluded inside narrow geographical confines and the same social classes. Marriage was an institution with the purpose of securing as well as possible through common work, production, and mutual help the survival of both partners and of their children. Today it is more a fellowship, which man and woman enter with the hope of intense emotional binding and closeness with the expectation that development and realization of self could be achieved with the help of the partner. A marriage should for the one part offer security and feeling of asylum, yet for the other part variety and stimulation in the drab monotony of everyday life. It should be both the familiar haven of relaxation and recovery and the scene of exciting emotional and erotic action. Marriage as an exclusive relationship of love is entered today not seldomly with *the hope of meaning to one another all things at all times in all situations of life* (Willi 1975). According to my experience exaggerated images of an ideal, and unrealistic expectations, which many men and women have of a partnership of two people, contribute strongly to the sexual dissatisfaction in and the failure of many marriages.

The situation of marriage and the family of the present time may be summarized in the following statements:

- Marital relations of couples endure an average of 45 years in our time, unless divorce intervenes earlier.
- The marital partnership, because of the smaller number of children, the shorter time of work, and the longer time of leisure, is influenced less by external factors than it was in earlier times.
- For the distribution of familial tasks and roles husband and wife have, in comparison with previously, a much larger range of decision.

- Marital relationships are today in a larger measure those of partners rather than of parents.
- The images of the ideal are related preponderantly to the domain of the intense emotional tie and satisfaction. They often are exaggerated, unrealistic, and contradictory.

Ideal of Marriage and the Reality of the Family

The limits of emotional intimacy and emotional harmony of a couple become especially clear during pregnancy and after the birth of a child. The tension that a couple enters to a various extent after the birth of a child could be circumscribed by the epithets "conflict of values" and "conflict of roles" (Ryffel-Gericke 1985).

A *conflict of values* arises foremost between for the one part the concept of achievement and for the other part that of quality of life. Whereas today still many men dedicate themselves to a mythos of achievement, career, and material standard of life, the women feel themselves obligated to a style of life in which the reasonable utilization of leisure time has priority before work. Additionally, enjoyment and pleasure of life and openess are esteemed as more important than achievement and possession of material goods. Conflicts of values occur most of all within a traditional structure of the family, that is one in which there are differences of education and profession between the partners.

Conflicts of roles occur most frequently in couples with an egalitarian structure in their relationship, i.e., those in which no or only slight differences of level of education and of profession exist. In any such case both the partners have the task of adjusting to one another most of all their professional goals of life and their ideal of marriage, and, as may be apt for them, of coming to a compromise.

Conflicts in couple relationships cause tensions in the domain of emotions, which often lead immediately to alterations of sexual desire and of the ability to experience sexual intercourse. In discussion with young couples who after the birth of a child soberly observe a worsening of their relationship, one comes regularly to the same topic, that young parents must accept impairments and unpleasant disappointments in regard to their relationship as a couple. The reality of ordinary daily life of a family with small children is far away from the adventure of a couple of lovers, who may play without concern with feelings and sexual reactions. Sobered and disappointed, young parents often confirm that their relations as twosomes become removed ever more distantly from the original ideal of marriage (Buddeberg 1987). Lessening of sexual desire is then frequently a perceptible signal of disappointments and frustrations for both partners.

Disorders of libido of men in middle age are induced usually by several causes. As a consequence of the reduction of production of testosterone, sexual drive of men decreases continuously as age increases. In addition to this biological factor, however, psychological reasons, too, play an essential role: professional stress and familial tensions for example through the separation of maturing children can lead many men into crises of identity, which can find their expression in sexual withdrawal and loss of libido. Women experience the middle years very variously as a function of how they have lived before and how satisfied they were with that. For the emancipated woman the separation of the children reveals new possibilities and vacant spaces for the realization of her own interests. Conversely women from traditional marriages do not seldom enter into crises of identity during the climacterium, as their husbands do.

Importance of Sex in Marriage

Undoubtedly the importance of sex for marital satisfaction has increased in the past decades; with this sexuality has become, too, more susceptible to frustrations which in the course of a lengthy marital relationship will affect both partners repeatedly. *It is not marriage that inhibits sexual desire, but rather our exaggerated expectations and images of the ideal of the relations of a couple.* Emotional harmony and happiness are beautiful, it is true, but not realistic or realizable as the enduring state of a marriage. To this extent we should perceive a deficiency of libido as not only a disturbing symptom, but rather also as a chance to confront critically the imperfections and limits within a couple relationship. Relationships of twosomes live from images of ideals. So that these may change and be congruent with the cycle of life of a couple, we must accept that these images fade ever again, become damaged, or are lost. To this extent disturbances of libido have a double signal effect: They characterize the end of previously valid motives and fantasies of mutual erotic attraction, and they are a challenge for the search for new sensual aims and ideals for a relationship of two people.

References

Buddeberg C (1987) Sexualberatung, 2nd edn. Enke, Stuttgart
Buddeberg C (1987) Familiäre Reifungskrisen. Praxis Psychotherapie Psychosomat 32:57–64
Buddeberg C, Furrer HJ, Sieber M (1987) 10 Jahre sexualmedizinische Sprechstunde am Universitätsspital Zürich, Switzerland. Unpublished paper
Clement U (1986) Sexualität im sozialen Wandel. Enke, Stuttgart
Elliott SA, Watson JP (1985) Sex during pregnancy and the first postnatal year. J Psychosom Res 29:541–548
Imhof AE (1981) Die gewonnenen Jahre. Beck, Munich
Levine SB (1987) More on the nature of sexual desire. J Sex Marit Ther 13:35–44
Ryffel-Gericke C (1985) Männer in Familie und Beruf. Ruegger, Diessenhofen
Willi J (1975) Die Zweierbeziehung. Rowohlt, Reinbek

V. Transsexualism

Harry Benjamin's First Ten Cases 1938–1953: Historical Influences

C. C. Wheeler and L. C. Schaefer

310 East 46th Street Suite 12-H, New York, New York 10017, USA

On 24 August 1986, our dear colleague Harry Benjamin died at the age of 101 ½. For all of his patients, he was concurrently an endocrinologist, a counselor, a psychiatrist, a referral service, and even an inspirer of networks. It would seem not too soon to begin to evaluate the formidable legacy which he left us.

For the past 5 years, my colleague (LS) and I have been priviledged to have the use of Harry Benjamin's entire gender dysphoria medical files for our clinical and research purposes. These files began in the 1930s and grew to over 1500 in number by the time of Benjamin's retirement (1979).

In the 15 years from 1938 to 1953, Harry saw his first ten gender dysphoric patients. In the next 15 years, from 1953 to the mid 1960s, Harry had seen approximately 350 patients; and in the final 15 years from 1965 to the late 1970s, Harry saw yet another 1200 patients.

We conjecture that this tripling of his practice in a similar period of years had to do with a combination of factors: primarily it was the outgrowth of his widespread fame which he initially acquired because of his unique approach and methods of treatment and, later on, more specifically, through the publication of his seminal work, *the Transsexual Phenomenon* (Benjamin 1966), and the attendant fame that motivated patients from all over the world to seek his care.

A primary function of clinicians and other professionals is to make a diagnosis, and so we asked, "In the beginning, how was it done?"

Our reason for studying Harry Benjamin's first patients is to learn how *they* described themselves, their feelings, and their lives before hardly any literature on the subject had been published... even before the phrase "trapped in the wrong body."

We were immediately struck by this realization: that even without any books to read, without any other source of information, with or without childhood conditioning, with or without dystonic families, assuming that he or she was alone and unlike anyone else in the world, Harry's earliest patients came to him self-diagnosed, describing symptoms and conditions exactly as his patients continued to describe themselves throughout his 30-year practice; and exactly as *we* continue to hear them describe themselves even today. Such descriptions as: the recognition of gender confusion *very early* in their lives; the attempts at cross-dressing; the secrecy, the isolation, the unsuccessful surpression of desires and feelings; and the guilt, mostly the guilt.

Being a true physician, Harry Benjamin treated each of these patients as people and by respectfully listening to each self-diagnosed individual; he learned from *them* what gender dysphoria was about.

Sexology
Eds.: W. Eicher, G. Kockott

Surely these early patients must be lauded for their courage in seeking a description and a solution for a phenomenon that had as yet *no* description and *no* solution. But also of importance is that they miraculously discovered a physician who was willing to try to treat their unusual condition in a way that had never been treated before.

A collective overview of these first ten people reflects a wide range of life circumstances and patterns. There were nine morphologic males and one female. (This ratio of 9:1 was considered representative until the mid 1960s).

First contact date with Harry Benjamin was from 1920 to 1953.

Ages at initial contact ranged from 23 to 54 years: three in their 20s, three in their 30s, three in their 40s, and one in her 50s.

Socioeconomic levels were exclusively middle class, with three from upper-class backgrounds.

Occupations varied: writer, office worker, scientific farmer, interior decorator, housewife, machinist, entertainer, military service, art student, chemist, and photographer.

Marital Status. Four never married; one married and separated over her transvestism; two married twice in the male role and were divorced or widowed; only one married in her new gender role, but had it annulled; and two already married to each other went through simultaneous gender changes and remarried *each other* in their reversed roles.

Offspring. Three among the ten had children, and only one reported grandchildren.

Physical/Phenotype. Three feminine, one hypogonadal androgynous, and six masculine (including a male to female transsexual with a massively tattooed body).

Sibling order. Two *only children* (both married to one another) and one *first born*. Three out of ten for only and first born is an amazing percentage. This ratio may also prove to be an accurate reflection of today's only and first born gender-transitioning children. More importantly, what might it tell us about this fascinating birth phenomenon? Other sibling orders ranged from the youngest of 2 to the 13th child of 14.

First evidence includes both "initial feelings" and "first contact with cross-dressing." Six reported feelings of "being the opposite sex from very early childhood"; one reported "having those feelings sporadically"; one reported "never having the feeling of wanting to be a girl"; the remaining two, whose feelings are not recorded, most likely had the feelings *early* as they both went through the surgery without regret. All ten had a history of cross-dressing from early ages into adult life.

Unusual *Childhood Conditioning*. Four were raised as boys, while three were raised as girls – one of whom was discovered at the age of 13 to have a birth anomaly; for three no information is available.

Sexual Orientation. Two *hetero*sexual, five *bi*sexual, and three *homo*sexual. Kinsey Scale ratings included a 1, a 2, two 3's, two 4's, no 5's, three 6's, and one "unknown." Added at a later date was Harry's famous *sex orientation scale*. Category designations: one genuine transvestite, six category V and VI transsexuals, and three category IV transsexuals. We were amazed to identify three out of ten as being transsexual IVs, i.e., the true transsexual who does *not* require genital reassignment surgery. This ratio may be as valid today as it was 30 years ago.

Known Family Attitudes. Five "sympathetic or permissive," two "opposition and lack of sympathy"; (only one out of ten divorced because of gender dysphoria); for three no information is available.

Hormone Medication. Seven received both oral and injections to increase feelings of femininity, one for feelings of masculinity, one used hormones for weight gain, and one received no hormones at all. All ten had psychologic help for their condition from Dr. Benjamin.

Surgery. Six of the ten were ultimately considered operated. Three had their first stage done abroad, while the other three had both stages done in the United States. Various stages were performed between 1945 and 1960. The female to male transsexual's surgery was both the earliest and the latest: a mastectomy in 1945, hysterectomy and plastic testicles in 1960.

Harry's seventh patient, Christine Jorgenson, was the first name to cause worldwide attention. Together, Harry Benjamin (a great creative genius) and Christine Jorgenson (a most successfully managed patient) brought hope and knowledge to thousands and changed the lives of countless people forevermore.

It is fascinating to realize how representative these first ten patients were of every combination and complexity known to the gender-concerned world today; the true cross-dresser; the female to male; a gender-changed couple; the true transsexual who does not require genital reassignment surgery; the very young and the very old, both seeking surgeries and both successful; the very public and the very private; from sympathetic and from rejecting families; those who maintained original spouses, and those who were ostrasized and abandoned; those whose transsexual conditions exist in addition to, or as part of, psychotic conditions; and much more.

Yet despite the varieties represented in these early cases, can it be coincidental that the characteristics manifested by all of them appeared at a very early age, or as far back as they could remember – with or without education, guidance, or conditioning – they were exactly the same symptoms we hear today? We do not think so. We think that Benjamin's early patients not only document the history of this unique field, but their stories make an exceptional argument in support of the belief that transsexualism is an in utero condition.

If this "uninvited dilemma" is indeed a birth phenomenon, then perhaps we should educate both the gender dysphoric and the professionals to treat it as such, in order to diminish the paralyzing guilt and negativity with which it is approached by most of the people in the world.

Reference

Benjamin H (1966) The transsexual phenomenon. Warner, New York

Follow-up Studies of Operated Transsexuals

Astrid Junge and Friedemann Pfäfflin

Department of Sexology, Psychiatric University Clinic, Martinistr. 52,
2000 Hamburg 20, FRG

Sex reassignment surgery (SRS) as a means of treating severely suffering persons has been performed and reported on in the medical literature for more than 60 years. The first documented operation took place in 1926 in Berlin. However, it was only after World War II and the spectacular case of the American GI Joergensen that such operations became widely known and were performed in larger numbers in many countries all over the world. When Ira Pauly (1965) published his literature review on the first 100 male-to-female transsexuals in 1965, he drew his information from 54 authors from 13 different countries.

Meanwhile, we know of SRS being performed in men and women from such divergent cultural backgrounds as the People's Republic of China, the Sheikhdom of Kuwait, Buddhist and Hindu cultures in the eastern parts of Asia, and catholic cultures like Spain and South American countries, as well as in people from highly industrialized cultures such as Australia, western European countries, and North America.

The first follow-up study that was not just an individual case report was that of Hertz et al. (1961). Since then, such studies have been performed in many countries and have dealt with various aspects such as surgical outcome and complications, rehabilitation and improvement, suicide ideation and attempts and suicides, psychic and social wellbeing, sexual functioning, and partner and family relations. The literature on follow-up studies has been repeatedly reviewed and summarized, for instance by Pauly (1981), Levine and Lothstein (1981), and Lundström (1981).

According to Levine and Lothstein (1981), by 1981 there had been at least 55 follow-up studies, not all of which, however, met the criteria required of proper research papers. That is why Lundström (1981) for example included only 18 studies from which exact data could be extracted in his excellent review. These studies included a total of 582 cases with follow-up times of up to 21 years. There were 124 female-to-male transsexuals and 458 male-to-female transsexuals.

Lundström et al. (1984) also compared the subsample of follow-up studies which both Pauly (1981) and Lundström (1981) included in their seperate reviews. They pointed out that with some of the reported results it was hard to judge whether they were a hit or a miss. Nonetheless, they agreed that suicide is a very rare event in operated transsexuals (less than 2%), even though they stated, that approximately 10%–15% of SRS procedures end up with unsatisfactory results. Putting the same statement more positively, this means that 85%–90% of SRS procedures are judged to be successful and beneficial for the patient in the long term.

Sexology
Eds.: W. Eicher, G. Kockott

Since Lundström's review in 1981 there have been a further six follow-up studies, one from Sweden (Lindemalm et al. 1986), one from the Netherlands (Kuiper and Cohen-Kettenis 1988), and four from Germany (Spengler 1980; Fahrner et al. 1987; Eicher 1984; Junge 1987) with another 331 subjects, 133 female-to-male transsexuals and 198 male-to-female transsexuals. A total of almost 1000 transsexuals have been studied postoperatively, 257 female-to-males and 656 male-to-females.

Even if it may be an oversimplification, it is generally correct to say that the overall results are good, and some are even excellent, especially when compared to the preoperative situation of most patients. Failures which end in suicide or in return to the previous gender role are very exceptional.

We will not here discuss in detail the criteria of success and outcome used by the various research teams. Within the scientific community there is an increasing trend towards standardizing diagnostic and evaluative measures. Instead, we want to address various agencies that are confronted with problems of transsexualism and gender identity and that often act either helplessly or even oppressively as far as SRS is concerned. Let us have a look at four examples:

1. There are still governments who do not allow their citizens to perform SRS. It is absolutely clear that prohibition of SRS does not prevent transsexualism and does not alleviate the suffering of the patients. It only provokes SRS tourism. And quite a few of the failures that have been reported in the literature are due to poor presurgical diagnosis and treatment or poor postoperative care.
2. There are still governments that do not allow operated transsexuals to have their birth certificates adapted and thus be socially fully integrated into their new gender roles. British, Yugoslavian, and Turkish citizens, for example, did not succeed in their home countries with their plea for a full legal sex change. They often did not want to change their nationality, but seemed to have no other choice. However, a shift in citizenship is similarly difficult and there are many preconditions which often cannot be met.
3. There are insurance companies that refuse financial support for any hormonal or surgical treatment, thus excluding poor people from the necessary help. The situation in the Federal Republic of Germany is, compared with other countries, by and large not too bad. Most of the court cases involving insurance companies have been won by the patients. A final ruling of the Supreme Court has been taken in August 1987 (Bundessozialgericht, 6.8.1987: 3 RK 15/86)
4. There are psychoanalysts and psychotherapists who refuse to support patients unless they give up their wish for an operation beforehand. From various studies it is well kown that counseling or psychotherapy before, during, and after SRS is essential for long-lasting good results. It is no longer useful to discuss somatic and psychological or psychotherapeutic treatments as exclusive alternatives.

On the other hand, it is beyond question but that there are failures now and again. These should remind us to address our own professions, medicine and psychology, to scrutinize our procedures. We want to put forward three important points:

1. The first prerequisite is to stick strictly to the Standards of Care issued by the Harry Benjamin International Gender Dysphoria Association (Archives of Sexual Behavior 14, 1985, 79–90). Our own data as well as many follow-up reports from other clinics clearly show that this is essential for good outcome. Premature hormonal treatment or premature operations usually do not pay off. Cooperation with colleagues who do not respect the Standards of Care should not be continued.
2. Research into effects and unwanted side-effects of hormonal treatment should be intensified. We often observe uncontrolled overdosage of hormones and little care being taken about side effects. As soon as the old fight about the pros and cons of SRS in general has stopped blocking all activities of doctors and patients, there will be more time to study thoroughly the hormonal part of treatment and to find more standardized and proven recommendations than are available today (Meyer et al. 1981).
3. The results of SRS have to be improved. Poor surgical results are closely linked to poor general outcome. There is no need to illustrate this point further as is well documented.

Statistical analysis is our most powerful tool in analyzing success and failure of treatment. It may, however, also sometimes be misleading, as may be illustrated in a very brief example:

A man whose gender identity syndrome could be traced back to kindergarden-age publicly adopted the female gender role in his twenties and lived successfully as a woman for approximately 5 years before he (or she) had the operation in Casablanca. For a while she continued to live happily as a woman. After conflicts with her partner and family, and after a close friend of hers had committed suicide, she became very depressed. As the dead friend had been an American Indian, she contacted an American Indian medicine man for treatment, and finally returned to the male gender role, hiding her breasts under large shirts and large pullovers just like a female-to-male transsexual. We met him 7 years ago when he had already lived in that way for another 5 years. He consulted us to be informed about the possibilities of reversal of SRS. Since that time we have been in contact irregularly. He did not undergo reversal surgery and was sometimes very depressed, sometimes even desperate. At the same time, he emphasized that he had never before experienced himself as a person in the same intensive way, and he felt happy about that. Although he sometimes thought life now might have been easier had he not had the operation in Casablanca, he was sure that he had had no other choice at the time of the operation and he did not regret it.

In objective statistical terms this is certainly a miss, a failure. After SRS the person was temporarily suicidal and later returned to the previous gender role. According to his own judgement, however, it was not a failure, but a complicated way to finally find access to a very rich emotional life.

References

Eicher W (1984) Transsexualismus – Möglichkeiten und Grenzen der Geschlechtsumwandlung. Fischer, Stuttgart

Fahrner E-M, Kockott G, Durau G (1987) Die psychosoziale Integration operierter Transsexueller. Nervenarzt 58:340–348

Harry Benjamin International Gender Dysphoria Association, Inc. (1985) Standards of care: the hormonal and surgical sex reassignment of gender dysphoric persons. Archives Sex Behav 14:79–90

Hertz J, Tillinger K-G, Westmann A (1961) Transvestism. Acta Psychiat Scand 37:283–294

Junge A (1987) Behandlungsverlauf und Katamnese von operierten weiblichen Transsexuellen. Diss Phil, Hamburg

Kuiper AJK, Cohen-Kettenis PT (1988) Sex reassignment surgery: therapeutically effective but no panacea. Arch Sex Behav (in press)

Lindemalm G, Körlin D, Uddenberg N (1986) Long-term follow-up of "sex-change" in 13 male-to-female transsexuals. Arch Sex Behav 15:187–210

Levine SB, Lothstein LM (1981) Transsexualism or gender dysphoria syndromes. J Sex Marital Ther 7:81–113

Lundström B (1981) Gender dysphoria. A social-psychiatric follow-up study of 31 cases not accepted for sex reassigment. University of Goteborg Press, Hisings Backa, Sweden (Report from Department of Psychiatry and Neurochemistry)

Lundström B, Pauly I, Walinder J (1984) Outcome of sex reassigment surgery. Acta Psychiat Scand 70:289–294

Meyer JK, Reter DJ (1979) Sex-reassigment. Follow-up. Arch Gen Psychiat 36:1010–1015

Pauly IB (1965) Male psychosexual inversion: transsexualism. A review of 100 cases. Arch Gen Psychiat 13:172–181

Pauly IB (1981) Outcome of sex reassigment surgery for transsexuals. Aust N Z J Psychiatry 15:45–51

Spengler A (1980) Kompromisse statt Stigma und Unsicherheit. Sexualmed 3:98–102

Social Aspects of Sex Reassignment Surgery

P. Cohen-Kettenis and A. J. Kuiper

Medical Faculty, University of Utrecht, Utrecht, The Netherlands
Free University Hospital, Amsterdam, The Netherlands

Introduction

In 1980 the Dutch Gender Foundation (the principal organization in the provision of care for transsexuals in the Netherlands) requested the department of clinical psychology to evaluate the sex reassignment surgery (SRS) that had been conducted by the Foundation for over ten years. Around the same time a commitee of the Health Council (which is the highest medical advisory body of the Minister of Public Health) advised the long-term therapeutic effects of SRS among transsexuals be investigated. The results were meant to contribute to a parliamentary decision to change the law so that it would allow for adding a note to the birth certificate. This note would make it possible to legally assume a different gender. Against this background, we have conducted the first Dutch study on the effects of SRS (Kuiper and Cohen-Kettenis, in press).

The main question of this study concerned the long-term therapeutic effects of SRS. The only criterium of success was an alleviation or abolishment of the gender dysphoria, as experienced by transsexuals before the treatment. It should be stressed that we differed deliberately in this respect from other follow-up studies, since in these studies other, more objective criteria (e.g., having a job) were also considered to be a relevant outcome criterion. It was felt it would be illogical to evaluate a condition that cannot be determined objectively, like transsexualism, by means of "objective" criteria. Although an alleviation of gender problems can be expected to go hand in hand with objective improvement, such improvement was not considered as a primary outcome but only a possible derivative from it. The principal result of the study was the finding that the majority of people interviewed reported feeling better in general, no longer experienced a discrepancy between their physical appearance and their gender feelings, and were more satisfied with their body. Nobody regretted the steps taken to the point of seeking crossgender reversal again. The therapeutic effect of SRS in our group was very obvious; however this is not to say no problems were mentioned.

In this chapter we will go over some data on the *social* consequences of SRS. Before presenting these data we will first give you some general information about the follow-up study.

Follow-up Study

All transsexuals treated by the Dutch Gender Foundation between 1970 and 1982 were contacted by letter. Altogether 153 subjects reacted positively. A few came

Sexology
Eds.: W. Eicher, G. Kockott

to us through newspaper advertisements, personal contacts, or some other way. This meant a (high) response rate of 74%. For several reasons ten persons did not take part in the study, so the following data concern 143 persons.

Data were gathered by means of a semistructured interview and several scales and questionnaires. The subjects were interviewed in their homes. The data relate to:

1. The general psychological and emotional situation and gender dysphoric feelings in particular
2. Physical condition
3. Sexual situation
4. Socioeconomic situation

This chapter covers only the last topic.

Population

The mean ages of our population were 37 for the MFs (male to female transsexuals, range 20–69) and 28.3 for the FMs (female to male transsexuals, range 19–50). The high ages of some of the MF's are probably due to the fact that they started treatment in the early seventies, at a much older age than is nowadays usual (Table 1).

As you can see from Table 2 the mean period between the beginning of the hormone treatment and the follow-up interview was nearly the same for FMs and MFs, i.e., slightly more than 4 years. Nearly a third of the MFs and 16% of the FMs were still in the phase of hormone therapy only. The others had undergone some form of surgery.

Table 1. Ages of the patients

Group	Patients (n)	Age (years)	
		$\bar{X}$	Range
M → F	107	37.0	20–69
F → M	36	28.3	19–50

F, female; M, male.

Table 2. Time between start of hormone treatment and follow-up interview

Group	Patients (n)	Time (years)	
		$\bar{X}$	Range
M → F	107	4.3	1–14.8
F → M	36	4.2	0.2–13

Employment

Half of the FMs and only a third of the MFs found a job (Table 3). Of the unemployed transsexuals 19% of the FMs and 42% of the MFs were unemployed for more than 2 years. More than half of the whole group reported a stable working history prior to the SRS (that is having the same job for an extended period of time, no heavy conflicts with colleagues or superiors, satisfaction with their work, etc.). A third of the whole group was still following courses and probably not old enough to have a working history. So it seems that a considerable proportion of the transsexual group lost their jobs temporarily or permanently, due to the SRS.

Table 3. Employment details in the FM group compared with those in the MF group

Employment status	F → M (n=36) (%)	M → F (n=107) (%)
Employment		
No	47.2	65.4
Yes	52.8	34.6
Duration of unemployment		
Irrelevant	63.9	39.6
Longer than 2 years	19.5	43.4
Shorter than 2 years	16.7	17.0

F, female; M, male.

Table 4. Incidence of prostitution in the FM group compared with that in the MF group

Prostitution	F → M (n=36) (%)	M → F (n=107) (%)
Before and after treatment	–	2.8
Only after treatment	–	4.7
Only before treatment	–	7.5
Never	100	85.0

F, female; M, male.

Financial problems as well as difficulties in finding a new job could be a reason to engage in prostitution. Only a small number of MFs had chosen this kind of work after treatment (i.e., five) while eight stopped after beginning their treatment (Table 4). Although the financial circumstances of the majority are not ideal they do not seem to do poorly in all respects. Around 80% report living on their own and being housed properly.

Partnership

Slightly less than 30% of the MFs and 14% of the FMs had ever been married) (Table 5). A few MFs were still living together with their spouse. A legal change of the birth certificate was not possible at the time of this study, so all marriages refer to the preoperative situation. Of the transsexuals, 27 had children. Nearly half of the FMs and 20% of the MFs were living together without being married.

An intriguing finding is that two FMs had a steady (homosexual) relationship with a man while a quarter of the MFs were involved in steady relationships with women (lesbian situation). Recently considerable importance has been attributed to the sexual orientation of transsexuals (e.g., the International Gender Dysphoria Association meeting held in June 1987 in Amsterdam). So-called transsexual homosexuality (that is postoperative lesbianism or male homosexuality) was said to correlate with a worse SRS outcome then postoperative heterosexuality. This

Table 5. Partnership in the FM group compared with that in the MF group

	F → M (n=36) (%)	M → F (n=107) (%)
Civil status		
Married	–	7.5
Cohabiting	47.2	20.6
Divorced	13.9	27.1
Unmarried	38.9	44.9
Steady relationship		
No	33.3	58.9
Yes, with a man	5.6	26.2
Yes, with a woman	61.1	15.0

F, female; M, male.

has some bearing upon the diagnostic phase of the treatment. According to some people the future "lesbians" or "gay men" should be approached more conservatively than the heterosexuals-to-be, in that permission for surgery should not be given too hastily. An analysis of our own data did not reveal any relation between postoperative "homosexuality" and the long-term outcome of SRS.

Social Contacts

Apart from a steady partner, other significant persons might be of help in the lives of transsexuals. Their lives are, as everyone understands, filled with more and more serious daily problems than those of most other people. From Table 6 you can see that the majority has a significant support system although the FMs are better than the MFs in all respects of the support system. It is probably due to this fact that satisfaction in FMs with social contacts in general is higher than in the other group. Another contributing factor might be that there is a higher level

Table 6. Social support system and satisfaction with social contacts in the FM group compared with the MF group

	F → M (n=36) (%)	M → F (n=107) (%)
Support system		
Significant support system	77.8	59.8
Some support system	19.4	17.8
Marginal or no support system	2.8	22.4
Satisfaction with social contacts		
Much satisfaction	80	55.7
Some satisfaction	17.1	19.7
Hardly any or no satisfaction	2.9	24.6

F, female; M, male.

Table 7. Acceptance of the FM group compared with that of the MF group

Acceptance by	F → M (n=36) (%)	M → F (n=107) (%)
Family	90	67.6
Friends	93.9	91.5
Neighbors	91.7	85.9
Shopkeepers	95.5	85.1

F, female; M, male.

of acceptance of the FM group of transsexual persons by other people (Table 7).

Most of the rejection reported by MFs seemed to come from the family. Whereas after treatment nearly half the FMs said that their contact with the family improved, only a quarter of the MFs said this. In fact 22% of the MFs even reported a deterioration of contacts with the family.

Concluding Remarks

Summarizing the aforementioned results we can say that many transsexuals loose their jobs, and therefore their social status. The financial situation worsens too. The standard of hausing goes down but stays at a reasonable level. Many postoperative transsexuals do have intimate (including sexual) relationships and other satisfying social contacts, but initiating those contacts and keeping them at a satisfactory level remains a problem for quite a few of them. The least acceptance and understanding seems to come from people who are thought to be the closest to the transsexuals: the family and the spouses.

What do the data on social consequences of SRS tell us? Firstly that daily worries and troubles are numerous. Moreover a lot of loss is involved. People loose jobs, relations, their house, money, and their children. Some handle these losses very well, others do it poorly. In the literature the attention is usually focussed on aspects of life not yet mastered by the newly transformed people (in my eyes even 10 years of living in the newly assumed role should not be considered a long period). Therapists need this information in order to deal with it in their therapy sessions. But once in a while it would be wise to wonder why some of them, in spite of all the stresses and strains that go with crossgender living, cope so wonderfully.

Reference

Kuiper AJK, Cohen-Kettenis PT (1988) Sex reassignment surgery: therapeutically effective, but no panacea. Arch Sex Behav, in press

Outcome of Persons Who Have Been Refused Sex Reassignment Surgery

B. Lundström

Klin I, St. Jörgens Hospital, 42203 Hisings-Backa, Sweden

During the period of 1962–1974, 92 patients were referred to the University clinic, St. Jörgens hospital, for evaluation of gender dysphoria. Fifty-two of these were considered transsexual and accepted for a sex reassignment program. Of the remaining 40 patients, 9 had no gender dysphoria syndrom and 31 had some form of gender dysphoria but for different reasons were not accepted as candidates for sex reassignment. This paper is a presentation of my follow-up study of the 31 patients, 26 males and 5 females, who were not accepted for sex reassignment.

Figure 1 shows the main reasons for the refusal of the patient's request for sex reassignment. In four males and one female with conditions bordering on homosexuality the reason was uncertain diagnosis. In six males with conditions bordering on transvestism the diagnosis was uncertain. Six patients, all males, were themselves ambivalent to sex reassignment due to the social or family situation. Social or mental instability was the reason in seven males and one woman, and finally in three males and three females the reason was a low-intensity gender dysphoria syndrome.

Many of the 31 patients showed conditions difficult to distinguish from effeminate homosexuality or from transvestism. Figure 2 shows the distribution of the patients according to the diagnosis transsexualism, effeminate homosexuality, and transvestism. Eight males and four of the five females were diagnosed as transsexuals, while in eight males and one female the condition was regarded as bordering on homosexuality; in ten males the condition was difficult to differentiate from transvestism.

	Males	Females
1. Diagnosis uncertain. Condition bordering on homosexuality	4	1
2. Diagnosis uncertain. Condition bordering on transvestism	6	0
3. Ambivalence on the part of the patient due to social or family situation	6	0
4. Social and/or mental instability	7	1
5. Low intensity of the transsexual symptoms	3	3
	26	5

Fig. 1. Main reasons for refusal of the patients' request for sex reassignment

Sexology
Eds.: W. Eicher, G. Kockott

	Males	Females
Transsexualism (TS)	8	4
Condition bordering on homosexuality (HS)	8	1
Condition bordering on transvestism (TV)	10	0
	26	5

Fig. 2. Distribution of patients according to main diagnostic criteria

	Males	Females	Males : Females
Accepted for sex reassignment	26	26	1/1
Not accepted for sex reassignment	32	8	4/1
Total	58	34	1.7/1

Fig. 3. Sex-distribution among patients who during the period 1962–1974 were referred for sex reassignment evaluation

The literature presents a greater or lesser male predominance for gender dysphoria. Various hypotheses have been suggested to explain this male dominance. In Fig. 3 I have divided our total material of 92 patients into two groups; *accepted for* sex reassignment and *not accepted for* sex reassignment. As you can see the sex ratio in the *group accepted* for sex reassignment is 1/1, while in the *group not accepted it is 4/1.*

In the two groups together the ratio is 1.7/1. It emerges that if we exclude patients who are not suitable for sex reassignment the sex ratio becomes 1/1. In this study the group who is considered not suitable for sex reassignment consists mainly of men with conditions atypical for transsexualism. Men seeking help to obtain sex reassignment represent a more heterogeneous diagnostic group than females with the same wish. This suggests that unselected material will show a male predominance. If we select from this material persons with the diagnostic features typical for transsexualism, the sex ratio will be 1/1. In 1967 Wålinder reported the sex ratio as 2.8/1. This figure was based on material in which assessment for sex reassignment had not yet been made. In a later study in 1971 the 1/1 sex ratio was based on persons who had been referred to the Board of Social Welfare for sex reassignment.

The follow-up time after refusal was at least 3 years. At follow-up one female had committed suicide. The other 30 (26 males and 4 females) were alive. Twenty-one (17 males and 4 females) of these 30 were personally interviewed. Nine, all males, either refused personal interview or did not answer my invitation to interview. Further information was obtained by register data. From social registers I obtained information on social security benefit and alcohol excess, from the central penal register information as to which of them had been convicted for crimes. From the member registers of public insurance funds I obtained information about disability pensions and sick certifications. Records from psychiatric clinics where the patients had been treated have given additional information. Register data were gathered for all the 31 patients in the study.

Four of those 21 patients had later received sex reassignment from other clinics. Two were biological females; both were doing excellently in their male roles. They had a very good working situation. None were married but both lived together with a woman and both reported good sexual adjustment. The other two patients were biological males. One of them lived after refusal under miserable conditions with daily compulsive cross-dressing, and was continuously unhappy, having great social and economic problems, and unable to work. In the female role after sex reassignment this patient did a lot better, having an acceptable appearance. She was not able to work and the prognosis for work in the future was not good. The situation at follow-up was better than before the sex reassignment but not quite satisfactory. The other man had not yet got any reassignment surgery, he lived in a satisfactory working situation in female role and had a good appearance.

Of the nine male patients who were not interviewed, three had after refusal received sex reassignment from other clinics. Thus a total of 7 patients (5 males and 2 females) out of the 31 patients had received sex reassignment from other clinics after the refusal from our clinic.

I will now present some result variables for the remaining 17 personally interviewed patients, 15 males and 2 females, who at follow-up still lived in their biological sex roles. Table 1 shows that 15 of the 17 patients still reported cross gender identity. Two, both males, denied gender dysphoria symptoms at follow-up. Both were young, 17 years, when they were first referred to our department. At the interview one of them was very reserved as to his actual life situation. He said he was now living quite a normal life, also denying homosexual activities. He said he regarded his earlier transsexual symptoms as silly ideas of his youth. The other one was somewhat confused as to his gender identity but denied clear transsexual symptoms. He now lived in harmony, regarding himself as a homosexual, having frequent sexual contacts. He had no trouble with work or economy.

Table 2 shows that eight males and the two females considered our refusal of sex reassignment as wrong. Five had the opinion that it was right to refuse sex reassignment. Two of them were the two who now denied gender dysphoria; one considered it right with regard to his wife and children; two now felt that they were too old when they first requested sex reassignment and furthermore their social and mental stability was poor, which would have made it difficult for them to adjust to the opposite sex role.

Four males and the two females still expressed a wish for sex reassignment. Five had given up the wish for sex reassignment but still practiced some form of

Table 1. Gender identity orientation at time of follow-up. Group I, $n=17$

	Males	Females
No or only occasional feeling of cross-gender identity	2	0
Permanent feeling of cross-gender identity	13	2
	15	2

Table 2. Patients' own opinions regarding refusal of request for sex reassignment. Group I, $n=17$

	Males	Females
Decision to refuse was		
Wrong	8	2
Right	5	0
Not assessable	2	0
	15	2

cross-dressing, while six patients had given up both their wish for sex reassignment and all forms of cross-dressing.

Four males and the two females had not needed any psychiatric care during the follow-up period. Five males had had outpatient contact with psychiatrists for depressive symptoms. Six patients had been admitted to hospital for psychiatric care, and three of them had been admitted several times, one for psychotic states, the two others mainly for symptoms associated with alcoholic excess.

One female committed suicide a short time after the refusal. Seven males had attempted suicide during the follow-up time. Two of them had made single apparently less serious, suicidal attempts. The other five had made serious or several attempts. Five males and the two females had an excellent working situation. In five cases the work situation was satisfactory; in two cases it was unsatisfactory. Three males received disability pension.

When a global assessment was made of the patients' situation at follow-up it was found that five patients, all males, had a very poor life situation. Three of these five practiced cross-dressing in a compulsive manner, which resulted in great social problems. Of the other two, one was severely addicted to alcohol and the other had recurrent psychosis, probably of organic origin. On the other hand, four patients, all males, scored the highest points in the global assessment. Three, who all had a diagnosis of gender dysphoria bordering on effeminate homosexuality, have gradually come to accept their biological sex role. The fourth, whose diagnosis was difficult to differentiate from transvestism, lived in a very good psychosocial situation but he had not completely accepted his biological sex role. The two biological women also scored high in the global assessment but they were extremely dissatisfied with their female role and they still requested sex reassignment.

Of the 31 patients in this study, seven (five males and two females) had been accepted for sex reassignment from other clinics after the refusal from our department. Figure 4 shows the gender dysphoria diagnosis for those who had been granted sex reassignment and for those who still lived in their biological sex role. Six of the seven accepted for sex reassignment belonged to the genuinely transsexual group; further, another three of the genuine transsexuals who had not undergone sex reassignment still requested this.

In summary:

- More males than females ask for sex reassignment.

	TS	HS	TV
Granted sex reassignment	6	0	1
Not granted sex reassignment	6	9	9
Total	12	9	10

Fig. 4. Number of patients who during follow-up have been granted sex reassignment. Division by subgroups, $n=31$. TS vs. HS+TV, $p<0.02$ (Fisher exact test two-tailed)

- The explanation might be that from the diagnostic point of view the male group is more heterogeneous than the female group.
- Only one of the patients originally diagnosed as genuine transsexuals had given up his wish for sex reassignment.
- On the other hand: The prognosis for continuing in the biological sex role seems to be rather good for the transsexual whose condition is bordering on homosexuality.
- Compulsive cross-dressing seems to be a prognostically bad sign for the patient who is not accepted for sex reassignment.
- These statements suggest that: Great weight should be attached to the question of differential diagnosis when sex reassignment is considered.

Reference

Lundström B (1981) Gender dysphoria. A social-psychiatric follow-up study of 31 cases not accepted for sex reassignment. Reports from the Department of Psychiatry and Neuro-chemistry, St. Jorgen's Hospital, University of Goteborg, Sweden, University of Goteborg Press, Hisings Backa, Sweden

Erotic Preference and the Prediction of Regrets in Postoperative Transsexuals

R. Blanchard, B. W. Steiner, L. H. Clemmensen, and R. Dickey

The Gender Identity Clinic, Clarke Institute of Psychiatry, 250 College Street, Toronto, Ontario, M5T 1R8, Canada

Homosexual transsexuals, in DSM-III terms, are those erotically attracted to members of their own chromosomal sex, and heterosexual transsexuals are those attracted to persons of the opposite chromosomal sex. Virtually all anatomical females who pursue sex reassignment are homosexual by this definition. A substantial proportion of male applicants, however, are heterosexual.

Stoller (1973), Lothstein (1979) and Wise and Meyer (1980) have all expressed the view that heterosexual (sometimes labeled *transvestitic*) applicants for reassignment surgery are likely to pose a particular risk of postoperative regrets. This view was weakly supported in a systematic study of prognostic factors by Wålinder et al. (1978). Neither Bentler (1976) nor Laub and Fisk (1974), however, found that their heterosexual transsexual subjects were more likely to regret reassignment surgery.

Given the irreversibility of reassignment surgery and the dearth of systematic data on contraindications for it, the need for further investigation of prognostic factors is self-evident. The present study examined a large sample of subjects to determine whether heterosexual (biologically) male transsexuals are more likely to regret reassignment surgery than homosexual transsexuals, male or female.

Subjects were 111 postoperative transsexuals who had been surgically reassigned for at least 1 year, representing a follow-up rate of 84.1%. The mean follow-up interval was 4.4 years (range = 1.0–13.6 years).

The male subjects were dichotomously classified as heterosexual or homosexual on the basis of chart data and diagnostic questionnaires. All the biological females were classified as homosexual. Subjects' feelings about surgery were assessed with self-administered questionnaires, which included items asking examinees whether they would undergo surgery again if they had it to do over again and whether they still preferred living as the opposite sex.

The results showed that none of the 61 biological females or 36 homosexual males consciously regretted the decision to undergo reassignment surgery. In contrast, 4 of the 14 heterosexual males (or 28.6%) expressed some regret or ambivalence. This difference in proportions was highly significant. Postoperative regret was not correlated with patients' education, age at surgery, age at follow-up, or length of follow-up, and it was not correlated with biological sex once erotic preference had been taken into account.

There was no significant difference between the regretful and nonregretful heterosexual transsexuals on any variable we examined. Three negative findings are of particular interest: The regretful and nonregretful heterosexuals were virtually

Sexology
Eds.: W. Eicher, G. Kockott

identical in mean follow-up duration and in the proportions who had been married and fathered children.

None of the four regretful cases had fully reverted to the male gender role at our last contact with them. Two of them had reverted to working as men in order to earn higher salaries, while apparently living otherwise as women. In both cases, employment in the male role ended when the patient developed medical problems; both were unemployed and living full time as females when last seen. It appears that a loss of income in the female role contributed to postoperative regrets in these two cases.

The third patient stated that surgery had failed to produce the coherence of mind and body that she had been seeking. The fourth patient, who continued to take great pride in her attractive appearance as a woman, stated: "I didn't feel it was a mistake; I felt I hadn't accomplished what I wanted to accomplish." It was unclear from her replies, however, what this had been. The interview data of these two cases suggest that the cause of their disappointment was the failure of surgical sex reassignment to satisfy some ineffable impulse peculiarly associated with heterosexual gender dysphoria.

In summary, this study showed that the heterosexual patients were more likely to regret surgery than either homosexual group. The actual number of regretful cases was only a minority of heterosexual transsexuals, however. This finding suggests that heterosexual applicants for sex reassignment should be evaluated with particular caution, although a heterosexual preference is not an absolute contraindication for surgery. Both our empirical result and our conclusion regarding clinical management agree with those of Wålinder, Lundström, and Thuwe.

References

Bentler PM (1976) A typology of transsexualism: gender identity theory and data. Arch Sexual Behav 5:567–584

Blanchard R (1985) Research methods for the typological study of gender disorders in males. In: Steiner BW (ed) Gender dysphoria: development, research, management. Plenum Press, New York, pp 227–257

Blanchard R, Clemmensen LH, Steiner BW (1987) Heterosexual and homosexual gender dysphoria. Arch Sexual Behav 16:139–152

Blanchard R, Steiner BW, Clemmensen LH (1985) Gender dysphoria, gender reorientation, and the clinical management of transsexualism. J Clin Psychol 53:295–304

Laub DR, Fisk N (1974) A rehabilitation program for gender dysphoria syndrome by surgical sex change. Plastic Reconstructive Surg 53:388–403

Lothstein LM (1979) The aging gender dysphoria (transsexual) patient. Arch Sexual Behav 8:431–444

Stoller RJ (1973) Male transsexualism: uneasiness. Am J Psychiatry 130:536–539

Wålinder J, Lundström B, Thuwe I (1978) Prognostic factors in the assessment of male transsexuals for sex reassignment. Br J Psychiatry 132:16–20

Wise TN, Meyer JK (1980) The border area between transvestism and gender dysphoria: transvestitic applicants for sex reassignment. Arch Sexual Behav 9:327–342

The Psychosocial Deviations of Transsexuals: A Study of 22 Cases

K.-L. Täschner[1] and G. A. Wiesbeck[2]

[1] Psychiatric Clinic, Bürgerhospital Stuttgart, Tunzhofer Str. 14–16, 7000 Stuttgart 1, FRG

[2] Psychiatric Clinic, Bürgerhospital Stuttgart, Tunzhofer Str. 14–16, 7000 Stuttgart 1, FRG

Between 1982 and 1984 we examined 22 persons, who had, according to the 1980 transsexuality law (TSG), petitioned for the changing of their first names or sexual status in the Register of Vital Statistics.

Of the 22 examined, 7 were biologically female (woman-to-man transsexuals) and 15 biologically male (man-to-woman transsexuals). Sixteen had already undergone sex reassignment surgery; the remaining six were trying to do so. In all 22 cases, the examined persons attempted hormonally to adjust their external sex characteristics toward the desired gender. The average age of the biologically male subjects was 31 years (21–65 years); of the biologically female subjects, 28 years (21–37 years).

Somatic symptoms existed in the cases of five of the examined, which did not seem to have any relationship to the maldevelopment of their sexuality. One male subject had a cleft palate from birth (cheilognathouranoschisis); another was abnormally tall, but despite endocrinal examination the cause remained unexplained. A further transsexual revealed residual paraplegia in the area of the hips, caused by poliomyelitis during childhood; in two cases there were thyroid gland dysfunctions, which had been compensated for by medication.

The case histories of our clients revealed that they had, already in childhood, imitated the behavior pattern of the respectively desired sex, which they perceived as typical of that gender. Biologically male subjects reported early incidents of wearing girl's clothing; biologically female transsexuals reported rowdy behavior. In the majority of cases, the subjects realized their desire for a sex-change operation before the age of 20, that is, during puberty and early adolescence. In the cases of three clients, there were traumatic childhood experiences: One had been abandoned by his mother directly after birth; two others were badly mistreated by their parents.

At the time of the examinations, the seven female transsexuals lived in stable partner-relationships with a woman, perceived themselves as heterosexual, adopted the male role in the sexual relationship, and decisively rejected homosexual contact. In contrast, of the 15 male subjects, only 5 lived in secure partner-relationships.

The majority had learned a trade; some had no occupational training and lived from temporary employment. Two subjects had been convicted of petty criminal offenses.

Sexology
Eds.: W. Eicher, G. Kockott

Psychological Status

The level of intelligence of our subjects was normal; two were marginally normal, one was feebleminded (IQ = 61), and one other was of above average intelligence (IQ = 133). In all cases, pre-histories showed depressive resentment; some were subdepressive at the time of the examination. In seven cases, the pre-histories revealed suicide attempts and, at times, even multiple attempts. These all took place before the sex-change operation; in some cases, the attempted suicides were meant to emphasize the patient's desire for the operation. In all cases, the depressions were of reactive nature, that is, they were related to the tense sexual situation.

In one case, sexuality was characterized by clearly sadomasochistic tendencies; however, for most of the transsexuals sexual fulfillment was of secondary importance. In one case, for years there had been absolutely no sexual activity.

Almost all of the transsexuals possessed secondary neurotic deviations. Especially impressive was the ostentatious character, through which their deviations were demonstrated and acted out. Their behavior gave the impression of inadequacy and exaggeration, indicating an underlying personality structure characterized by showing off, infantilism, and hysteria. Strains of narcissism and psychological insecurity and pressing for compensation complete the personality picture. In every case, the goal-conscious vehemence to which the sex-change operation was aspired was impressive and connected with a curious, fanatic-paranoid impersonation of the subjectively experienced sexual identity. None of the examined saw his deviation as an illness.

Discussion

There was a series of psychological disturbances in all 22 examined individuals, which were not directly related to their deviant sexual identity. Despite a number of psychopathological peculiarities, the transsexual syndrome in no way concerns a typical neurosis or a specific psychopathia, although secondary neurotic deviations and also seemingly primary personality disorders were abundant.

In particular, all transsexuals, who found themselves still in the preoperative "struggle phase," showed compulsive character structures with paranoid intimations in reference to the absolute certainty of their contrary sexuality. We could not find a typical, transsexual personality structure.

We are inclined, along with Springer (1981), to classify transsexualism less in the sense of sexual deviations as in relation to other psychological disorders. Transsexualism concerns primarily neither a deviation with sexual instinctive motivations (as with transvestism or fetishism), nor is homosexual partnership predominant. Of the 22 examined transsexuals 21 perceived themselves as heterosexuals and moreover lived, in fact, according to heterosexual criteria. The behavioral sexual peculiarity of the group appears to us to be far more but one symptom among many, which must be viewed within a framework of an encompassing process. That this one symptom is the most evident it becomes pars pro toto, that is, a single symptom signifies the total clinical picture.

If one seeks related clinical models, so one at first comes upon *addiction*. Those whom we examined had in common the same, decisive progression of the development of the will, which Giese (1971) termed "addictive progression." The sthenic character with which the afflicted persons advanced toward the realization of their goal was remarkable. The goal, once chosen, was striven for compulsively and without compromise, despite all the discrimination and opposition of the environment.

There also exist certain structural relationships to *anorexia nervosa*. By the way, in German we speak of this disease in terms of *Magersucht*, which contains the word addiction. In the cases of both transsexualism and anorexia nervosa, the existing sexual role and the sexual characteristics cannot be accepted. Again, in both cases the disturbance begins during puberty.

Parallel to an unsuccessful search for sexual identity, we also found in some of our clients psychotic identity disturbances. This aspect would be interesting to explore.

Why we have made the sexual moment of transsexualism its central and signifying deviation is questionable. For in the cases of those clients examined by us, sexuality was rather of subordinated function. It only became significant where it was, to a certain extent, a means to an end: namely to confirm the newly desired sexual role or as a means of self-confirmation and of securing ones self-consciousness. On the other hand, one-third of our sample had no partner relationship. One-half of them did not even have the wish to enter a sexual relationship and rather conducted themselves asexually. Here it becomes clear that the sexual aspect of disorders of sexual identity is indeed secondary.

On the Question of Sex Reassignment Surgery

Sixteen of our 22 cases had already undergone sex reassignment surgery. The majority of the operations had only been recently performed, making a reliable evaluation of success impossible. In any case, the clients had come to a certain mental calm and stabilization. Within the literature, however, the conclusions appear contradictory: on the one hand Benjamin (1969) speaks of a 75% success rate among 125 cases; König (1978) and Pauly (1981), who give the broadest overview, report similar results. On the other hand, more recent studies are to be found by Beatrice (1985) or by Lindemalm (1986). They judge the success rate of sex reassignment surgery with much reservation.

It is clear that even after the operation most transsexuals retain psychopathological traits: a personality structure, established from years of struggling for recognition and realization, cannot be corrected overnight by an operation. An operation lessens suffering and offers the chance of a more tension-free life. But it cannot replace psychotherapy. Therefore, the surgical correction of primary sexual characteristics cannot be the treatment of choice. Yet if a surgical resolution is planned or desired, then it should be preceded by an at least 2-year period of probation including psychotherapy. We view surgical intervention as ultima ratio, not as the treatment of choice. Even more important, it appears to us, is psychiatric examination and counseling of transsexuals, before surgical intervention is an accomplished fact.

References

Beatrice J (1985) A psychological comparison of heterosexuals, transvestites, preoperative transsexuals and postoperative transsexuals. J Nerv Ment Dis 173(6):358–365
Benjamin H (1969) Newer aspects of the transsexual phenomenon. J Sex Res 5:135–144
Giese H (1971) Die Sexualität des Menschen. Handbuch der menschlichen Sexualforschung. Enke, Stuttgart
König MP et al. (1978) Transsexualismus. Schweiz Med Wschr 108:437–444
Lindemalm G et al. (1986) Long-term follow-up of "sex-change" in 13 male-to-female transsexuals. Arch Sex Behav 15(3):187–210
Pauli IB (1981) Outcome of sex reassignment surgery for transsexuals. Austr New Zealand J Psychiatr 15:45–51
Springer A (1981) Pathologie der geschlechtlichen Identität: Transsexualismus und Homosexualität. Springer, Vienna New York

VI. Sexual Therapy – New Trends

Sexual Therapy: New Trends – Critical Remarks

M. Springer-Kremser [1] and A. Springer [2]

[1] Institut für Tiefenpsychologie und Psychotherapie der Univ. Wien, Währinger Gürtel 18–20, 1090 Wien, Austria
[2] Ludwig Boltzmann Institut für Suchtforschung, Mackgasse, 1230 Wien, Austria

This presentation concentrates on three issues concerning new trends in therapy of sexual dysfunction and further on certain activities of the therapist, which occur more frequently in therapeutic interactions with patients with sexual dysfunctions.

Etiology of Sexual Dysfunction

Four interacting factors may be involved in the etiology of sexual dysfunction:
- Organic factors, such as somatic diseases and hormonal imbalance
- Sociocultural factors (ethical problems, religious bonds)
- Style of interaction (communication) of a couple
- Personal psychodynamic factors

Sexual dysfunction may be the expression of:
- A particular outcome of the oedipal triangle and castration anxiety
- Early developmental impairment of affective life and body awareness
- Inhibition of psychosexual maturation (pregenital disposition)
- Faulty or defective symbolization of the sexual function and/or the genitals
- Excessive structural control (superego neurosis) and excessive reaction-formation (shame, repulsion)

Depending on the degree of involvement of each of these four factors in the sexual dysfunction, there is a continuum, ranging from superficial expectation anxiety and fear of failure to far-reaching psychopathological dynamics, which causes the sexual reaction to gain an ominous symbolic meaning at an unconscious level (Springer-Kremser 1983). This may just as well apply to the subjective interpretation of sexual dysfunction of organic origin, such as some forms of erective failure, based on circulatory disorders.

Consequently, effective therapeutic intervention may be described as resting on a continuum which begins with sexual education and counseling and leads, via brief psychotherapy, to extensive psychoanalytical treatment. Somatic forms of treatment, such as surgical intervention or prescription of drugs, also call for psychotherapeutic attention or guidance.

Sexual dysfunction may be associated with a somatic disease, a neurosis, or another mental disorder. However, this is not necessarily the case.

Sexology
Eds.: W. Eicher, G. Kockott

Various Impulses for Treatment

Recent Therapeutic Approaches in Cases of Somatic Etiology

The development of new examination techniques in urology/andrology has enlarged our knowledge of the somatic conditions of sexual function, thereby permitting us to recognize disturbing somatic factors, which had not been spotted previously or had been ignored. Radical supporters of the new approach maintain that 90% of all erectile dysfunctions are of organic origin and can and should therefore be treated with the methods of somatic medicine.

There is no doubt that today we know more, although not everything, about the physiological processes and conditions of erectile function. On the basis of this increased knowledge a better understanding of the pathological situation has developed. This applies primarily when hemodynamic disturbances or lesions of the vascular system are under suspicion of being the causative factors. We know today that in the case of erectile function we must differentiate between tumescence and rigidity: in the light of this knowledge, previously practiced examination techniques, especially the checking of nocturnal tumescence, appear rather inexpedient.

One advantage of modern somatic examination methods is that they have enlarged the spectrum of noninvasive techniques: hemodynamic disturbances can be detected by ultrasonography, and the differential diagnosis between erection disturbances predominantly caused by mental inhibitory processes and those of somatic (vascular) origin can be established with the help of intracavernous administration of papaverine/phentolamine or prostaglandin, or local administration of nitroglycerin.

Consequently, new methods of somatic treatment of somatogenic erectile dysfunction involve an improvement of the hemodynamics necessary for erection. Supporters of somatic therapy consider microsurgical techniques, implantation of penis protheses, but also the self-administration of the vasodilators mentioned above to be the treatment of choice today.

Against the euphoria of some adherents of somatic treatment it must, however, be pointed out that in this field of research and therapy any kind of one-dimensional approach will produce considerable problems. The same is true if someone maintains that 90% of all erectile dysfunctions could be traced back exclusively to psychological causes. Specifically in this area body and mind cannot always be neatly separated in their effects. Quite often, for instance, a somatic disorder is the cause of acute sexual dysfunction. After removal of this somatic source of irritation, however, psychic reactions and fixations are exclusively responsible for the chronicity of disturbed sex life. Erectile dysfunction in men and dyspareunia in women are paradigmatic examples of multiple causation of certain complaints.

Iatrogenic impotence has gained increasing importance, and since the situation is not likely to improve in the near future, we want to draw particular attention to this form of impotence as a „borderline" somatic condition of sexual dysfunction. A considerable number commonly used and definitely necessary drugs have side effects which may impair the patient's sex life. This concerns primarily almost all the usual psychotropic drugs, but also hypnotics and antihistamines, as well as substances with cardiovascular action (e.g., clonidine, aldosterone antagonists). Frequently the patient is not given the necessary information about these „side effects."

Assistance Offered when Sociocultural Causes Predominate

The liberalization of the late 1970s and the influence of the feminist movement have prompted many women to take a more critical view of their sexual problems. This means that women themselves – thinking in terms of lay etiology – consider their life situation to be responsible for the development of dysfunctions; they describe themselves as *disturbed* but not as mentally ill. Another consequence is that the barriers of shame surrounding traumatizing experiences suffered by women are increasingly broken down.

One field where social awareness and psychoanalytical research meet is in the „women counseling women." As a psychoanalyst I am interested in the direct or indirect impact of current social processes on psychoanalytical work. An example of such a process is the closure of the sex counseling center of the Viennese Psychoanalytical Association in the 1920s under the pressure of social issues (housing shortage, unemployment, antisemitism, etc.). Following Parin, however, the significance analysts attach to realistic problems in their psychoanalytical work varies a great deal (Parin 1975). Therefore, there has always been a minority of analysts in the history of analysis who have tried to integrate contemporary problems into their clinical and theoretical work. In connection with the feminist movement and in an attempt to associate the concept of the feminist movement with psychotherapy of women, guidance centers were established in several places (Zurich, Vienna). These guidance centers normally have three functions, which are stated by the Zurich Guidance Center to be the following (Buess et al. 1985):

- Place of documentation: information and addresses are put on record.
- Place of clarification: women have the chance of identifying and expressing their problems, frequently sexual problems, in one or two sessions; they can understand their situation and consider further steps.
- Place of crisis intervention, where group therapy, various body-related treatment forms, and focal therapy are offered.

Credit must be given to such institutions for collecting those women whose sexual dysfunction is not markedly interlocked with their psychodynamics and therefore has no symbolic significance, but represents a complex reaction to life events. This means that such institutions help to prevent unnecessary stigmatization through illness.

Another example is the increasing readiness in some countries to accept the fact that the trauma of rape or other sexual assault shapes the whole future life of a girl/a woman, influences her psychosexual development, and is a frequent cause of sexual dysfunction, more frequently than generally assumed, since a very large number of cases remain in obscurity. This realization has prompted the establishment of „Rape Counseling Centers," following a Swedish example. Such facilities are preventive institutions, or at least they represent an attempt to prevent late sequelae of such a trauma. The necessity of deepening the theoretical concept of focal counseling and brief therapy arises automatically.

A More Critical View of the Systemic Approach in Treating Sexual Dysfunction in Couples

The following illustrates the escalation of sexual dysfunction in a partnership (Springer/Kremser 1974):

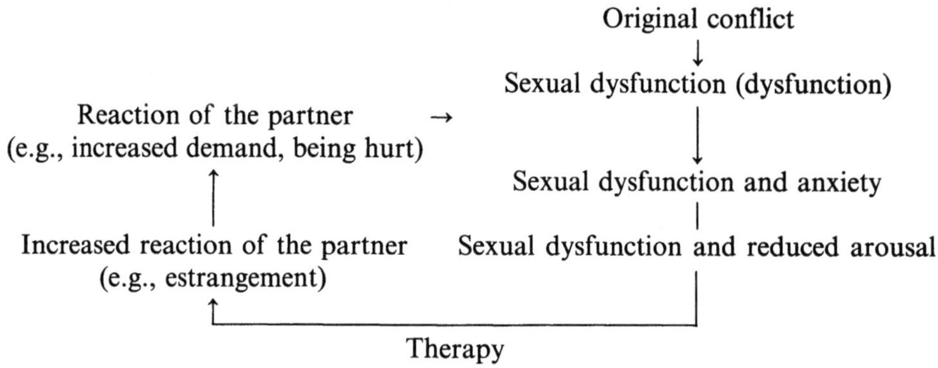

Systemic interpretation strives to elucidate sexual dysfunction in terms of partner contact and to make the partner relationship understandable. Basically, this approach sees sexual desire, sexual behavior, and sexual expression as a form of communication, it ascribes communicative significance and value to any form of sexual expression, and any disturbance in this process is interpreted as one aspect of a more comprehensive disturbance of human interaction. We explained this concept many years ago.

It must be pointed out that there should be strict indications for undertaking couple therapy and unrealistic demands must not be made on the partner. This happens now more and more, after the initial phase of euphoria, which accompanies any kind of new therapeutic method, has abated.

Recent Findings on Female Psychosexuality

According to psychoanalytical interpretation, disturbances of the instinctual sphere as well as of the ego structure (symbiosis/separation; narcissism) may be responsible for the development of sexual dysfunction. The recognition that femininity is associated with cavity, receptacle and not with deficiency, defect – as expressed by Chasseguet-Smirgel: "not for deficiency, but primordially for receptacle" (1984); that the primacy of the phallus is no longer valid has been well substantiated in recent years. Consequently, the psychoanalytical ideas of "penis envy" have become more understandable and more easily integrated into treatment programs, because they draw attention to the "suffering from idealization," which plays such a central role in anorgasm and other female sex problems.

Envy is never related to the organ as such, but to the idealization of power and control associated with the organ. Women tend more toward idealization than men. Partly as a reaction to the anatomical difference and partly as a reaction to social reality, many women grow up in a climate in which men are idealized, and they are either unrealistically overestimated or underestimated. Idealization is always associated with envy, envy of something which we do not have. Moreover we always transfer idealization to ourselves: we cultivate a definite image of ourselves; this image is unrealistic and we attach unrealistic expectations and wishes to it. When we compare the expectations and wishes with reality, we see the deficit and feel disappointment. This disappointment is a constant source of depressivity, vulnerability, and subsequently sexual dysfunction (Torok 1974). Important ideas of the nature of female sexuality are related to the work of Luce Irigaray, author of *Speculum de l'autre femme*. She pointed out that female sexuality is to be defined out of its very specific nature, isolated from the male's definition, from a different point of view, not primarily genitally orientated. She demands the enthronement of a *femme dieux,* not a déesse a female god. Neglecting this autonomic status of female sexuality the discourse of sexuality is incomplete.

Critical Remarks on the Activity of the Therapist

Instructions for Sexual Activities

It often appears to be indispensable that within the framework of therapy specific instruction for activities to take place outside the therapeutic session are given. This may be the case in individual as well as in partner therapy. The aim is either that the individual achieves a better knowledge of his/her own body, or that a couple develops physical-sexual communication. Particular attention should be paid to the emotional reaction of the patients to the recommendations given during the session, sensitivity on the part of the therapist being an absolute prerequisite in this connection, so that he or she may judge whether an individual will be in a position to accept a certain recommendation, or whether shame, fear, etc., will prevent him or her from doing so. It is often difficult to find the right balance between necessary therapeutic intervention on the one hand and keeping one's distance from the patient's intimacy on the other. Therefore, it is of particular importance in this type of therapy to pay attention to counter-transference reactions on the part of the therapist. Self-reflection, e.g., in Balint groups, may be a help in controlling unintentionally seductive behavior and thereby avoiding it. This leads to a further critical topic, i.e.:

Sexual Contact Between Patient and Therapist

Frequently this subject is considered to be taboo; however, it seems well worth mentioning, since the women who have become the victim of an activity – hypocritically labeled as „liberal" (therapeutic as empathic) – suffer considerable damage from it. A review by Apfel and Bennett (1985) describes the effects of such breeching of boundaries in a therapeutic setting. The authors describe the following consequences for female patients (as a rule, these cases involve female patients and male therapists):

1. Patients question their own sense of reality and their sanity. This happens in particular if the therapist offers an elaborate therapeutic justification for his behavior instead of admitting honestly that his motive was simple human need for sex.
2. Pathogenetic childhood situations are being repeated, e.g., the oedipal drama.
3. Extreme bonding to the therapist. The dependance is often a mutual one; the therapist may also feel enslaved by his patient. The only possible consequence is the abrupt withdrawal of one party, usually the therapist, which leaves the patient hurt, betrayed, and abandoned.
4. The original symptoms, including sexual dysfunction, which brought the patient to therapy, persist or even worsen. There may be illusory gains so that the patient believes she can now enjoy sex, but only with the therapist and not with any other person. Other symptoms are thereby circumvented.
5. Problematical relationships with men are a characteristic result. Difficult marriages become even more difficult.
6. Rage and desire for revenge on men are a frequent result, particularly if the sexual relationship with the therapist is broken up. In some instances psychotic defense mechanisms may be mobilized, such as splitting, in order to spare the therapist. Shame and guilt cast the patient into a deep depression.
7. Excessive shame and guilt are always present in women who have been party to such sexual relationships. Frequently shame has much to do with infantile sexual activities, since therapists mostly display pregenital needs, facilitating the association with children's play.
8. Realization of the sexual contact precludes the employment of fantasies to a large extent. The object of psychotherapy, which consists in demonstrating to the patient the either-or mentality of her neurosis, thus gets lost.
9. Dramatic and abrupt endings (by overreaction from outside) leave the patient stranded in a severe crisis.

The instances of transgressing boundaries described above show clearly the difficulty in the management of transference and counter-transference, specifically in the treatment of patients with sexual dysfunctions. In my opinion the most important conclusion to emerge is to demand from the therapist that he continuously monitors transference and counter-transference, that he practices self-reflexion, and that he „feels at home" in his own set of values. I would like to conclude by quoting Freud on a special issue which has been mentioned already in this volume: the unhappy love affair between C. G. Jung and his Russian patient Sabina Spielrein. Commenting on this affair in a letter to Jung, Freud referred to his own experience with a female patient, stating „I had a narrow escape," meaning that a seductive situation may emerge out of therapeutic interaction, but nevertheless countertransferential emotions have to be watched carefully.

References

Apfel RJ, Bennett S (1985) Patient-therapist sexual contact: I. Psychodynamic perspectives on the causes and results, II. Problems of subsequent psychotherapy. Psychother Psychosom 43:57–68

Buess MI, Freye M, Güntzig-Seebronner M, Gubelmann M, Koch B, Wandeler-Deck E (1985) In: Leuzinger-Bohleber M (ed) Psychoanalytische Kurztherapien. Westdeutscher Verlag, Opladen

Chassguet-Smirgel J (1984) The feminity of the analyst in professional practice. Int J Psycho-Anal 65:169

Greenacre Ph (1950) Special problems of early female sexual development. The Psychoanal Study of the Child 5:112–138

Gremal P (1963) Dictionnaire de la Mythologie Grecque et Latine. Presses Univ France, Paris

Irigaray L (1980) Speculum – Spiegel des anderen Geschlechts. Suhrkamp, Frankfurt

Laufer EM (1982) Female masturbation in adolescence and the development of the relationship to the body. Int J Psychoanal 63:295

Parin P (1975) Is psychoanalysis a social science? The annual of psychoanalysis III, 371–393. Int Universities Press, New York, N.Y.

Roiphe H, Galenson E (1972) Objectless and early sexual development. Psychoanal Q 42:73–90

Springer A, Kremser M (1974) Die symptomatische Spirale. Sexualmedizin 7:353–358

Springer-Kremser M (1983) Psychosexualität und Gynäkologie. Deuticke, Wien

Torok M (1974) Die Bedeutung des Penisneides bei der Frau. In: Chasseguet-Smirgel J (ed) Psychoanalyse der weiblichen Sexualität. Suhrkamp, Frankfurt

Ethics and New Therapeutic Techniques in Sexology

A. Merguy and P. Blachere

3, Place du Revard, Le Gr. Hotel, 73100 Aix les Bains, France

Introduction

After the discoveries of Krafft-Ebing, following the theoretical lead of Sigmund Freud, sexology has had to wait 60 years to become recognized as a science. Indeed, it is only with the sexual dysfunction concept and in studying human sexuality like any other behavior that Masters and Johnson have enabled sexology to become a science in its own right. Since 1980 new medically oriented investigative techniques and therapies have evolved (vascular exploration, intracavernous injections, etc.). Such scientific evolution has brought about a radical change in our day-to-day therapeutic attitudes. It is in reflecting upon what has evolved from these new ways of treating patients that we have attempted to develop an ethical position stemming from our personal work as sexology consultants.

The most spectacular aspect of this technological revolution is probably the significant rise in the use of intracavernous injections. For those sexologists dealing with feminine orgasm difficulties, science has not yet given us the "ultimate cure" against the absence of pleasure; we need to recognize, however, that two promising research paths exist at the moment in this area: Many teams are currently working on neuromediators and it seems that certain antidepressant medication would be effective against frigidity (we refer here to the work on Trazodone). Other researchers are studying the use of laser on vulvar blood circulation, and certain studies have produced interesting results (Waynberg).

One cannot comment on these techniques without considering what sort of relationship develops between the patient and the therapist when these new methods are either used or suggested for use. These techniques are in fact a "direct intervention" in the sexuality of the patient; it is in this respect that they are radical; up until now, outside rare surgical cases (transsexual penial protheses or the exceptional case of sexual relations between patients and therapists) the sexotherapy relationship operated on a psychotherapy mode, and the therapist's advice only had a symbolic effect on the patient's mind and not concretely as is the case with intracavernous injections. What we have just mentioned enables us to underline the first danger of these new techniques; the first ethical obstacle. Doctors today can use several options (injections, drugs, etc.), allowing them to reply *immediately* to the patient's needs without necessarily taking the time to reflect upon the meaning of the patient's request for a cure. The irrational and above all systematic use of these methods will therefore oppose the teachings of sexology, whether behaviorally or psychoanalytically inspired.

Sexology
Eds.: W. Eicher, G. Kockott

These new techniques raise questions about the sexual dysfunction concept of Masters and Johnson, the concept that structured the sexology issue. Therefore with these new "aphrodisiacs" we can not only reply to the immediate needs of the patient but equally make abstraction of the dynamics of the couple on which Masters and Johnson placed emphasis. Certain patients functioning in an operative system will probably be pleased to find that we can now give an immediate response to their requests concerning their performance, without having to question the quality of their relationship with their partner. One cannot help questioning the therapeutic value of our medical intervention in a psychoanalytical sense. Wanting to respond without delay to patient's needs prevents us from taking the time to listen to the patient, to the real suffering that lurks behind the symptom.

If we now try to adopt a theoretical approach that we may qualify as metasexology, we notice a strange similarity between the evolution of sexology, which abandons the concept of sexual dysfunction (to come back to a more individualistic concept of the symptom), and Western society of the 1980s, which favors that which is individual to the detriment of relationships with others. It is the concept of "self-concern" developed by Michel Foucault some months before his death which now seems to govern the way people act today. This concept makes possible therefore (and necessary) the development of "social phenomena" unthinkable only 10 years ago, and we will cite among the more caricatured examples the intense way in which the upper classes involve themselves in marathon races, extending themselves to the limit, or the use of Walkmans, favoring a return to narcissism. The new sexology techniques in reducing the individual to his or her bare symptom tend to diminish the importance that the relationship used to play in sexuality in recent years. Consequently they coincide perfectly with the evolution of Western civilization. The emphasis is placed therefore on intimate ties, which brings together sexology and "power," that is to say what forms the evolution of our behavior. One should not interpret our work, however, as a rejection of sexology nor a refutation of these new techniques that we in fact use each day in our team work. Our ethical reasoning has simply allowed us to understand how a scientific discovery could modify the very concept of science, and why the media are so interested in it.

Conclusion

In conclusion we note that the development of these new sexology techniques marks a radical change in the very principles of sexology since it refutes the concept of dysfunction. We can no longer consider as fortuitous this evolution of our science which adheres so well to those fundamental changes which our society is undergoing. This no doubt will give more weight to the arguments of those who have always criticized us. In the face of these objections and if sexology wishes to remain credible, it is vital for us to avoid at all costs ethical obstacles and the principal danger awaiting the sexologist inclined to give too quick a response, prescribing medication without taking the time to analyze the meaning of the patient's request. More than ever the sexologist cannot remain specialized and sexology can only exist in the future if it is amenable to all disciplines, philosophy, sociology, and psychoanalysis. This is in fact the current wish of our French Association (the SFSC) and I hope that I have convinced you of the importance of keeping it this multidisciplinary science.

A Program of Brief Psychotherapy for the Treatment of Psychosexual Dysfunctions

F. Manara

University of Brescia, Via Valsabbina, 19-25123 Brescia, Italy

As the attention of everyone is becoming fixed to an ever-increasing degree on the various etiopathogenetic analyses of psychosexual dysfunction, it seems to me more opportune to speak of sex dysfunction therapies rather than limiting myself only to the term "sexual therapy." The link between sexual pathology, on the one hand, and psychiatric pathology, or even serious hidden psychic problems on the other, confronts us with the choice of a possible therapy which could range from psychopharmacology (preferably backed up by psychotherapy) to psychoanalysis. Nevertheless, the cases in which brief sexual therapy should be applied are still numerous. In particular, our research in the field of couple-oriented psychotherapy has focused around those dysfunctional situations where the sexual dysfunction and the pathology of the relationship were most closely tied together.

The prerequisites for putting such a therapy into practice obviously include the motivation of the patients to accept the treatment and their desire to function as a stable couple, as well as the exclusion of psychoses or severe intrapsychic conflicts. The pathology of the relationship is certainly not to be understood as a single entity, but instead as having an essentially binary character, for the simple reason that in these cases the individual needs of each member of the couple play a large part as each one looks for satisfaction in the relationship. In these cases we have designed a program of couple-oriented sex psychotherapy to be executed by a single therapist, and aimed at resolving the symptom while setting for itself the limited goal of clarifying the couple's relational problems.

This type of therapy, while remaining basically within the realm of brief sex therapy, is designed to liberate the latter from, firstly, the use of repeated prescriptions and, secondly, to avoid as much as possible the use of psychodynamic material. This strategy, perfected during the course of the past 3 years, has been utilized in those cases where the prevalence of relational problems, that is, conflict, hostility, struggle for power, aggressiveness (usually expressed on a metacommunicative level), etc., have been diagnosed as being the root of the sexual dysfunction. This type of therapy utilizes three levels of intervention aimed at bringing forth and building a maieutics of communication:

Level 1. This concerns the pathological elements relative to communication, to messages which are more or less contradictory, aggressive, etc. They are finalized to the treatment of relational conflicts and their expression.

Level 2. This concerns the relational and sexual skills which the couple had previously put into practice in their relationship. They are aimed at helping the

Sexology
Eds.: W. Eicher, G. Kockott

couple recover the relational and sexual skills previously experienced in same period in the relationship.

Level 3. This could be called "integrative" in that it is aimed at enlarging the skills which the couple has been able to acquire and put into practice through the work of the first two levels. They are dedicated to direct treatment of the sexual dysfunction.

I would now like to outline the techniques and theoretical presuppositions connected with these three levels in greater detail:

Level 1

In this level use is made of the videotape technique, following the indications of Alger, Hogan, and Berger. Actually, this technique is immediately proposed to the patients even during the diagnostic phase. The evaluation, after the first session with the couple, is carried out during the next two sessions, the first of which serves to interview each member of the couple (in order to collect information about their personal histories) and a second session with the couple (which is videotaped) aimed at examining the material which has emerged up to that point. The videotape is then proposed to let the partners see how they interrelate. In this phase the videotape is used only to get feedback from the couple, without any active intervention on the part of the therapist, except to refer to elements which could be useful better to define the therapeutic contract.

The entire first phase of the treatment (five to six sessions) makes use of the videotape technique, and focuses mainly (but not entirely) on reopening channels of communication more suitable to an intimate relationship. This technique may also be useful in later phases of the treatment but usually only in a much less structured fashion.

Many, if not all, couples exhibit in how they interrelate aggressiveness, passivity, or competitivity, or whatever else might come to light in a situation of latent or manifest conflict, or a situation of power struggle, or role acquisition. Whoever works with couples knows just how much time is usually spent in dealing with these dysfunctional modes of interrelationships.

Our experience has shown us that the practice of videotaping the session (during which there is the tendency to bring out the relational difficulties which are present) makes it much easier for the therapist to intervene on the subject of conflict or the dysfunctional elements of communication, without having to rely on interpretations, or external interventions, as he or she can work directly on a scene where the interpreters are none other than the patients themselves. This makes the work of the therapist less intrusive and reduces the risk of creating resistances which can be often difficult to deal with and, in any case, lengthen the time necessary for the treatment.

Level 2

At least in construction, this level is contextual with the first, and is designed to confront the patients with their relational and sexual skills, both past as well as present. To reach this goal the situations which touch off conflict for the patients are compared with those in which they have the possibility of experiencing pleasure from their life together and something good from sex. We begin from the hypothesis that there is an a priori that has, up to now, never evidently been seriously considered in the field of brief sexual therapy whether it be a Masters type or an integrated sexual therapy. What I mean is that every couple, except for a few rare exceptions for whom, however, brief sex therapy is usually not suitable, have experienced, at some time in their relationship, something positive from the sexuality they have shared. This aspect is often ignored beginning from the sexual anamnesis itself, which is principally, if not entirely, aimed at the dysfunctional area, in spite of the fact that clinical work has demonstrated the importance of these moments which, even though they may arrive from far in the past, are spontaneous, and should be looked into and evaluated regardless of how big or small they are as this is the best way to begin to give a concrete direction to the dialogue.

In this way the prescription will not be an abstract "one-size-fits-all" type of approach, but instead will spring from the couple itself, who will thus be able to proceed along a course which they already know to be pleasurable. In fact, the material which emerges in this manner will be manipulated in prescriptions that can propose experiences of a similar nature to those the patients have referred to.

Typical prescriptions of the common brief sex therapies can be utilized, but it is often necessary to assign tasks specifically designed for the particular situation in question. In this way it will be, especially in the first sessions, much easier for the therapist to keep the patients' level of anxiety within the required limits, by avoiding the monologue of canonical prescriptions and therefore reducing the risk, as I said before, of building up heavy resistance, and, at the same time, helping rapidly to solidify the therapeutic alliance.

Level 3

This level is based on several of the classical prescriptions of brief sexual therapy, prescriptions, however, which are not, at this point, aimed at rebuilding a sexuality that had been previously erased by the therapist, but which are to be inserted into others arising directly from the positive experiences of the patients themselves. In this way the use of these prescriptions, chosen not only in relation to the dysfunction in question, but, more importantly, in relation to the particular clinical situation, can meet the needs of maintaining at the best possible level the gap between the prescriptive content and the discretional content, intrinsic in the assigned tasks, as long as the former is not overly binding and that the second is not so wide as to generate an unbearable anxiety.

The setting for carrying out this treatment is as follows. The couple meets with the therapist usually on a weekly basis, but in the first phase of treatment, in particular during the use of the video, there can also be two sessions per week. Each ordinary session lasts 1 h, while those dedicated to watching the videotape of the previous session last for 2. The basic therapeutic method is the same in form as

Table 1. Statistical data (49 couples)

	Drop outs	No variation of symptom	Improvement of symptom	Resolution of symptom	Clarification of communication problems	Improvement of relationship problems
	12 (24%)	4 (8%)	8 (16%)	25 (51%)	33 (67%)	35 (71%)
Inhibition of sexual desire (21)	5	–	5	11	16	16
Premature ejaculation (9)	3	–	1	5	6	6
Female orgasm inhibition (5)	1	2	1	1	3	4
Male excitement inhibition (8)	1	1	–	6	6	6
Female functional dyspareunia (6)	2	1	1	2	2	3

that of integrated sexual therapy, where the use of psychodynamic interventions is always in relation to the architectural, and not the archeological, project.

The cases we have examined with this method come to a total of 49 couples, ranging in age from 24 to 42 years and who for the most part have a secondary school education.

The sexual dysfunctions treated fall into the following categories:

Inhibition of sexual desire	21 couples
Premature ejaculation	9 couples
Female orgasm inhibition	5 couples
Male excitement inhibition	8 couples
Female functional dyspareunia	6 couples

Those couples who completed the treatment came for a total of 20 sessions. Twelve couples withdrew without having finished the therapy, and in each instance this happened between the fourth and eighth session, i.e., two to four videotape sessions. Of these 12 couples, 5 fell into the category of inhibition of sexual desire, 3 had premature ejaculation, 1 female orgasm inhibition, 1 male excitement inhibition, and 2 dyspareunia.

The results of our research are shown in Table 1. The symptom was not modified in spite of the complete development of the treatment in four cases (8% of total and 10.8% if we consider only the cases – 37 – treated during 20 sessions). We have so far showed an improvement of the relational problems in all the cases and in three of them a clarification of the causes of conflict. This goal was not reached in one case of dyspareunia. We obtained an improvement in the sexual symptom [1] in 16% of the total cases (21.6% if we consider the completed therapies). In all cases the therapy had a notable benefit on the relationship. We also obtained the same results in the 25 cases with resolution of the sexual pathology (51% of the total and 67.6% of the completed therapies).

We feel that the results obtained with the couples who completed the treatment, as well as with the 12 therapy dropouts, are due to the fact that this strategy of obliging the patients to "watch" with their own eyes the inner workings of their relationship requires a high degree of motivation toward the treatment. Such a motivation is, however, a fundamental necessity to achieve any therapeutic success, whether it be partial or complete.

I believe what I have shown up to this point demonstrates that couple-oriented sex therapy should not have as its sole objective the resolution of the symptom, but must also present the couple an occasion to help them diminish the areas of conflict in their relationship. It should nevertheless be stressed that the therapeutic program proposed here can be successfully applied to those couples whose psychosexual dysfunctions are not tied to serious hidden psychic problems or important or structured psychopathological conditions, but for whom the prevalent factor is a situation of relational conflict.

I would now like to conclude with a general consideration, namely, that a successfull therapy in sexology does not depend solely on the intrinsic effectiveness of any particular instrument used in the cure, but also to a large part on the preliminary diagnosis and the consequent therapeutic choices, and that only in this way can there be a reasonable guarantee of obtaining satisfactory results.

References

Alger I, Hogan P (1970) The use of videotape recordings in conjoint marital therapy. In: Berger MM (ed) Videotape techniques in psychiatric training and treatment. Brunner/Mazel, New York

Berger MM (1970) The use of videotape in the integrated treatment of individuals, couples, families and groups in private practice. In: Berger MM (ed) Videotape techniques in psychiatric training and treatment. Brunner/Mazel, New York

Carani C, Manara F, Marrama P (1985) La diagnostica delle disfunzioni sessuali. Libreria Cortina, Milano

Kaplan H (1974) The new sex therapy. Brunner/Mayzel, New York

Kaplan H (1983) The evaluation of sexual disorders. Psychological and medical aspects. Brunner/Mayzel, New York

Malan DH (1963) A study of brief psychotherapy. Tavistock Publ Ltd, London

Manara F (1983) Le disfunzioni psicosessuali. SIRFS, Brescia

Masters W, Johnson VE (1970) Human sexual inadequacy. Little Brown, Boston

[1] As improvement of the sexual symptom we define the unsteady lack of sexual pathology for at least 3 consecutive weeks during the treatment.

Treatment of Sexual Disorders: A Systemic Point of View

L. R. Gindin and L. L. S. Caldiz

Center for Education, Therapy and Research on Sexuality, Darregueyra 2247 Dto. B, (1425) Buenos Aires, Argentina

This presentation aims to contribute to the diagnosis and treatment of sexual disorders based on the application of the general systems theory. Such an approach has been implemented by our working team at CETIS (Center for Education, Therapy, and Research on Sexuality) in Buenos Aires, Argentina. In the past 8 years of clinical work, the institution has received about 60 patients/month. A short time after starting our work with this consultant population, we began to realize that the classic approaches of sex therapy were not enough to give an answer to the complexity of the present sexological consultation, at least in our country. The problems of inhibition of sexual desire, courtship disorders, sexual phobias, and sexual incompatibility connected with marital disadjustments have changed the present profile of our patients and made the traditional approaches less useful.

Our team is composed of 20 professionals: psychologists, clinical physicians, urologists, gynecologists, endocrinologists, neurologists, etc. A few years ago, we began to learn about and use the different variants of the systemic model which was already being applied successfully in the resolution of various conflictive situations, particularly in family therapy.

Probably the most significative concepts introduced by the systems theory in its therapeutic application are vinculated with the substitution of a lineal explanation of events (cause-effect equations) for a circular causality perspective both of the origin as well as of the persistence of the symptomatic situation, introducing the concepts of wholeness, dynamic interaction, organization, and relationship.

As we have pointed out in previous presentations a therapeutic approach will be successful only if it gives an accurate response to the needs of the sociocultural context in which it develops. This statement applies both to the sexual habits of society as well as to the ideology of the professionals from the different fields of science who interact in this environment. The beliefs, assumptions, hopes, and prejudices of the sexual therapist have profound effects on the interaction with his/her subjects of study or treatment and have clear consequences in planning therapeutic interventions.

Conceiving sexual disorders as the surface of a deeper problematical situation or thinking that they are only the result of miss-learning will channel therapies in different ways. If the sex therapist thinks that the removal of a symptom should irreversibly lead to its displacement, his or her theoretical pattern necessarily makes him or her suppose that the sexual problem "is not real." Otherwise in the frame of therapies based on the systems theory or the learning theory, the

Sexology
Eds.: W. Eicher, G. Kockott

manipulation of the symptom turns out to be coherent with the theoretical premises which justify the different interventions. From our point of view the persistence of the sexual problem and even its appearance depend not only on consideration of the patients as individuals, but also on the marital, familiar, and social systems in constant reciprocal interaction and feedback.

Our approach highlights three aspects:

1. Integrative diagnosis of sexual problems
2. Systemic therapeutic intervention in cases with both organic and functional predominance
3. Active participation of the interdisciplinary team with the consequent influence on the characteristics of the treatment

It is not our intention to present here the body of theoretical principles on which we are working, but only to focus attention on some of the theoretical and practical aspects which specifically make up the suggested approach.

Diagnosis

We regard diagnosis as a most important process which also makes up part of the treatment of sexual dysfunction. The variants we take into account are: sexological, medical, psychological individual, familiar, social, and the interviewer-patient relationship. On the other hand, the patient and his or her partner are considered part of the diagnostic team, including them in the system. Diagnosis may be understood as a process with multiple actors directed by the sexologist. Urologists, gynecologists, marital therapists, etc., appear on the scene in diagnostic interviews or laboratory tests. We consider the diagnostic interview in itself operative. So much so that in some cases it may, by itself, untie certain mechanisms which lead to sexual disorder, such as lack of information, lack of experience, or myths and false beliefs. The therapeutic interaction begins at the very moment the diagnosis stage starts. The auxiliary, resources for diagnosis (NPT, Doppler, arteriography, vaginal myograph studies, etc.) are carried out when a clear organic predominance appears. It must be clarified which are the behaviors that contribute to the maintainance of the problem and which are the possible goals of our treatment. Stating therapeutic goals at the end of the diagnostic stage acts as a positive suggestion about the possibility of change and provides a measurable criterion of therapeutic success or failure.

Treatment Format: Basic Premises

Sexual symptoms persist if they are maintained through the habitual behavior of the patient and of his/her environment: the people he/she generally interacts with. The "other," is a fundamental part of the system which produces and maintains the sexual disorders. Therefore, he or she has great possibilities of resolving the problem. We center our interventions on what is indicated by the consultant as the principal problem. A permanent sexual symptom always responds to a situation of the system or systems surrounding the patient, which is handled in a stereotyped way. People must be seen interacting with the environment, affecting it, and being modified by it.

Treatment Procedures

Deliberate and active interventions are required to challenge the prevailing sexual system. Whenever possible, the therapeutic process is carried out by the couple. Attention must be focused on the present and observable sexual and nonsexual behaviors. The learning of new effective sexual behaviors needs to be encouraged to replace those which lead to disorder. The solution of sexual problems means, essentially, changing variables of the ecosystem to replace the feedback circuits which maintain the symptom. The problems must be limited to those likely to be changed. This strategy favors the therapist's influence to induce changes. Once the goals to be achieved have been established, interventions are limited to those goals. The couple can modify themselves, allowing the appearance of new sexual behaviors whenever the context has been modified. Moreover, for the individual changes to take place, the interpersonal system must be modified.

Therapeutic Process

The emphasis is placed in the present more than in the past. The interpretation is habitually used to "relabel" rather than to produce an insight. Generally the therapy cannot progress directly from a dysfunctional stage toward a stage of cure without passing through one or more intermediate stages which, superficially, may also appear as dysfunctional. The therapy tends to be brief and does not last for more than 4 months. The sexual assignments characteristic of sexual therapies are used as an answer and as a way of acting on the couple system, not merely as a method of learning. The design of such specific assignments is based essentially on a pragmatic approach to the sexual problem. We create these assignments in each case according to the nature of the consultation. Our prescriptions include nonsexual assignments aimed at solving individual, marital, family, social, or psychological conflicts which contribute to maintain the disorder. A distinctive characteristic of our therapeutic procedures is the possibility of intervention of another professional of the team during the sexological interview, watching through a videocamera. These participations are part of the therapeutic process because they tend to modify the therapist-patient system at the very moment of consultation. The therapeutic contracts are arranged with the patients, so they deal with the problem and the objectives of change. Resources are used to promote changes in relation with the sexual symptom.

Preparation of Operators

We consider the accurate preparation of the operators in this kind of sexual therapy most important. This involves:

- Adequate specific background in the sexological and systemic fields.
- Intensive training in the psychological, medical, marital, and social conflicts which affect sexuality.
- Operative knowledge of the general systems theory with its correlation of adequate therapeutic interventions.

The training of the sexologist must include indispensable help from professionals with experience in the field. That is why we include "in vivo" supervision in our interventions, which at the same time allows therapy of the consulting couple and improvement of the professional's training.

Conclusions

Both the sexological medicine as well as the research in the field of interpersonal relations show us a very complex panorama of contemporary sexuality. We cannot deal with it only from a reductionistic/mechanistic perspective. The organization of the relationship system, the circulation within a family structure, and the relations with the socio-cultural environment must be considered in an evaluation of the sexual problem. Facing the complexity of the contemporary sexological consultation, we understand it is necessary to include alternative models of therapeutic procedures which contribute to *enlarge the sexological field.* We find that the systemic model provides a useful resource for the sex therapies adapted to the reality of this problem according to the nature of the present relationship and conflicts. This paper has aimed to present a series of ideas which we have found operative all through these years of clinical work and investigation on sexual disorders.

Anxiety and the Treatment of Sexual Dysfunctions

W. Everaerd

Psychological Laboratory, University of Amsterdam, Weesperplein 8,
1018 XA Amsterdam, The Netherlands

Introduction

To look into the role of anxiety and the treatment of sexual dysfunctions, two sets of data have been considered in this paper: firstly, the anxiety profile of sexually dysfunctional patients, to see whether anxiety is characteristic of these patients; and secondly, anxiety reduction and the treatment of sexual dysfunction, to see whether reducing anxiety is necessary to improve the dysfunction.

Anxiety Profile of Sexually Dysfunctional Patients

In contrast to the hypothesized primary role of anxiety in both the etiology and maintenance of sexual dysfunctions, the treatment literature has failed to provide data on this subject. So far, two questions have been addressed in the sparse studies that have been reported. First, general psychopathology in sexually dysfunctional subjects have been screened by psychological tests and clinical interviews. The availability of short-term sex therapy methods has been met with the suspicion that deeper causation was being disregarded. Schumacher and Lloyd (1976) analyzed Minnesota Multiphasic Personality Inventory (MMPI) data on 302 patients with sexual problems and did not find specific distress in their sample. Derogatis and Meyer (1979) have reported data in a comparison of 87 dysfunctional males and females and 200 heterosexual normals. On the Derogatis Sexual Functioning Inventory (DSFI) both male and female dysfunctionals showed more psychological distress and dysphoric affect. Psychological symptomatology in DSFI profiles was elevated for depression, anxiety, and interpersonal sensitivity. It seems reasonable to expect some distress in individuals suffering form sexual dysfunctions. It is as yet impossible to provide a clear perspective on the contribution of psychopathology in the etiology of sexual dysfunctions. Munjack and his co-workers (Munjack and Kanno 1979; Munjack et al. 1981) have reviewed evidence of psychological characteristics and male sexual dysfunctions. They also report more psychopathology in dysfunctional than in sexually normal males. In discussing their data they carefully stipulate that it is not possible to explain the nature of the relationship between male sexual dysfunction and psychological characteristics. Their clinical observations showed that some severely disturbed psychiatric patients functioned well sexually. Therefore they propose that psychological disturbance was the result of sexual dysfunctions, and not the cause.

Sexology
Eds.: W. Eicher, G. Kockott

Anxiety seems to be linked with the onset of several dysfunctions. These include acute erectile failure, premature ejaculation, dyspareunia and vaginismus, and some cases of orgasmic dysfunction (Heiman and Hatch 1981). Anxiety in the initial stages of arousal seems to be linked with cognitive interference, which prevents the development of the sexual reponse. Specific fears of being touched, pregnancy, pain, and intimacy: all these may reduce or inhibit sexual arousal and orgasm.

Anxiety may develop as a consequence of the experience of sexual failure. Worries about sexual performance will diminish sexual response, which may eventually result in avoiding sexual interactions as an anxiety-provoking situation and in some cases in loss of sexual interest or desire.

Anxiety Reduction and the Treatment of Sexual Dysfunctions

Treatments that aim at reducing (sexual) anxiety can provide evidence on the role of anxiety in sexual dysfunction. Most informative are those studies that have compared anxiety reduction and other interventions that are not specifically aimed at reducing anxiety in order to alleviate sexual dysfunctions.

Wolpe's reciprocal inhibition approach to anxiety disorders (Wolpe 1958) has instigated the application of systematic desensitization in the treatment of most of the sexual dysfunctions. Wolpe (1973) essentially holds that inhibition of sexual arousal results from conditioned anxiety responses. Anxiety, in Wolpe's conception, thus inhibits the physiological sexual response. For reciprocal inhibition it is necessary that both the events, anxiety and sexual arousal, occur simultaneously (Wolpe 1978). Some studies on the role of induced anxiety and sexual arousal have used temporal sequences, where anxiety was induced prior to or after induction of sexual arousal. In Everaerd (1987) these studies have been reviewed. Other studies were carried out where anxiety and sexual arousal were induced simultaneously (epinephrine chloride, shock threat). Regardless of the temporal sequence it seems that in sexually functional subjects anxiety prior to or simultaneously with sexual arousal either does not affect or may even serve to enhance sexual arousal. In dysfunctional subjects anxiety is detrimental to the sexual response. Thus far, it seems that anxiety prevents dysfunctional subjects from attending to the erotic content of sexual stimuli and so decreases or inhibits sexual arousal.

Outcome of systematic desensitization has been reported in several studies. A large number of case studies and group treatments claimed success for systematic desensitization. Although these studies did not use control groups, the results reported are consistent with those reported in studies that used no-treatment controls or comparison treatments (Norton and Jehu 1984; Lopiccolo and Hogan 1979). The exposure to anxiety-provoking situations under simultaneous control of anxiety responses through relaxation is essential in systematic desensitization. Cooper (1969a, b) reported two studies where relaxation alone was part of the treatment program for different sexual dysfunctions in men. Less than 40% of the dysfunctions improved.

Kockott et al. (1975) compared systematic desensitization with "routine therapy," consisting of medication and advice, and with a waiting-list control condition. Twenty-four men with erectile dysfunction were treated, eight in each treatment condition. Outcome was measured on three levels: behavioral, subjective, and physiological. Behavior measurement consisted of ratings on answers during pre- and posttreatment interviews. For the subjective index, subjects rated how well anxiety-related adjectives described their feelings. Penile plethysmography was used to measure genital responses to imagined sexual scenes. On the subjective measure desensitization subjects rated less anxiety than those in the routine and waiting conditions. On the behavioral measures erections increased both in the desensitization and routine group. The groups did not differ in genital response, but only 10 out of 24 patients had been measured. It was concluded that systematic desensitization is of limited help in the treatment of erectile dysfunctions.

Wincze and Caird (1976) compared systematic desensitization, using standard videotaped sexual stimuli, with a no-treatment control group. Subjects were all women with complaints of sexual arousal or orgasmic dysfunctions. Systematic desensitization helped to reduce sexual anxiety on self-report measures. All subjects rated themselves as improved, although there was no major improvement in orgasmic functioning. Sotile and Kilmann (1978) reported that group systematic desensitization reduced coital anxiety and increased overall satisfaction with sexual function. This was also demonstrated by Anderson (1981). In a comparison of group and individual desensitization, O'Gorman (1978) used patient self-ratings of improvement and a sexual interest questionnaire. The outcome as measured with self-ratings favored the group method, but sexual interest increased in favor of the individually treated patients.

Everaerd and Dekker (1982) compared desensitization with sex therapy modified after Masters and Johnson. They combined desensitization and sex therapy, and a waiting-list control group. Forty-eight women with orgasmic dysfunction, 12 in each condition, were treated together with their partners. Outcome was measured with a sexual experience scale, a relationship satisfaction scale, and a scale that measured anxiety for several forms of sexual interaction. Desensitization and sex therapy showed more improvement as compared with the combined treatment and the waiting-list control group. Only the women and men in the desensitization condition reported a significant decrease in anxiety.

In another study, Everaerd and Dekker (1985) compared systematic desensitization with sex therapy in the treatment of male sexual dysfunction. With the exception of the anxiety scale, the same scales were used as in the female dysfunction study (Everaerd and Dekker 1982). In this study another anxiety scale was used which measured social approach versus social avoidance in various situations. In addition, an independent rater judged clinical improvements from the treatment protocols of the therapists. Although subjects in both the treatments showed improvement on the scales, near or complete recovery of the sexual dysfunction was achieved only in a limited number of subjects according to clinical judgment.

From the controlled studies it seems likely that systematic desensitization at least decreases subjective anxiety and helps to improve some of the sexual dysfunctions. Improvement, however, was reported by the patients themselves. An independent judgment of outcome might show discrepancies as in the Everaerd and Dekker study (1982). Further, female dysfunctioning showed more improvement than male dysfunctions. Anxiety is mentioned most often in connection with male erectile dysfunctions in cases of performance anxiety.

More important, however, is the fact that no data are available on physiological measures both of anxiety and sexual arousal with respect to desensitization outcome studies. The concomitant decrease in sexual anxiety and the improvement of sexual functioning supports the usefulness of systematic desensitization for the treatment of some sexual dysfunctions. Wolpe's contention (Wolpe 1978) that conditioned anxiety is etiological in the development of sexual dysfunction and causal in the maintenance thereof has not been corroborated.

Evidence of the role of anxiety in sexual dysfunctioning may also be derived from studies about treatments that do not explicitly aim at improving sexual functioning by means of reducing (physiological components of) anxiety. It is important to observe that during systematic desensitization, anxiety, as a source of sexual malaise, will be extensively discussed with the patient(s). Sexual interactions are rated according to their anxiety-provoking qualities, each step in the treatment process being accompanied by an evaluation of feelings of anxiety. In contrast with this focus of attention on anxiety, several other methods of treatment do not focus on anxiety but on sexual feelings, as in the approach by Masters and Johnson (Kolodny et al. 1979). One consequence of this difference in approaching anxiety may be that reports about anxiety feelings are biased. Systematic desensitization subjects do report changes in anxiety while sex therapy subjects do not report such changes, although they show the same degree of improvement (Everaerd and Dekker 1982). Different approaches to sexual dysfunctions not only seem to result in differences in self-reported changes, but it is likely that different aspects of sexual functioning may be improved. Comparisons between treatment approaches with respect to long-term treatment follow-up (Dekker and Everaerd 1983) suggests that, in retrospect, every patient or couple solved their sexual problems in accordance with the very specific approach they had learned in a particular therapy. This was true for all approaches: systematic desensitization, Masters and Johnson's approach, communication training, rational emotive therapy, and masturbation training. Furthermore, rational emotive therapy and masturbation training, for example, did improve orgasmic dysfunction in both males and females, whereas with systematic desensitization this was not achieved. In most of these approaches skills training and communication exercises are the primary goals of treatment technique. This suggests that the essential ingredient does not reside in anxiety reduction.

Reports on psychological treatment studies have not provided data that are informative about physiological aspects of anxiety reduction. Pharmacological approaches in the treatment of sexual dysfunctions have been used to reduce anxiety directly. Here too, the evidence is indirect, since no physiological data on anxiety have been reported in this respect.

Matthews (1983) referred to the use of diazepam in the treatment of female sexual dysfunction. It appeared that the drug alone did not significantly improve the dysfunction but seemed to have a dampening effect on positive feelings. This observation corroborates remarks by Kolodny et al. (1979). In their opinion drugs which lower anxiety are difficult to evaluate. The effect on sexual function may be paradoxical, because reductions in anxiety may enhance sexual performance, whereas sedation usually diminishes sexual responsiveness and sexual desire (Kolodny et al. 1979, p 330). Hypnotics, sedatives, and anxiolytics have been insufficiently studied in relation to their effects on sexual function. In a recent review, Davies and D'Mello (1986) reported that they were unable to find reports in the literature on the effects of these drugs on sexual function.

Conclusion

A tentative conclusion from reviewing studies that relate anxiety and sexual dysfunction is that many but not all males and females complaining of sexual dysfunction report sexual anxieties. Psychological induction of anxiety does not affect or enhance subsequent or simultaneous sexual arousal in sexually functional subjects (for review see Everaerd 1987). In dysfunctional subjects this same induced anxiety causes sexual response to deteriorate.

The pharmacological induction or drug-induced alleviation of anxiety has been studied insufficiently to warrant a conclusion as to the effect of drugs on sexual functioning. Psychological treatment studies aimed at anxiety reduction certainly have positive outcomes for some sexual dysfunctions. In most instances effects on anxiety have been measured as changes in the self-report of patients. Thus far, it seems that anxiety interferes with sexual response by preventing the relevant cognitive processes from taking place in the development of the sexual response. Although many authors subscribe to this tentative position, there may be serious flaws in the data base which has been used to formulate this position.

References

Anderson BL (1981) A comparison of systematic desensitization and directed masturbation in the treatment of primary orgasmic dysfunction in females. J Consult Clin Psychol 49:568

Cooper AJ (1969a) A clinical study of "coital anxiety" in male potency disorders. J Psychosom Res 13:143

Cooper AJ (1969b) Disorders of sexual potency in the male: a clinical and statistical study of some factors related to short term prognosis. Br J Psychiatry 115:709

Davies MA, D'Mello A (1986) Drugs and sexual function: a pharmacological approach. Ridge Publications, Herts

Dekker J, Everaerd W (1983) A long-term follow-up study of couples treated for sexual dysfunctions. J Sex Marital Ther 9:99

Derogatis LR, Meyer JK (1979) A psychological profile of the sexual dysfunctions. Arch Sex Behav 8:201

Everaerd W (1987) Anxiety and sexual dysfunction. In: Burrows, Noyes R, Martin, Roth (eds) Handbook of anxiety. Elsevier Biomedical, Amsterdam (in press)

Everaerd W, Dekker J (1982) Treatment of secondary orgasmic dysfunction: a comparison of systematic desensitization and sex therapy. Behav Res Ther 20:269

Everaerd W, Dekker J (1985) Treatment of male sexual dysfunction: sex therapy compared with systematic desensitization and rational emotive therapy. Behav Res Ther 23:13

Heiman JR, Hatch JP (1981) Conceptual and therapeutic contributions of psychophysiology to sexual dysfunctions. In: Haynes SN, Gannon L (eds) Psychosomatic disorders. Praeger, New York

Kockott G, Dittman F, Nusselt L (1975) Systematic desensitization of erectile impotence: a controlled study. Arch Sex Behav 4:493

Kolodny RC, Masters WH, Johnson VE (1979) Textbook of sexual medicine. Little Brown, Boston

Lopiccolo J, Hogan DR (1979) Sexual dysfunction. In: Pomerleau OF, Brady JP (eds) Behavioral medicine, theory and practice. Williams and Wilkins, Baltimore

Mathews A (1983) Progress in the treatment of female sexual dysfunction. J Psychosom Res 27:165

Munjack DJ, Kanno PH (1979) Retarded ejaculation: a review. Arch Sex Behav 8:139

Munjack DJ, Oziel LJ, Kanno PH, Whipple K, Leonard MD (1981) Psychological characteristics of males with secondary erectile failure. Arch Sex Behav 10:123

Norton GR, Jehu DJ (1984) The role of anxiety in sexual dysfunctions: a review. Arch Sex Behav 13:165

Noyes R, Clancy J, Hoenk PR, Slymen DJ (1980) The prognosis of anxiety neurosis. Arch Gen Psychiatry 37:173

O'Gorman E (1978) The treatment of frigidity: a comparative study of group and individual desensitization. Br J Psychiatry 132:580

Schumacher S, Lloyd CW (1976) Assessment of sexual dysfunction. In: Hersen M, Bellack AS (eds) Behavioral assessment. Pergamon, New York, p 419

Sotile WM, Kilmann PR (1978) Effects of group systematic desensitization on female orgasmic dysfunction. Arch Sex Behav 7:477

Wincze JP, Caird WK (1976) The effects of systematic desensitization and video desensitization in essential sexual dysfunction in women. Behav Ther 7:335

Wolpe J (1958) Psychotherapy by reciprocal inhibition. Stanford University Press, Stanford

Wolpe J (1973) The practice of behavior therapy. Pergamon, New York

Wolpe J (1978) Comments on "A test of reciprocal inhibition" by Hoon, Wincze and Hoon. J Abnorm Psychol 87:452

Sexuality: Intimacy or Illusion?

B. Apfelbaum

2714 Telegraph Avenue, Berkeley, CA 94705, USA

The paradox is that sex is perhaps among the most nonintimate of human activities, yet, at least in the West, it is idealized as the ultimate form of intimacy and even as the best form of communication. (I would be interested to learn how widespread this idealization is in other cultures.)

Not only is sex often solitary, such as masturbation, but sex partners typically are silent and are likely to resent it when the silence is broken, unless it is by expressions of desire and pleasure. "Sex talk," when it does occur, is highly stylized – limited to flattery and encouragement. When the real partner is not responsive in this way, we are likely to turn to a mental picture of someone who is. (This raises a question that has not yet been addressed in the literature: what does sexual arousal have to do with flattery? This is taken for granted, yet not accounted for, especially by those who think of sex neurohormonally.)

My impression is that both historically and cross-culturally sex is typically an act of masculine possession. It is taken as a test of male adequacy and is a subject for male boasting, with the strong potential for humiliation that the term "impotence" indicates. (I would be interested to learn whether there are cultures in which the word used to describe erection problems does not carry the meaning of weakness or inadequacy.)

Thus, sex represents both a male prerogative and a male performance demand. This appears to be even more true in the few cultures that are thought of as sexually free. Thus (Marshall and Suggs 1971, p. 124, 126), in central Polynesia it is said that the name of an island "travels on a man's penis." Polynesian men do not wish to let the name of their island "fall." Where women's wishes are included in sex, this does not change the picture:

> The Polynesian woman takes an immediate demonstration of sexual virility and masculinity as the first test of her partner's desire for her and as the reflection of her own desirability... One virility test used by Mangaian women is to require a lover to have sexual intercourse without making contact with any part of the partner's body other than the genitalia.

In most cultures women are subordinated and the sex act is much like rape. As Davenport (1977, p. 149) summarizes it:

> In most of the societies for which there are data, it is reported that men take the initiative and, without extended foreplay, proceed vigorously toward climax without much regard for achieving synchrony with the woman's orgasm. Again and again, there are reports that coitus is primarily completed in terms of the man's passions and pleasures, with scant attention paid to the woman's response. If women do experience orgasm, they do so passively. In the Ojibwa, a North American Indian group, it is reported that women are passive

Sexology
Eds.: W. Eicher, G. Kockott

during intercourse and orgasm; however, they may take the lead in initiating coitus. In the Guinea survey of young single adults from several African ethnic groups, the women overwhelmingly reported passivity during coitus, embarrassment at expressing satisfaction during intercourse, distaste for caressing and many admitted an inability to achieve orgasm.

We have recently become aware of how widespread sexual harassment is, child sexual abuse, and the degrees of rape, with new terms appearing like "acquaintance rape" and "marital rape" that indicate our increased consciousness, at least in the United States, of sexual coercion. (And rape, of course, can be homosexual as well as heterosexual.)

It therefore seems reasonable to conclude that the sex act, when it includes a partner, is often an act of male dominance and aggression, an act of possession. It appears to have little to do with sensual pleasure, much less intimacy, but is a celebration of male status and a demonstration of role adequacy.

We should keep the social context in mind. Most societies, both historically and worldwide, are authoritarian, with highly ritualized relationships. Arranged marriages are the rule. I believe that the best indicator of the presence of male dominance and sexual ritualization is the concern with bridal virginity, and this concern is almost universal.

All this appears to be obvious and yet not recognized, or at least not acknowledged, in the sex field, neither in the professional nor in the popular literature. Not only that, but we have the stunning paradox that I began with, that in the West sex is often referred to as the ultimate form of intimacy and even as the best form of communication.

Of course, the Church, at least in the West, has reflected some recognition that sex can be "dirty," although the churchly emphasis on *lust* is, I believe, misleading, since it completely misses the extent to which men are required to prove their sexual adequacy.

I would say that the most direct acknowledgement of sex as nonintimate and even as coercive is in our use of profanity, at least in English. Thus, the English word "fuck" is our most emphatic way to express one-sidedness or being cheated. When we want to find the strongest way of saying someone has been used, we say that he or she has been *fucked* or *screwed.* There also is an idiomatic expression in English, being "ripped off," that in the past 2 decades has become an even stronger way of expressing the same thing. Most people appear to be unaware that this is a condensation of the original expression which was "to rip off a piece," which in turn was condensed from "to rip off a piece of ass," a violent reference to coitus. (I would be interested to learn how much it also is true in other cultures that profane words refer to sex in this way.)

Thus, when we want to find the most extreme metaphor to express one-sidedness, we refer to sex. This practice is obviously not limited to English, although I do not know how general this usage is. It is done quite innocently and, as far as I know, it has not been noted that this picture of sex conflicts with the picture of sex as *two*-sided, even as the ultimate form of mutuality.

This split image of sex can be seen to reflect a familiar habit of thought: the process of idealization. Accordingly, we can say that when people think of sex as highly intimate, they mean that this is what sex should be. They then dismiss nonintimate sex as not what sex *really* is. Nonintimate sex can thus be disqualified as an aberration, as in effect a *distortion* of sex. I am not entirely satisfied with this explanation and I hope that others will apply themselves to this question and offer a better answer.

The next question is where the idea came from that sex is highly intimate. Fortunately, this question is not entirely unfamiliar. First, it should be clear that this idea can only exist in cultures that have the concept of intimacy. This concept is quite recent, being not more than 2 centuries old, and is confined to those postindustrial societies in which the ego has begun the process of individuation, as contrasted with the more typical group-centered anthill or beehive social organizations. In the area of sex, it can be thought of as following the appearance of the idea of romantic love in the fourteenth and fifteenth centuries.

This involved a revolutionary change in the status of women, from household property to highly admired images of perfection. Perhaps, once cut off from the comforts of a group (and extended family) identity, the individual (male) needed some other ennobling and affirming reference point. However this may be, the appearance of relationships based on feeling choices and the attempt to create sexual encounters in which women played a larger role triggered a quantum leap in the image of women from the household slave (or concubine) to the love object.

My way of putting this is to say that we have been trying to find a way to have two-sided heterosexual encounters, but our first attempts are just new forms of ritualization. The sex-as-possession model is highly ritualized. The sex-as-intimacy model is still ritualized, but there is much less commitment to ritual. Indeed, it is part of the intimacy model that sex be spontaneous.

As I have mentioned, "sex talk," when it does occur, is highly stylized – limited to flattery and encouragement. In romantic sex, the partners are typically extravagantly complimentary and ritually avoidant of criticism, disagreement, or dissatisfaction of any kind. It is as if when we still do not know how to include another person in sex, and that what has happened so far is that the older version, in which one partner is forced to submit, has led to this recent version in which we must *voluntarily* enact a ritual of submission.

Now why do we bother? For one thing, women are of course now much less content with thinking of England, at least in England. That is, submitting for the good of the social order and one's place in it is no longer so compelling. But, more importantly, I think is the fact that the two-person version of sex offers, for the first time, the possibility of *passion*.

If the process of what I call "romantic induction" (to point up the parallel with hypnotic trance-induction) is successful, it results in a trance state in which the partners experience an extraordinary sense of mutuality: the merging experience. It is to this experience that we must look to find why sex can be thought of as the ultimate form of mutuality.

There of course are difficulties associated with this trance state. It can require a special effort at concentration (bypassing), which can make people highly distractible, and it is vulnerable to any distractions, with the effect that this experience of mutuality can suddenly evaporate, often evoking mutual recriminations in its stead, as well as extremely opposite states of detachment, alienation, and self-condemnation.

However, for all its present drawbacks, this new script offers much more than does the older one. As I have suggested, the sex-as-possession model appears to have little to do with sensual pleasure, much less intimacy, being a celebration of male status and a demonstration of role adequacy. It can be an exciting experience to prove one's adequacy and to force a partner to submit, but the threat of inadequacy still looms and the potential for passion created by a responsive partner is typically absent.

However, in the present stage of development of the human ego, there still are formidable disadvantages to sex-as-intimacy, not the least of which is that we have no clear picture of what intimacy is. Unfortunately, most people still think of intimacy as an experience of intense positive rapport, akin to courtly love and to what in the West we think of as the "honeymoon" period that can occur at the beginning of an individually chosen relationship.

This conception is in conflict with another recent Western innovation, the concept of *authenticity*. Thus, more avant-garde thinkers in the West conceive of intimacy as an exchange of vulnerabilities and a disclosure of experiences that feel threatening, especially to the partner. Hence, from this point of view, intimacy is a threat to eros, even of the apparently intimate kind.

What makes this a problem is the fact that when the merging experience develops, people think that they *discovered* mutuality rather than that they *created* it. People who are unable to create the experience are seen as *not allowing it to happen*, as unable or unwilling to *let go*. This overlooks all the work at saying yes and making things happen smoothly that it takes to create this experience. It also overlooks how fragile it can be and how it takes a special mental set which not everyone is capable of or motivated to create.

Unfortunately, much of sex therapy is based on this view. People are being asked to focus on sensation and fantasy in the service of letting go. Intimacy and mutuality are taken as a natural outcome of sexual arousal rather as an objective that we are only beginning to try to reach and to understand.

Among other problems this approach creates is that it makes it difficult to recognize how much the sex-as-possession model is still with us and how the sex-as-intimacy model has simply redefined our tests of adequacy. The job of proving one's adequacy is now more difficult. It means satisfying your partner. It means trying to be spontaneous and not to think of sex as a performance, while being threatened with humiliation and rejection in the event of failure. Since we are still so ruled by duty, it becomes a special problem when the pursuit of pleasure itself becomes a duty.

We also now have to contend with guilt about wanting a partner to be sexually accommodating and so sexual coercion has become much more subtle, now being likely to be verbal and psychological rather than to take the form of overt threats and physical violence.

Finding ways to recognize and to tolerate the lack of mutuality in sex and to tolerate real communication, as of "negative" experiences, rather than "sex talk," while still feeling the acceptance (ego support) that appears to be vital to passion is what I consider the frontier of sex therapy to be and is yet largely uncharted territory. One encouraging finding is that when people can work out relatively safe ways of expressing even minor worries and insecurities in sex, this can create an experience of *genuine* acceptance which makes them feel included, with the effect that even such a slight degree of actual mutuality can be an aphrodisiac (Apfelbaum 1980, 1984a, b, to be published; Apfelbaum and Apfelbaum 1985).

References

Apfelbaum B (1980) The diagnosis and treatment of retarded ejaculation. In: Leiblum SR, Pervin LA (eds) Principles and practice of sex therapy. Guilford, New York

Apfelbaum B (1984a) The ego-analytic approach to individual body-work sex therapy: five case examples. J Sex Res 20:44–70

Apfelbaum B (1984b) Ego-analytic sex therapy: the problem of performance anxiety anxiety. In: Segraves R, Haeberle EJ (eds) Emerging dimensions of sexology: proceedings of the fifth international congress of sexology. Praeger, New York

Apfelbaum B (to be published) An ego-analytic perspective on desire disorders. In: Leiblum SR, Rosen RC (eds) Clinical perspectives on desire disorders. Guilford, New York

Apfelbaum B, Apfelbaum C (1985) The ego-analytic approach to sexual apathy. In: Goldberg DC (ed) Contemporary marriage: special issues in couples therapy. Dorsey, Homewood, pp 439–481

Davenport WH (1977) Sex in cross-cultural perspective. In: Beach FA (ed) Human sexuality in four perspectives. John Hopkins Press, Baltimore, pp 115–163

Marshall DC, Suggs RC (1971) Human sexual behavior: variations in the ethnographic spectrum. Basic, New York

Tannahill R (1980) Sex in history. Stein and Day, New York

Intimacy-Based Sex Therapy

C. R. Ellison

39 Park Way, Piedmont, CA 94611, USA

In the 1970s most sex therapy modalities focused on *dysfunctions* and sexual performance (i.e., on erections, ejaculatory control, orgasms). Phrases like "function," "dysfunction," "achieve" orgasm, or "achieve" erection were so common that most of us never even noticed that their origins are in the language of mechanical performance and work.

With notable exceptions, like other authors in this volume, most 1970s sex therapists addressed the sexual problems of partnered individuals in terms of individual functioning goals rather than in terms of the enjoyment and satisfaction of *both* partners. The criterion of success was typically better functioning, not mutual satisfaction.

Unfortunately, this therapy model, which I have called "manufacturing-orgasms-sex," sometimes led to functioning "achieved" at the expense of intimacy, as in the case of the woman who learned to be orgasmic by herself in a women's group and because of that was called a "therapy success." She and her husband came to me for couple's therapy because she was unable to use that new skill in a *satisfying* sexual experience with him: he had begun to experience performance anxiety because of her therapy, their sexual times together had become awkward, and sex had begun to feel like work instead of fun for both of them.

By 1980, as self-help information became widely available, fewer of the couples who came to therapy needed basic sexual skills. More and more couples came to therapy whose problems of desire and arousal reflected the dynamics of their relationship and their yearnings for deeper intimacy. In that year Bernie Zilbergeld and I published a delineation of the sexual response cycle that included not only interest, arousal, physiological readiness, and orgasm, but also a fifth phase: satisfaction (Zilbergeld and Ellison 1980).

It is now my belief that most couple problems, whether with sexual functioning, arousal or desire, are best treated in an intimacy-based therapy mode.

In *intimacy-based sex therapy* [1] I focus on self-esteem, intimacy, satisfaction, and *mutual* pleasure.

I regard a couple as a therapy success when they are able to: create erotic experiences that conclude with each feeling good about himself/herself and the other and that they had a good time.

In the first session I ask a couple if they will make this a therapeutic goal. Most find this definition of success liberating because they are immediately relieved of old performance goals.

---

[1] This descriptive phrase has been used by others. While preparing this paper, I was given a copy of an article entitled *Intimacy-based sex therapy* (Travis and Travis 1987).

Sexology
Eds.: W. Eicher, G. Kockott

With consent to this goal they adopt a *mutual intention*. Now, if they "get off the track" in any of the "experiments" I assign them, they can focus their attention back on creating a good time together rather than on issues of blame or right and wrong. They can find creative solutions to get "back on track" once again.

Ruth and Kevin, a newly wed couple, both therapists, did a lot of things together that could be fun, but which often were not because, as they said: "For a couple of therapists, our communication skills are terrible." They found that while they were working on changing their communication patterns, paying attention to the intent of creating a good time helped them avoid getting caught up in their old negative communication scripts and enabled them to have more fun together.

Because *intimacy based sex therapy* is a holistic model that acknowledges the four dimensions of an individual: the physical, mental, emotional, and spiritual/transpersonal, I note the presence and significance of physiological factors, of various emotional states such as anger, depression, and anxiety (including "performance anxiety"), and of concerns about such issues as trust, monogamy, and commitment. However, in the rest of this paper I am going to focus on the idea that:

Intimacy thrives on separateness – and togetherness and talk in particular about techniques for facilitating experiences and feelings of togetherness.

I often think of the members of a couple as two separate energy systems – each with a separate boundary. In sex, they seek to merge those boundaries into one pleasurable field of shared arousal.

Talmadge and Talmadge (1986) have noted that a paradox of intimate relating is that intimately to merge requires some autonomy, some separate delineation of the individuals. "Intimacy requires 'an established sense of personal identity and ego-strength' – that separate boundary I describe – and at the same time 'a preservation of the capacity for dependence'" (Dicks 1967). We can be too merged, too dependent, and lose ourselves, or too independent and lose our loved one. The emotional bond of a couple is based on being able to negotiate and maintain a delicate balance in the conflict between wanting to be one with another and the desire for an independent, autonomous self (Talmadge and Talmadge 1986).

As one of my graduate students wrote of this conflict in her term paper this spring, "Even though we seek a union of intimacy as our ultimate goal, at the very innermost core of our being what we want most for ourselves is to have our own way" (Lucero 1987).

Since intimacy requires that each individual maintain and develop a separate Self, a therapist needs to think of such *diagnostic questions* as: Do these two people need to increase their nonsexual intimacy, increase separate time, or both? Is each getting the individual nurturance and recognition necessary to maintain a high level of self-esteem?

Some couples can immediately begin both to increase intimate activities and fill needs for more separateness through individual activities; others will need to focus first on either more intimacy or more separateness.

Often a strength of the relationship is how good a couple are at creating intimate feelings in some nonsexual way(s). They may share interests in music, hiking, or reading aloud to each other, for example. I find that asking about activities they have enjoyed together in the past but have not done for awhile is often a useful reminder.

Activities that increase their relaxed time together and feelings of intimacy outside of sex tend to keep the boundaries between a couple open and thereby make it easier for them to turn on with each other at sexual times. Here are some of the activities I suggest:

I recommend *a date night once a week* that is kept sacred for creating good feelings; no gripes or dealing with conflicts allowed. I instruct the couple that if they get off the track into negative issues, they should recall their mutual intent to enjoy each other and let those negative issues go for the moment.

If they are unable to do this, we deal with the problem in subsequent sessions. When a couple wonder how they can possibly find time or money to have weekly dates, I remind them that they are finding time and money to see me, that there are many free and inexpensive activities, and that baby sitters charge a lot less than I do.

A gripe session once a week is as important as the evening set aside for good times. Many couples are so busy with work, children, and other responsibilities that they have a limited amount of time to have each other's undivided attention. It is almost impossible consistently to have positive dates if they are not balanced by opportunities to deal with the conflicts in the relationship. If necessary the couple is instructed in communication skills and fair fighting techniques.

Evening walks before bedtime are another recommended activity. These allow a couple to step outside their roles of home, shed the day's tensions, and end their day with a special time together.

Consenting to be intimate. A typical intimacy issue of couples who present the complaint of low sexual desire is not knowing how effectively to enter into *mutually consensual* sexual intimacy.

Knowing how successfully to make, accept, reject, and negotiate sexual invitations is critical in creating consistently intimate and satisfying sexual experiences. Being able to say "No" or "As soon as I finish what I'm doing..." is as important as knowing when and how to say "Yes." Roger, who knew his partner Denise would never say "No" or negotiate for what she genuinely wanted, had no way of knowing when Denise genuinely consented to sexual intimacy. Because she was often half-heartedly having sex when she did not really want to, resentment had built on both sides and their sensual pleasure was blocked. The partner who is unable to say "No" typically begins to avoid sex, and this was true of Denise. Roger seemed to be after sex all the time, but at times he would withdraw, too, and if the problem remained untreated, he might have withdrawn altogether. In therapy, Roger and Denise learned to give and deal more effectively with sexual invitations and to negotiate for mutually consensual intimate interaction.

Transitions and "Intimate Trance." In creating *truly satisfying* and *intimate* sexual experiences, the time of coming from separateness into sex is critical. Each of the partners needs to become psychologically and physically ready for arousal and good feelings to occur. As a couple they need to focus attention on each other and form a bond in which, at some point, their readiness and arousal synchronize.

As they focus more and more on sensations, emotions, mental images, and each other in sexual interaction, a state I call the "*intimate trance*" can unfold. Their movements and arousal synchronize and a rhythmic, continuous feedback loop is established; awareness of separateness can merge into a sense of "oneness" or unity (Ellison 1986). When appropriate, I give couples exercises and techniques that shift their interaction from an active, outward-oriented, linear mode toward a receptive, mutual, couple-focused one.

Sex that feels *intimate* and *satisfying* most readily evolves out of feeling psychologically close before touching and genital contact begins. Stimulation that is too specifically sexual before consent and some relaxation have occurred can feel unpleasant, cause one to pull away, and inhibit instead of facilitate arousal.

I may suggest that each individually *warm up for sex* by taking a shower or bath, stretching, and breathing deeply – or that as a couple they bathe or shower together. I might also suggest that they take a walk, do an errand together, put on music while they sit down and drink a glass of wine, or exchange massages. One couple I saw had their most satisfying sex in several years just after they finished cleaning out their garage.

"*Simmering*" (Zilbergeld and Ellison 1980, p. 79), i.e., lighting a pilot light of arousal and keeping it fueled, is another technique I recommend. For example, I instructed Dave, an attorney, to call his wife Ann at work one afternoon and suggest sex later that evening. His call let them both begin to let arousal build. I told them to greet in a sexually suggestive way when he got home, have a glass of wine with dinner, and, of course, not to stay up too late!

I teach couples *to focus on pleasure* and *to recognize cues* that let them know when their partner is focused enough into sexual activity to perceive sexual or genital stimulation as pleasurable. I also suggest ways to facilitate their partner's relaxation and receptiveness and may recommend that they take a massage course.

Since many people find that allowing arousal to build and diminish a number of times enables them to create more intense feelings than they get when they pursue constant stimulation to orgasm, I suggest to couples that they *experiment with intensity of arousal*, that they play with different rhythms and patterns of stimulation and with allowing the intensity of their arousal to wax and wane. I also sometimes suggest that they *make love to music*, and experiment with various styles of music to find out if changing the style of music changes their sexual experiences.

But above all, for each couple, I focus on – in whatever appropriate form their lovemaking may take – enabling them to create experiences in which each feels good about herself or himself and the other and that each has a good time.

References

Dicks HV (1967) Marital tensions. Basic, New York, p 29

Ellison CR (1986) Using intimate trance to increase sexual satisfaction. In: Zilbergeld B, Edelstien MG, Araoz DL (eds) Hypnosis questions and answers. Norton, New York, pp 210–218

Lucero W (1987) Discovering and treating barriers to intimacy. Student paper, John F. Kennedy University, Orinda, California, USA, 5/5/87, p 1

Talmadge LD, Talmadge WC (1986) Relational sexuality: an understanding of low sexual desire. J Sex Marital Ther 12:3–21

Travis R, Travis P (1987) Intimacy based sex therapy. J of Sex Education Ther: 21–27

Zilbergeld B, Ellison CR (1980) Desire discrepancies and arousal problems in sex therapy. In: Leiblum SR, Pervin LA (eds) Principles and practice or sex therapy. Guilford, New York, pp 65–101, p 71

Treatment of Inhibited Sexual Desire in the Woman by Trazodone

G. Tordjman

Paris Hospital System, Société Française de Sexologie Clinique,
21 Boulevard Boune, 75014 Paris, France

Introduction and Definitions

On the basis of clinical experience, inhibited sexual desire is the commonest and most difficult dysfunction encountered in a sexology outpatient clinic. Forty percent of patients make reference to the problem.

The clinician comes up against two major difficulties from the outset:

- The difficulty of defining sexual desire
- The difficulty of evaluating it from a quantitative standpoint

From a scientific point of view, the definition of desire suffers from lack of a common vocabulary. A large number of almost interchangeable synonyms are used to describe it: impulse, libido, lewdness, interest, appetite, excitement, passion, etc.

Do we take sexual desire to mean ability to take the initiative in touching and sexual stimulation? Anglo-Saxon biologists refer to this under the name "proceptivity." Or is it better defined as a response to the advances of a possible partner, corresponding to the "receptivity" component?

The man in the street often confuses desire with the urgent need to relieve sexual tension. In this respect, pelvic congestion seen in women during the phase of ovulation or premenstrually would be an equivalent to heat, which renders the female receptive to the male during kinds of rut in the animal kingdom.

It is not today possible for anybody to state that sexual desire can regularly and invariably reduce the threshold of excitement of genital erogenous areas in man. However, sexual desire encourages search for erotic stimulation by a partner, fantasies, or masturbation.

In the animal kingdom, under the influence of estrogens the female secretes pheromones which attract and stimulate the male. Although pheromones have been isolated in the human species, there is no evidence of such an interaction in the woman. However, it is known that in man, as in the animal, sexual behavior is controlled by cerebral centers.

Physiology of Desire

We enter into desire with our entire personality. This no doubt occurs on the basis of special imprinted information harking back to mental experiences in childhood. A partner is selected without any other apparent reason than that of pleasure. This is a complex personalization process into which we cannot enter here.

Sexology
Eds.: W. Eicher, G. Kockott

However, it is known that certain neurotransmitters and certain hormones at least govern the erotic background.

Dopamine (DA) and Prolactin (PRL)

Dopamine has been described as the primary hormone of desire (Vincent 1986). It is certainly true that a rat deprived of DA is indifferent to any sexual stimulation and becomes uninterested.

- In the elderly man, fall in desire is linked to a fall in DA.
- Antidopaminergic drugs often have the iatrogenic effects of inhibiting sexuality (neutropic and hypotensive agents, sulpiride) and increasing plasma prolactin levels.

  Hyperprolactinemia is today a recognized cause of problems with erection and loss of sexual interest in man. It causes a state of hypogonadism with a risk of reducing testosterone levels. It no doubt also acts by directly inhibiting cerebral centers concerning sexual function.

Hyperprolactinemia in woman causes disturbance of menstrual cycles and infertility. However, on the basis of a study concerning prolactin adenomas (Tordjman 1981), we feel that hyperprolactinemia is commonly accompanied by a reduction in desire in the woman. This has been confirmed by the study by Fioretti et al. (1977). In such cases both bromocriptine and metergoline are capable of improving sexual desire by normalizing PRL levels.

Twenty percent of patients seen for lack of sexual interest showed evidence of hyperprolactinemia, if not directly at least by the LHRH+TRH test (PRL exceeding 50 ng/ml in this test).

Prolactin may disturb sexual function by different mechanisms:

- As in the male, it may cause a reduction in plasma testosterone levels as a result of hypogonadism.
- It may also have a direct inhibitory effect on cerebral centers of sexual function. Thus, certain women with hyperprolactinemia suffering from ISD show evidence of normalization of plasma testosterone levels and recovery of desire only after PRL levels have been successfully reduced.
- Finally, hyperprolactinemia may only reflect imbalance in cerebral neurotransmitters. For example, an increase in (5-hydroxytrpytamine) (5-HT), a serotonin precursor, increases the secretion of PRL and tends to inhibit erotic function in the woman.

5-Hydroxytryptamine and Serotonin

Animal experiments suggest that 5-HT inhibits sexual behavior in the female. In contrast, depletion under the influence of parachlorophenylalanine (PCPA) increases sexual activity in the female rat. This same phenomenon would appear to happen in women. Of obese women treated with an anorexic drug, fenfluramine, which increases 5-HT secretion, 85% reported a fall in libido (Pinder et al. 1975).

Alpha-Blockers

At least when administered by intracavernous injection in man, alpha-blockers are powerful vasoactive agents facilitating rapid and prolonged erection (Tordjman 1984).

There is every reason to suppose that they have a similar action in the woman, favorizing vaginal lubrification.

Testosterone

Testosterone has long been recognized as the clinical messenger of desire in both men and women. The increase in desire seen in certain women on the day prior to ovulation is believed to be due to an increase in male hormones secreted by the adrenal glands which have receptors in the brain. This could also explain why women who have undergone hysterectomy and ovariectomy generally retain a normal libido.

There has been recent evidence of a significant correlation between plasma testosterone levels and three parameters of sexual response in the woman:
- Erogenicity of the clitoris
- Sexual excitation threshold
- Capacity for orgasm (Bailey 1973)

As we have emphasized, it is reasonable to consider that reduction in PRL levels at least increases the receptivity of cerebral centers to testosterone. These considerations led us to an experimental trial of trazodone, which has the profile of the aphrodisiac drug which we were seeking.

Use of Trazodone in the Treatment of ISD

We had the idea of using trazodone in the treatment of ISD because of its clinical, iatrogenic, and pharmacological properties.

Clinically, trazodone is an antidepressant drug although it is not chemically related to the tricyclic imipramine antidepressant family nor monoamine oxidase inhibitor (MAOI), known for their possible negative iatrogenic action on sexuality. Furthermore, it is known that one of the essential clinical manifestations of depression is lack of sexual desire. From an iatrogenic standpoint, there have been recent reports of priapism in depressed men treated with trazodone. Trazodone has a large number of pharmacological actions which suggested a potentially favorable effect upon sexual behavior:

Action on the Serotoninergic System

Trazodone inhibits the uptake of serotonin by the platelets, which are the representative model of the serotoninergic neuron.

Alpha-Blocker Action

Alpha-blocker action on alpha-1 and, to a lesser degree, alpha-2 receptors. This action would probably account for the cases of priapism reported after administration of the drug.

Desensitizing Action

Desensitizing action on the postsynaptic beta-receptors.

Decrease in Blood Prolactin Levels

Decrease in blood prolactin levels and binding of 5-HT2.

Trazodone was therefore studied in inhibited sexual desire in women and in premature ejaculation in men. The results of the first experiment are reported below.

Trial Inclusion Criteria

The following were included in the study:

Cases of nonselective ISD of obviously organic origin (16 cases):

- ISD accompanying depression (ten cases)
- ISD with hyperprolactinemia (two clear-cut cases + four cases by LHRH+TRH test)
- ISD with reduced plasma T levels (one case)
- ISD related to genetic abnormalities (Turner's or Kallman's syndrome) (one case)
- ISD secondary to chronic illness (two cases of renal failure with exchange transfusion)

Nonselective ISD related to stress (14 cases), such as:

- Occupational problems
- Severe marital conflict
- Illness in a close family member
- Post-traumatic ISD, e.g., after rape

It is known that stress is extremely likely to produce hyperprolactinemia.

The following were excluded from the study:

- All cases of situational selective ISD
- Selective loss of interest in partner
- Loss of interest in masturbation only, or for a particular erotic stimulus
- Specific or overall aversion related more to phobia than to lack of desire

Method

Trazodone was prescribed at the progressive dose of three to four 25-mg tablets for 3 months in 30 women aged 20–40 years.

Sexual Desire from a Clinical and Biological Standpoint

An attempt was made to evaluate sexual desire from a twin clinical and biological standpoint. The major difficulty lay in the fact that sexual desire is difficult to quantify. Frequency of sexual intercourse or masturbation only very distantly and indirectly reflects the degree of sexual desire which may not find a way to express itself. Furthermore, the sex act is not an indicator of true desire. We therefore used laboratory tests and subjective methods of evaluation which were quantified on an arbitrary basis.

With regard to laboratory parameters, the following were measured in all our patients: LH, testosterone and PRL levels, and LHRH + TRH test (where applicable, tryptophan and serotonin).

Such evaluation is more difficult in women than in men in view of interference with hormonal balance by episodes in reproductive life: menstruation, pregnancy, contraceptive pill.

The following tests were used clinically:

- Frequency of sexual intercourse during the month
- Frequency of orgasm, although bearing in mind that there is no significant correlation between the degree of sexual desire and capacity for orgasm

Above all, subjective evaluation of sexual desire was quantified on an arbitrary basis.

In practice, hypnotized patients were presented with an erotic fantasy recorded on a cassette, using the method of Mosher and White (1980). This fantasy included two parts: a sexual invitation sequence followed by a coital experience sequence.

Studies over the past 15 years have disproved the belief that only men react to erotic stimuli while the rise in female desire necessarily involves the precursor of a romantic context (Kinsey et al. 1983; Berger et al. 1971). Studies of female responses to erotic literature in a laboratory in Hamburg (Institute of Sex Research) as well as those carried out by the Commission on Obscenity and Pornography (Abelson et al. 1981) have virtually reversed the above statements. Even in women, erotic stimuli independent of any relational affective context are found to be more exciting than romantic fantasies.

At any event two types of specific fantasy were used in evaluation of desire in our patients:

- In one case erotic fantasies were integrated in a relational affective context.
- In the other the suggested fantasy involved a brief erotic sequence without any affective investment.

Three variables shown by questioning were taken into account in deciding the preferred material:

Level of sexual guilt feelings

Extent of previous erotic experience

Affective reaction to masturbation, which is a good projective index of erotic availability in the woman.

In those women who had practiced masturbation for a long time, who had extensive erotic experience, and who appeared to be relatively free of guilt feelings (12 out of 30), the cassette involving brief fantasies without any affective investment was used. Fantasies integrated in an affective context were used in the other 18. Three types of subjective evaluation of sexual desire using the slightly modified method of Mosher et al. (Mosher and Abramson 1977; Mosher and O'Grady 1979) were used, before and after treatment with trazodone, on our patients previously hypnotized and exposed to one of the above-mentioned erotic sequences.

1. Subjective evaluation of desire ranging from 0 to 5
2. Perception of genital responses, heat, lubrication, and orgasm from 0 to 5 in relation to their degree.
3. Quantitative evaluation of fantasy emotional reactions. The evaluation scale was made up of 6 headings which the patient was asked to score from 0 to 5 in an attempt to define her emotional reaction: passion, sensuality, excitation, loss of control, desire, eroticism. The score of the scale was provided by the arithmetic sum of the responses to the six adjectives.
4. Qualitative emotional evaluation. In addition, the patients were asked which of the following ten emotions appeared best to coincide with their fantasy experience: interest, joy, surprise, distress, anger, disgust, fear, guilt, contempt, or shame.

In practice, hypnotic inductions lasted for 15 min with extension of Schultz-type relaxation. A transition led to the fantasy sequence.

"Now that you are as relaxed as possible, you are going to identify yourself with the heroine of this fantasy. As completely as possible you are going to see, hear, and feel what this woman sees, hears, and feels in the story which you are about to hear."

Results

Under the influence of trazodone, in 18 patients out of 30 there was a notable increase in libido, coinciding in 6 of them with the remission of depression. No improvement was seen in 12 patients. Among these there was remission of depression in two though without any accompanying notable modification in libido.

Discussion

During the first presentation of the prerecorded fantasy before treatment, qualitative emotional reactions were all negative, distributed by order of frequency between "disgust," "anger," "contempt," "shame," and "fear." In the 18 women who were improved, emotional reactions seen most often were interest, joy, and surprise. Their quantitative subjective assessment of desire and their genital and emotional reactions increased significantly.

Certainly the physiology of female desire remains in great part unknown. However, up to the present time experimental studies have demonstrated the stimulant action of androgens and the inhibitory action of prolactin.

Estrogens are usually beneficial even if they are effective via indirect routes. However, the no doubt decisive influence of cerebral neurotransmitters remains to be explored and discovered. It can nevertheless be stated, as the author wrote several years ago, that future aphrodisiacs should combine cerebral actions on neurotransmitters, notably an antiprolactinemic, antiserotoninergic, and alpha-blocker action. This is the very profile of trazodone.

References

Abelson, Cohen, Heaton, Suder (1971) National survey of public attitudes toward and experience with erotic materials. Technical Report of the Commission on Obscenity and Pornography, vol 6. US Government Printing Office, Washington DC

Bailey (1973) Studies in depression: II treatment of the depressed frigid woman. Med J Australia 1:834–837

Berger, Gagnon, Simon (1971) Pornography: high school and college years. Technical Report of the Commission on Obscenity and Pornography, vol 9. US Government Printing Office, Washington DC

Fioretti, Corsini, Murru, Medda, Genazzini (1977) Depression and sexual behaviour in hyperprolactinaemic amenorrhoea. Effect of bromo-ergocriptine treatment. Acta Endocrinol 85:141

Kinsey, Pomeroy, Martin, Gebhard (1953) Sexual behavior in the human female. Saunders, Philadelphia

Mosher, Abramson (1977) Subjective sexual arousal to films of masturbation. J Consult Clin Psychol 45:796–807

Mosher, O'Grady (1979) Sex guilt, trait anxiety and females subjective sexual arousal to erotica. Motivation and emotion, vol 3, pp 235–249

Mosher, White (1980) J Sex Res 16

Pinder, Brogden, Sawyer, Speight, Avery (1975) Fenfluramine: a review of its pharmacological properties and therapeutic efficacy in obesity. Drugs 10:5, 6

Tordjman G (1981) Prolactine sexualité bromocryptine et adénomes à prolactines. Cahiers de Sexologie Clinique, vol 7, No 42

Tordjman G (1984) Action des alphabloquants sur l'éjaculation prematurée et sur l'érection. Contraception-Fertilité-Sexualité, vol 12, No 9

Vincent JD (1986) Biologie des passions. Seuil, Paris

Hypnosis as a Form of Treatment for Sexual Disorders, Particularly Those Resulting from Sexual Violence

F. Bruinsma and R. Stichting
Regentesselaan 101, 3571 CD Utrecht, The Netherlands

Introduction

The concept of sexual dysfunction is relatively new. Masters and Johnson published their research data in 1966 and their treatment model in 1970. The sex therapy, later developed, based on their model, is actually a specific form of behavior modification.

In the study of sexual behavior and sexual dysfunctions, cognitions are also considered important factors, and their biological determinants also represent a central focus for current research.

In the scientific literature hypnotherapy as a specific form of treatment is generally referred to in the context of a case study or via clinical anecdotes. Publications on the combined use of hypnosis and behavior therapy appeared in the 1970s, particularly for the treatment of vaginismus (Frutiger 1981; Fuchs 1973). Crasilneck (1982) also reported the use of hypnotherapy for problems of impotence. With respect to the importance of cognitions regarding the causes of sexual dysfunctions, Araoz (1982) described some of the hypnotherapeutic techniques used to influence the ideas of the client with regard to sexuality. He first coined the term "negative self-hypnosis" to refer to all the imagined and irrational ideas that may cause or maintain the client's symptoms. Sexual violence can have a great negative impact on the sexual functioning within or outside of an intimate relationship. Hypnosis can help diagnostically to reveal the consequences of sexual violence, and it can contribute to its treatment.

In this paper I will present a decision tree for the use of hypnotherapy with sexual dysfunctions, especially those resulting from sexual violence. Brown and Chaves (1980) did a detailed study and review of the scientific literature in this field. They came to the conclusion that hypnotherapy does not stand up to the test of critical investigation. Nevertheless, because the use of hypnosis in a clinical context continues to be promising, I would like to give my experience as a clinician.

Sexual Dysfunctions

As you all know, psychosexual disorders are divided into different diagnostic subgroups such as paraphilia and sexual dysfunctions. With regard to the latter the DSM-III distinguishes:
- Inhibited sexual desire
- Inhibited sexual excitement

Sexology
Eds.: W. Eicher, G. Kockott

- Inhibited female orgasm
- Inhibited male orgasm
- Premature ejaculation
- Functional dyspareunia
- Functional vaginismus
- Atypical psychosexual dysfunction

This classification is more or less based on the sexual phases physiologically defined. Diagnostically speaking the behavioral and biological aspects of sexual dysfunction are more important than the way the patient subjectively experiences his or her symptom. To my knowledge Everaerd et al. (1977) were the first to point to the relationship between sexual phase and the way it is subjectively experienced. In a very simplified way it can be said that disorders of sexual desire have their roots in the cognitive field, while those of sexual arousal are relationally based and those of the orgastic phase are more individually grounded (anxiety, loss of control).

Hypnotherapy

In my opinion hypnotherapy cannot be seen as isolated from the clinical relationship in which it occurs. Within a psychotherapeutic relationship or in a medical setting it can be a useful technique, but not more than that. Excessive expectations on the part of the client or the referral source or on the part of the therapist himself may in the long run cause or increase distrust in the client. While hypnosis can provide a good short-term means to build the sound therapeutic working alliance, necessary for adequate change, initial disappointment of unrealistic expectations can have an adverse affect on this process. That is also the case if the desired change is only symptom oriented. Various hypnotherapeutic techniques can be seen both as symptom oriented or as explorative and insight oriented in nature.

The following classification should be seen as a continuum:

- Reduction, shifting, or displacement of the symptom
- Ego-building techniques of emotional conditioning, like the "clenched fist" technique
- Fantasies of the future, reframing, or other "ideal self" techniques
- Age regression such as the affect bridge or ideomotor responding
- Ego state therapy

At the Rutgers Foundation, when a patient presents his or her symptom in isolation, we generally choose a symptom alleviation approach. If we decide to use a hypnotic technique more exoploratively, we regularly evaluate our hypothesis as to the effects the chosen methods have diagnostically and/or therapeutically. In this way we adjust our methods according to the treatment goal.

Sexual Dysfunction and Hypnotherapy

Is it possible to speak of a treatment indication where hypnotherapy is the treatment of choice for specific sexual dysfunctions? Are there specific hypnotherapeutic techniques for specific sexual problems? In my opinion the answer to both these questions is generally negative. Still it is possible to give some guidelines. While not always consciously experienced as such, disorders of *sexual desire* are defined cognitively. It is advisable therefore to have a clear understanding of the cognitions at play in a given case. Hypnotherapy, especially the more explorative techniques, can be of value here. In these cases I use techniques such as "reframing," "ideal self," age regression, "silent abreaction" (Edelstein 1981), and "ego-state" therapy (Watkins 1966). Disorders of sexual *arousal* tend to be relationally based, although remarkably enough it is men with impotence problems who generally do not recognize this relational aspect of their complaint. Owing to this relational context disorders of sexual arousal are better treated by couple therapy. Unfortunately this treatment model is often not possible or cannot be worked toward. Reassurance, counseling, or sex therapy, using for instance the stop-start technique or masturbation training exercises, suffice for treatment of disorders of the *orgastic phase*. If necessary hypnotherapy can be used as a technique for relaxation or ego-strengthening. The same applies to the treatment of patients with *functional dyspareunia or vaginismus*, where in addition to the above-mentioned techniques those of symptom reduction, shifting, or displacement are also used. More explorative techniques diagnostically useful are also used in these cases, for instance when repressed or partially repressed underlying psychotraumatic events in the past are suspected. Hypnosis is essentially an individual therapy, although it can be applied very well in the presence of a client's partner. In general hypnotherapy is especially indicated for primary and/or global symptoms, that is, when the symptom is long-standing and/or is present in every situation. If the sexual problem is more secondary and/or situationally bound, then the relational context is more important.

Men and Women

Many men experience their sexuality as an unrelated feeling by itself. "Spontaneous" sexual arousal gives a sexual meaning to the situation associated with the arousal, instead of the other way around. Moreover, men can experience their sexuality as very compelling, sometimes exceeding any conscious control of their sexual emotions. So, the subjective experience that men have of their sexuality can be felt as very compelling. Woman have told me they experience similar obsessive feelings less in the sexual field but more with regard to eating or buying clothes. I wonder whether these differences might be related to the male-female occurrence ratio of syndromes like sexual paraphilia and delinquency on the one hand and anorexia and shoplifting on the other. Paraphilias occur almost exclusively in men. The actual paraphilic behavior often takes place when there is a sudden loss of impulse control. Sometimes this happens under the influence of alcohol; most of the time these men experience themselves in some kind of trance state (Money 1976). In my opinion, it is very important when treating these men to allow them to regain a sense of control over their own behavior. Besides a functional analysis of their behavior, techniques of self-control with or without the support of hypnotherapy are very helpful. Symptom-oriented techniques can be especially useful, stressing the fact that all hypnosis is actually self-hypnosis.

Sexual Development

Sexual development in puberty is mostly accelerated by biological factors. This is different for boys and girls. For girls this sexual development is psychologically better balanced that it is for boys, whose sexual development can be considered to evolve dichotomously. The so-called "madonna-whore-complex" is an artifact of this dichotomy. On the one hand we see an asexual chivalrous attitude, on the other a crude sexual one. As a consequence of imprinting processes during masturbation this rough sexual orientation, sometimes associated with parafilic fantasies or events, may become autonomous and compulsive. It depends on the process of internalization, occurring at a more and more unconscious level as adolescence proceeds, whether or not a man will later experience his sexuality as a feeling with a life of its own. The result is that men tend to speak of sexual functioning or achieving, while women experience their sexuality in more emotional terms.

Because of this process men are likely to present their sexual dysfunction in a more symptomatic way, even though sexual impotence has a relational background most of the time, from a psychological point of view. In such cases a symptom-oriented treatment approach is indicated. I use the techniques of changing the symptom and ego-strengthening. A general induction procedure can be applied, but the use of metaphors or the induction of arm catalepsy in combination with a quite authoritarian attitude on the part of the therapist works best in these cases. In this way, Crasilneck (1982) succeeded in attaining a 87% success rate for men with psychogenic impotence after a 1-year follow-up. Regaining control of one's own body is an important aspect of the treatment.

Performance Anxiety

Masters and Johnson introduced the well-known concept of performance anxiety leading to sexual dysfunction. On the other hand anxiety can sometimes increase sexual arousal (Beck and Barlow 1984; Norton and Jehu 1984), especially for men with paraphilias (Stoller 1976). Barlow et al. (1986) researched cognitive influences on sexuality. Like Herman and Rowland (1983) they compared sexually dysfunctional men with functional men. Results indicate that anxiety can increase the sexual arousal of the functional group, while it greatly weakens that of the dysfunctional one. Sexually functional men are sexually stimulated by the arousal of their partners, while the dysfunctional group is negatively influenced by the partner's arousal. In short, performance anxiety produces much sexual trouble in the sexually dysfunctional group, but it does not in the other. Sexually functional men are able to integrate feelings of anxiety in their sexual arousal pattern, even under stressful conditions. On the other hand, neutral distraction like reading or doing arithmetic induces a decrease of sexual arousal in the functional group, while it does not affect the dysfunctional man. The latter is already distracted by his performance anxiety.

Finally, in comparing these two groups, it is important to note how the men in each group evaluate their own sexual arousal. Dysfunctional men subjectively experience their erection as being less than it is in reality; the sexually functional man overestimates his reaction. These cognitions are very important for sexual functioning, in fact even more important than the arousal itself. In looking at these findings I would also like to refer to the work of Briddle and others (1978), who came to the conclusion that the disinhibiting effect of alcohol on sexual behavior is not due to the alcohol itself but to the idea the person had about having imbibed alcohol.

What does all this mean therapeutically? Barlow suggested the use of neutral distraction for men with strong performance anxiety, so that attention is shifted away from sexual performance. Translated into hypnotherapeutic terms (and that seems a good thing to do) this means a symptom-oriented approach will suffice, but one should be indirectly structured and make use of metaphors, reframing, or guided imagery. Recently, Gilmore (1987) published a report about hypnotic embedded metaphors (Lankton and Lankton 1983) and sexual dysfunction.

Sexual Violence

Sexual violence and its sequels are presently the order of the day. This may be limited to a single occurrence, but it can also go on for a long time. We see this continuing process going on within an existing relationship of dependency. The offender is nearly always an older man, the victim mostly a younger woman, although we are lately also seeing more and more male victims in The Netherlands. The feminist movement has made clear that sexual violence takes place within a society where men have the power to establish the rules. Many writers (Lukianowicz 1972; McGuire and Wagner 1978; Tsai and Wagner 1978; Tsai et al. 1980; Becker et al. 1982) wrote about sexual dysfunction as a delayed effect of incest, especially disorders of sexual desire, disorders of arousal, and situational anorgasmia. The last symptom can be understood in terms of anxiety for loss of control in the presence of a sexual partner. The negative aftermaths of a single incidence of sexual violence, like rape, are also evident for sexual functioning (Burgess and Holmstrom 1974; Rose 1986). Male victims of sexual violence react differently than woman. They identify more with the male agressor through acting-out behavior or by becoming sexual delinquents themselves. Female victims are more likely to be victimized again. Many mothers of incest victims have been sexually molested themselves in the past. Nevertheless some women react by showing the same acting-out behavior that men do in the form of promiscuity or prostitution. In this way sexuality becomes a functional way for them to suppress the pain felt in the past at the time of the sexual abuse.

Sexual Violence, Post-Traumatic Stress Syndrome, and Dissociation

Sexual violence can result in the so-called post-traumatic stress syndrome (Burgess and Holmstrom 1974; Tsai and Wagner 1978). The syndrome consists of reliving traumatic experiences. Patients relive experiences in a dissociative way, that is, feelings of estrangement toward oneself, toward others, or toward the world in general (Gelinas 1983).

Frankel (1976) has pointed out the adaptive aspect of dissociation as a coping mechanism. In my opinion it is a mistake without forethought to remove this dissociation or amnestic barrier for the traumatic events. If the client is unable to cope in another way, this pseudoreintegration can result in a psychotic decompensation.

Janet (1889) mentioned the term dissociation for the first time. His hysterical patients showed this sign. DSM-III no longer mentions hysteric disorders, but places them under the somatization disorders, conversions, dissociative disorders, dysthymic disorders, post-traumatic stress disorders, and disorders of the personality. Diagnostically the overlap is large. Janet (1898) in his book *Les Obsessions et la Psychasthénie* wrote about the dissociation connected with obsessive compulsive disorders. The so-called *ideés fixes* are not totally suppressed as they are in the hysterical patient. As far as sexual traumas are concerned women seem to dissociate more in the "hysterical" way, men more in the "obsessive compulsive" way. Maybe Janet was more correct than we realize when he supposed that dissociation could be caused by "biological stress" in puberty. Androgens seem to lead to an upheaval of the obsessive compulsive type of dissociation with sexually acting-out behavior, while estrogens have a more smoothing effect, producing an internalized suppressing kind of dissociation.

Dissociation and Hypnosis

The hypnotic trance is a specific form of dissociation. Trance experiences of everyday life, described by Erickson (1975), can be accompanied by more or less consciously experienced phenomena of dissociation. On the other hand, certain precipitating events, the so-called triggers, can lead to spontaneous dissociative experiences. Flashbacks during sexual behavior are examples of these. There are many similarities between the dissociation of hypnotic trance and sexual arousal or orgasm. The trigger to paraphilic behavior is experienced quite often in a state of dissociative trance (Money 1981).

Sexual Violence, Sexual Dysfunction, and Hypnotherapy

A sex therapist should be aware of his position in the therapeutic relationship when he is dealing with the sequels of sexual violence. Symbolic or actual repetition of the abuse can happen all too easliy. This is even more so in the context of the hypnotic relationship. Formal trance inductions should be handled carefully because loss of control can be very threatening. Spontaneously occurring trance experiences with dissociation occur quite often in victims of sexual violence. Working through the trauma means that these experiences should be taking place under the control and at the pace of the client. Emancipatory treatment consists of getting control of the overwhelming feelings of dissociation. A well-knit scar will ultimately remain as the result of successful treatment. That means associative triggers will no longer bring about the automatic reactions of the post-traumatic stress syndrome. Vaginismus or dyspareunia as the aftermaths of sexual violence are experienced by the woman as something apart from herself. The sense of the body has been trespassed. I talk about *the* sense and *the* body instead of *her* sense and *her* body, on purpose, because a sexually violated woman does not experience her body as her own. Yet, in her own time and under her own control it is possible for her to visualize her body in fantasy or in vivo. Hypnosis can help her recover her own body in this way. She can decide very consciously later on whether she wants to remain "vaginistic." Her vagina has become a part of her body and it is a mistake to "break through" this control like some gynecologists are inclined to do. In regard to male victims it is very important to intervene as soon as possible, just as for females. The internalization of the trauma in the personality has not yet completely taken place in puberty or adolescence. The shame felt by the male victims is extreme (Porter 1986; Gianotten 1987). So male victims desparately try to hide these experiences. On the other hand, if they are able to disclose what happened to them, the largest part of the therapy has been done. A "hypnotic therapeutic relationship" per se works better in these cases than a formal induction or a hypnotic trance. The anxiety for loss of control can be overwhelming. The same holds true for offenders of sexual violence. They are quite sensitive to authority generally and to the hypnotic relationship specifically. The intimacy of the therapeutic relationship determines the extent to which particular content can be worked through. The male sexual offender experiences his sexuality in a very obsessive way. At the same time his emotional and intimate life is very restricted. In these cases it is sensible to use suggestive distraction as I explained earlier with respect to the therapy of male impotence. Metaphors around the question of performance anxiety should be used creatively. Especially fantasies of driving cars stimulate their imaginative faculties without affecting this sense of ego strength and self-esteem. The hypnotic approach should be symptom oriented because the client is generally quite suspicious.

When the sequels of sexual violence have led to disorders of sexual desire, more explorative hypnotherapeutic techniques may be considered. Finkelhor and Browne (1986) have written about the effects of sexual abuse in childhood. At the level of dynamics, of psychological impact, and of behavior they distinguish four clusters: traumatic sexualization, stigmatization, betrayal, and powerlessness. In my opinion it is necessary to assess a victim diagnostically in this respect before performing therapy. If the traumatic sexualization has been great it carries with it the risk of an untreatable sexualization of the hypnotherapeutic relationship. When the effects of stigmatization are in the foreground, thematic group therapy is indicated. In the case of betrayal, building up a good and trustful relationship is very important. Counseling the patient feeling overwhelmed by a sense of powerlessness needs to emphasize his or her own control and pace. Working with this last cluster of powerlessness the therapist should be able to recognize the signs of dissociation.

References

American Psychiatric Association (1980) Diagnostic and statistical manual of mental disorders, 3rd edn. DSM-III, Washington DC

Araoz D (1982) Hypnosis and sex therapy. Brunner/Mazel, New York
Barlow DH (1986) Causes of sexual dysfunction: the role of anxiety and cognitive interference. J Consulting Clin Psychol 54:140–148
Beck JG, Barlow DH (1984) Current conceptualization of sexual dysfunction: a review and an alternative perspective. Clin Psychol Rev 4:363–378
Becker JH, Skinner LJ, Abel GG, Tracy EC (1982) Incidence and types of sexual dysfunctions in rape and incest victims. J Sexual Marital Ther 8:65–74
Briddle DW, Rimm DC, Caddy GR, Krawitz G, Stoles E, Wunderling RJ (1978) Effects of alcohol and cognitive set on sexual arousal to deviant stimuli. J Abnorm Psychol 87:418–430
Brown JM, Chaves JF (1980) Hypnosis in the treatment of sexual dysfunctions. J Sexual Marital Ther 6:63–74
Burgess AW, Holmstrom L (1974) Rape trauma syndrome. Am J Psychiatr 131:981–985
Crasilneck HB (1982) A follow-up study in the use of hypnotherapy in the treatment of psychogenic impotency. Am J Clin Hypnosis 25:52–61
Erickson MH, Rossi EL (1979) Hypnotherapy. Irvington, New York
Edelstein MG (1981) Trauma, trance and transformation. A clinical guide to hypnotherapy. Brunner/Mazel, New York
Everaerd W, van Naerssen L, Cohen-Kettenis P (1977) Anders Denken over Seksualiteit. van Loghum Slaterus, Deventer
Finkelhor D, Browne A (1986) Initial and long-term effects: a conceptual framework. In: Finkelhor D et al. (eds) A sourcebook on child sexual abuse. Sage Publications, Beverly Hills, pp 180–199
Frankel FH (1976) Hypnosis. Trance as a coping mechanism. Plenum, New York
Frutiger AD (1981) Treatment of penetration phobia through the combined use of systematic desensitisation and hypnosis: a case history. Am J Clin Hypnosis 23:269–273
Fuchs K, et al. (1973) Hypnodesensitisation therapy of vaginismus. Int J Clin Exp Hypnosis 21:144–156
Gelinas DJ (1983) The persisting negative effects of incest. J Psychiatr 46:312–332
Gianotten WL (to be published) Een jongen met incest
Gilmore LG (1987) Hypnotic metaphor and sexual dysfunction. J Sex Marital Ther 13:45–57
Heiman JR, Rowland DL (1983) Affective and physiological sexual patterns: the effects of instructions on sexually functional and dysfunctional men. J Psychosom Res 27:105–116
Janet P (1889) L'automatisme psychologique. Felix Alcan, Paris
Janet P (1903) Les obsessions et la psychasthénie. Felix Alcan, Paris
Lankton S, Lankton C (1983) The answer within; a clinical framework of Ericksonian hypnotherapy. Brunner/Mazel, New York
Lukianowicz N (1972) Incest: paternal incest. Intern J Psychother 120:301–313
McGuire LS, Wagner NN (1978) Sexual dysfunction in women who were molested as children: one response pattern and suggestions for treatment. J Sex Marital Ther 4:11–15
Money J, Bennett RG (1981) Postadolescent paraphilic sex offenders: antiandrogens and counseling therapy follow up. Intern J Mental Health 10:122–133
Norton GR, Jehu D (1984) The role of anxiety in sexual dysfunctions: a review. Arch Sex Behav 2:165–183
Porter E (1986) Treating the young male victim of sexual assault: issues and intervention strategies. Safer Society, Syracuse, NY
Stoller R (1976) Sexual excitement. Arch Gen Psychiatr 33:899–909
Tsai M, Feldman-Summers S, Edgar M (1979) Childhood molestation; variables related to differential impacts on psychosexual functioning in adult women. J Abnormal Psychol 88:407–417
Tsai M, Wagner NN (1978) Therapy groups for women sexually molested as children. Arch Sex Behav 7:417–427
Watkins J, Watkins H (1979) The theory and practice of ego state therapy. In: Grayson H (ed) Short term approaches to psychotherapy. National Institute for the psychotherapies and human sciences press, New York

VIII. Sexuality and Illness (Including Cancer)

Sexuality and Depression

W. Pöldinger and F. Labhardt

Psychiatrische Universitäts-Klinik, Wilhelm-Klein-Str. 27,
4000 Basel, Switzerland

Throughout the literature on depression you will find that depression impairs libido as well as potency. It makes a major difference whether or not these limitations of sexual needs are registered by the partner. While a woman can easily pretend to be sexually aroused, or even fake an experience of orgasm, a man obviously has greater difficulties in this regard.

It is not well enough known that the reduction of libido and potency including orgasmic potency often occur very early in a depressive phase, distinctly before the disturbance has fully manifested itself. As depressive patients, due to their feelings of guilt, tend to interpret their state not as an illness, but rather as a punishment for a real or imagined guilt, they generally tend not to speak about it and do not seek help in therapy. This can lead to a state where the partner of a depressive or subdepressive patient starts believing that the desire for him or her has diminished although it is all caused by depression.

The more severe depression becomes, the more libido and potency diminish. As the patient is plagued by feelings of guilt already, these tend to increase due to his or her fear of no longer being able to satisfy his or her partner. This factor will be all the more serious with a problematical intimate relationship. It can happen that a strained relationship has just survived, but falls apart under the difficulties and tensions added by the depression of one partner.

Difficulties in the relationship of such partners also arise because the men orient their sex life merely toward orgasm and show too little care for their partner. Many men do not know or only learn during the relationship that the arousal curves for men and women are different, slower for women with the formation of plateaus, whereas men need less time from the onset of arousal to orgasm and show an immediate decrease of sexual interest thereafter. It is therefore necessary for men to prolong foreplay according to the needs of the partner and to continue to exchange tenderness after orgasm. The purely orgasm-centered patients as depressives have a lack of regard for their partner. The male patient wants to reach a climax as fast as possible; then it is over for him. A corresponding behavior also exists for depressive women.

Another intriguing phenomenon is the frequently observed fact that orgasm is strived for purely for the sake of a reduction of anxiety, but is not reached due to impotence. For women the corresponding phenomenon is that she cannot experience orgasm, although or because she strives so hard for it. This can lead to disappointment and anger, which is aggressively discharged either against the partner or against the self in the form of increased suicidality, which tends to be present anyway.

Sexology
Eds.: W. Eicher, G. Kockott

Youths in particular are prone to such "degrading" experiences e.g., in the case where a man is impotent at his first attempted sexual intercourse. In his depressive attitude he considers himself not a man but a hopeless case, which again can sharply increase suicidal tendencies.

Another problem with these difficulties is whether the partner recognizes the depression at all. Frequently the depression is hidden behind somatic symptoms – we then speak of a "masked depression" – or the depressive patient tries to maintain his dignity, not to show his suffering. There are patients who know how to do this very well, who hide their depression behind a smiling mask. In this case we speak of a "smiling depression." For couples who get together relatively infrequently, it can happen particularly easily that the partner oversees an initial or sustained depression.

At that we must realize that many couples have great difficulty in speaking about their relationship; and this holds particularly true for the whole field of sexuality.

Occasionally increased sexual activity is noticeable among depressives, particularly in the early phase and again toward recovery. This can have various reasons. It occurs that while becoming depressive some people try to have more sexual adventures as a distraction. Others notice if they are still capable of an orgasm that their mood brigthens up substantially and that fear is reduced after an orgasm. This phenomenon of reduced anxiety and tension after orgasm is similar to the experience induced by Jacobson's relaxation technique, which is frequently used for desensitization, a central behavioral modification technique. Various groups of muscles are repeatedly first tightened intensively and then relaxed. The relaxation is incompatible with tension or fear; in physiological terms it is known as "reciprocal inhibition." This procedure can be used in sexual therapy as well, as many symptoms appear as a result of the anticipation or fear of the symptoms. Therefore fear in general needs to be reduced. To desensitize a patient, he or she is requested to write down everything he or she is afraid of in the context of sexuality. In a second step the patient ranks these fears in a hierarchy: the least anxiety provoking items first, the most anxiety provoking items or situations last. With the help of relaxation techniques – e.g., the one by Jacobson, which has the advantage of being learned rapidly, but also the widely used autogenic training and others – a relaxed state is induced first. In this state the patient is asked to imagine the least fear provoking item, here some kind of intimacy. When no fear arises the next item in the hierarchy can be presented. As soon as fear arises, the thoughts have to be stopped immediately and replaced by more relaxation exercises. In this way it is possible gradually to overcome fear, fear of the symptom, and at last the symptom as such. This technique is first limited to mental images. Only in a later phase is the actual behavior modified, again along the same hierarchy. The method used by Masters and Johnson is nothing else but the application of the general behavior modification to the field of sexual disorders: The partners are only allowed to share intimacies up to the point where the partner can support them absolutely fearlessly. Again, as soon as anxiety arises the contact is interrupted and followed by more relaxation analogous to the imagination phase.

To summarize this point: The increased desire for sexuality in depressives during certain phases of their illness can originate from the fact that they experience less anxiety and less bad mood after an orgasm.

This can have two consequences: on one hand a fast striving for an orgasm without much regard for the sexual arousal of the partner. Frustration and tension will be the consequences for the partner. In their self-centeredness and with their reduced perceptual capacity the depressives are frequently not aware of the existence of this bad mood and these tensions. On the other hand this need for relaxation by orgasm may lead to a search for additional partners, even though they are accustomed to a faithful relationship, just to reach rapid sexual relaxation. This will happen particularly when the experience of the brightening of mood, immediately after the orgasm is paired with the desire to be active, again as a distraction from the depressivity.

Under similar circumstances, particularly bisexually inclined persons engage in a homosexual affair, which in these guilt-ridden depressives increases their feelings of guilt, ultimately leading to or supporting suicidal tendencies.

The same holds true for sadomasochistic actions which are occasionally seen during an initial depressive phase. These desires arise when libido is present and requires immediate relief of tension by an orgasm, but the potency is lacking. Out of this personal incapacity an aggressiveness may develop which is turned against the partner in the sense of sadism or against the self in the sense of masochism.

Such sexual problems within depression will always be influenced by the treatment of the depression as such. Monocausal depressions being relatively rare, independent from the nosological category, biologically based treatment such as pharmacotherapy, sleep deprivation, and possibly light therapy need to be combined with psychotherapy. There is a choice between the analytically oriented short therapy or crisis intervention and the use of behavioral modification techniques. Recently the cognitive elements within the behavioral technique have gained importance. However, particularly the sexuality clearly illustrates the necessity to include the social context in the treatment of depression, first of all the intimate partner. The early recognition and the corresponding treatment of the depression will simultaneously lead to an alleviation of these disorders. On the other hand, it needs to be mentioned that sexual difficulties, the neurotically induced ones in particular, can lead to a decompensation of the neurosis leading to the impression that sexual problems were the cause of the depression. In fact there are also psychoreactive depressions following sexual difficulties, especially among young adults who have not been so fortunate in their first intimate affairs. Impotence, e.g., which is most frequently caused by fear during first intercourse, can lead to the impression in a man that he is no real man and never will be potent. Such an experience can lead to the most severe depression and to a substantial suicidal risk.

References

Eicher W (1979) Psychosomatische Aspekte in der Gynäkologie. In: Uexküll TV (ed) Lehrbuch der psychosomatischen Medizin. Urban und Schwarzenbach, München Wien

Hole G, Poeldinger W (1968) Larvierte Depressionen und vegetative Symptome bei der Depression. Monatskurse f d ärztl Fortbldg 18:526–530
Kielholz P, Poeldinger W, Adams C (1981) Die larvierte Depression. Ein didaktisches Konzept zur Diagnose und Therapie somatisierter Depressionen. Deutscher Ärzteverlag, Köln
Nikolowski W, Poeldinger W, Spechter HJ (1978) Kompendium der Kohabitations- und Fertilitätsstörungen. Karger, Basel
Pöldinger W (1974) Larvierte Depressionen. Deutsch Ärzteblatt 71:1317–1324
Pöldinger W (1977) Sexuelle Störungen aus psychosomatischer Sicht. Z Allg Med 53:86–91
Pöldinger W (1981) Die Psychosomatik der sexuellen Störungen des Mannes. In: Jores A (ed) Praktische Psychosomatik, 2nd edn. Hans Huber, Bern
Pöldinger W (1981) Psychosomatosen und larvierte Depressionen. Ärztl Praxis Psychother 6:4–13
Pöldinger W (ed) (1984) Somatisierte Angst und Depressivität. Karger, Basel
Pöldinger W, Wider F (1986) Die Therapie der Depressionen. Deutsch Ärzteverlag, Köln

Sex After Myocardial Infarction

M. J. Halhuber

An der Gontardslust 17, 5920 Bad Berleburg, FRG

Survival, quality of life, and the management of all situations after an acute myocardial infarction are dependent on the *biography* of the patient, i.e., his behavior in the past, his present conditions, and how the patient anticipates his future. This is my basic experience as a cardiologist and rehabilitation expert after 20 years. My hypothesis in this paper on sex after myocardial infarction is based on this comprehensive psychosocial and biographical concept of cardiac rehabilitation, because the individual sexual behavior of the patient is an important symptom of the patient's biographical background.

The Patient's Past

The sexual life of the patient after a myocardial infarction also depends on the understanding or attitude the patient had regarding sex *before* the attack, on somatic and psychosocial risk factors, on the accepted attitude of the surroundings (especially of the spouse) and on many cultural influences. (As physicians we tend to neglect the influence of cultural values in the thinking and feeling of our patients and in our own judgment.) For example, when a man's sexual relationship with his wife was not a happy one, then it may be the wife who avoids relations after the attack with the excuse of them being a possible danger for the patient.

It is important to discover such subconscious reactions in the partnership to find the right kind of medical counseling.

Organomorphologically caused disturbances of potency were proven by Virag et al. at the Centre d'Etudes et de Recherches d'impuissance à Paris. One hundred percent of all patients with three to four established long-term standard risk factors such as smoking, diabetes, hyperlipidemia, and hypertension have sexual disorders, even without myocardial infarction. I think these findings are not well enough known to physicians and patients.

The cardiologist Friedman (Friedman et al. 1982) characterized infarct patients as follows: introvert, anxious to control all situations, obsessively responsible, performance oriented, and disciplined (type A). In the modern world a man endowed with such personality traits is influenced by several factors:

1. His sexual education, which is determined by sexual taboos
2. The dogma that performance and achievement are the key to being accepted
3. Social norms expecting males to hide their feelings

Sexology
Eds.: W. Eicher, G. Kockott

4. Advertising, which puts the male under achievement pressure: he is expected to be good-looking, young, dynamic, sexually active, imaginative, athletic, adventurous, etc.

The infarct patient is particularly haunted by a fear of failure in his career, his marriage, and in sports. To him this is tantamount to the fear of not being able to live, that is dying. If the sexual act is understood as a task to be achieved rather than as an expression of feeling toward his partner, the male will count each functioning sexual intercourse as a victory and the alternatives of masturbation or impotence as a defeat, since he does not prove his ability to perform. Some men react to just a single failure in an intimate situation with fears of renewed failure in the next coitus and with anticipatory conflicts. Their fears inhibit them in intimate situations. Hence, it is is not unlikely that their secret fears are self-fulfilling just because of their worries. The only way out of this vicious circle lies in a change in the patient's attitude toward failure. This change must be aided and supported by his partner.

If the female partner finds no fulfillment in the mutual sexual experience and has made the coronary patient aware of this before his illness, it can lead to feelings of guilt and depression in him. The depressive man tends constantly to check himself and observe his own sexual conduct, because he strives for sexual achievement for fear of being deserted by his partner. This intensive self-observation blocks spontaneity and prevents natural devotion. A wife hardly ever leaves her husband because of his impotence, least of all if their relationship has been intact otherwise. It is my impression that the wife may take the infarction of her husband as an excuse for the termination of all sexual intercourse. She does so under the pretext of being concerned about his health. But at the bottom it can frequently be found that she has not had a happy sexual life for decades. This is a kind of revenge the wife takes especially during menopause, when she feels a desire to withdraw anyway.

The Patient's Present Sexual Situation After the Acute Attack

Levy et al. (1985) examined the influence of myocardial infarction and bypass surgery on sexual relations and the perception of health and happiness at three levels:

1. At the symptomatological level as expressed by the frequency and severity of anginal pain
2. At the sexual level as expressed by the frequency of sexual relations
3. At the psychological level as expressed by the feelings of health and happiness

An estimate of the state of the patient in these fields was made both from his and from his spouse's viewpoint. According to the results of this study, a coronary artery bypass graft (CABG) contributes to an alleviation of symptoms and also to an improvement in the subjective feeling of health and happiness. According to the patients there is a decrease in the frequency of sexual relations, but according to the spouses there is a slight increase after CABG surgery. By contrast, there is a deterioration in the state of the myocardial infarction (MI) group in all parameters examined both from the point of view of the patients and from that of their spouses. In conclusion, CABG is not only beneficial in the alleviation of symptoms but also has a positive action in improving the quality of life of the patient.

What is the reason for the diminution of sexual relations after a heart attack, observed in the majority of patients? The most important reason is without doubt *anxiety*, the fear of dangerous reactions of physical activity by sexual intercourse, dangerous arrhythmias, angina pectoris, and sudden death. There is also a lack of information by the physicians about encouraging statistics. I would like to cite a paper from Garcia-Barreto et al. (1987): "Sexual Intercourse in Patients Who Have Had a Myocardial Infarction." "Thirteen men and ten women who had had a myocardial infarction were studied by 24 h ambulatory electrocardiographic (ECG) monitoring, during which time they had sexual intercourse. No statistical difference was found between male and female patients in peak heart rate, percent of maximum-age-calculated heart rate, or duration of sexual intercourse. Peak heart rate did not exceed, in any case, that caused by slight to moderate exercise. Four female patients experiencing sexual intercourse for the first time after infarction showed the lowest percentage of maximum-age-calculated heart rate. A marked increase was recorded in these patients during a second experience 15 days later, during which time they underwent physical and psychologic rehabilitation. Of 11 patients (nine men and two women) with premature ventricular contractions (PVCs) before coitus, only one man maintained arrhythmia during sexual intercourse. Of the 11 patients with PVCs, five recorded a lower PVC rate after sexual intercourse, during sleeping hours, compared with the rate they had before sexual activity. Two female patients had anginal pain and ST segment depression during sexual activity, accompanied by a heart rate lower than or equal to the peak heart rate reached during intercourse, suggesting a coexisting vasospastic component in their angina." (They needed nitrates before intercourse.)

The last statement provokes the question about the interaction of drugs and sexual intercourse of coronary patients. It is well known that nitro preparations (nitrates), especially when taken as a prophylactic, have a positive effect. It is also well known that hypotensive drugs, tranquillizers, and antidepressants have a negative effect on potency. Beta-blocking agents have a negative reputation, but it is probably not justified.

The Patient's Anticipated Future as an Emotional Cause of Sexual Problems After Myocardial Infarction

As regards sexual dysfunction men are mainly dominated by the fear of failure. They equate physical and/or emotional weakness with the loss of virility, which leads to a shattered sense of self-worth, depression, and isolation. I have observed anxiety, nervousness, and disturbed sleep in male patients who deny the existence of these problems and are excessively motivated to force themselves back to their former levels of performance. The anticipation of death and the imagination of hurt feelings arising from failure in sexual activity can provoke either partner to withdraw from personal intimacy and change their normal behavior. As a result of feelings of helplessness and dependence, these patients experience increased sensitivity and a desire for security, all of which surprises them. Unsophisticated blue-collar workers have particular difficulty in articulating and realizing such desires. Tensions within the family may arise and accumulate especially if the male patient loses his job, and has financial problems and demanding attitudes.

If the wife goes to work, the husband feels degraded in his role as a house husband; he turns aggressive and/or depressive. If he fails to do the regular housework, his wife will be irritated as a result of the double burden. The loss of money, image, and recognition often creates an atmosphere of latent aggression in which the partners blame one another.

Aims of Therapy and Counseling

Sexual counseling is an important component of the rehabilitation of all coronary patients, although to date there are no published data substantiating its effectiveness. A current research project, however, has shown that patients who receive appropriate sexual counseling return to a precoronary level of sexual activity more quickly than patients who do not receive such counseling. More research needs to be done in this area.

In instructing about sexual activity, as in other areas involving rehabilitation following an MI, a multidisciplinary approach and follow-up of the patient and his/her spouse are essential. Discharge often activates issues and concerns not felt during the period of hospitalization, and effective sexual counseling then occurs in the outpatient setting. This means that nurses working in expanded roles in community settings must be as knowledgeable as their colleagues in acute care settings about the issues and techniques of doing sexual counseling with coronary patients.

References

Friedman M et al. (1982) Feasibility of altering type-A behavior pattern after myocardial infarction. Circulation 66:83–92

Garcia-Barreto D et al. (1987) Sexual intercourse in patients who have had a myocardial infarction. J Cardiopul Rehab 6:324–328

Levy MJ et al. (1985) Sexual relations and the perception of health and happiness among patients following coronary artery bypass grafting and myocardial infarction. In: Walter PJ (ed) Return to work. Springer, Berlin Heidelberg New York

Sexual Disturbances in Diabetes Mellitus

H. R. Henrichs

Abteilung für Diabetologie, Evangelisches Krankenhaus, 4570 Quakenbrück, FRG

Following chronic renal failure and coronary heart disease, diabetes is a further cause of trouble with male sexuality. The common factor of these chronic diseases is their effect on well-being and self-esteem which might produce reactive psychogenic disturbances, e.g., erectile dysfunctioning. So far a common etiological view has led to common remedies: special sex counseling or the wide range of further psychological management.

But what is special with diabetes? Besides the mentioned nonspecific form, diabetic impotence represents a distinct entity that is an isolated erectile dysfunction, with the libido remaining normal. First mentioned in 1798 by Rollo, the latter specific form has seen greater interest in the past 10–20 years (Henrichs 1985). Reasons for this late development might be the prolongation of life and relative well-being of diabetics, which are paradoxically the prerequisite for the recognition of impotence symptoms. That follows the general improvement of the treatment of diabetes, its acute metabolic and its chronic functional consequences.

As this erective disorder is globally understood to be part of the diabetic complication syndrome, this automatically implies the idea of prevention. We believe the complications of diabetes to be the result of metabolic control of the disease, with no development of impotence as far as normoglycemia is established. This could be the basis of the solution of the problem in the future.

What is the incidence, severity, and prognosis of diabetic impotence today? Focussing on the fate of men with diabetic impotence, Podolsky (1982) stated: "It is not generally recognized that loss of erectile function is more threatening to many diabetic men than blindness or loss of a lower extremity due to gangrene." Rollo (1798 – some 189 years ago – described a 30-year-old man: "He is the father of several children, but since he has been seized with diabetes – coitus nullus. Erigitum numquam: Ne quidem semel regescit."

From a numerical point of view, the prevalence of impotence among diabetics gained from everyday clinical impression on the one hand and statistical data compiled from epidemiological or clinical studies on the other differ widely. From these sources, it can be estimated that 20%–60% of diabetic men will develop or complain of impotence to some degree throughout their sexual life, more often and much earlier (10–15 years; Lehman and Jacobs 1983) than nondiabetic men do. The astonishing wide range of the cited data reflects differences in the degree of impotence itself; differences in the degree of individual complaints; differences in the method of evaluation, interview or questionnaire, open or anonymous; and differences between the specialists performing the examination or study – urologist or diabetologist, psychologist or priest, psychiatrist or epidemiologist.

Sexology
Eds.: W. Eicher, G. Kockott

To obtain an impression of the difficulties involved in this area, we compared the figures of impotence noted in 224 of our male inpatient files with its presence or absence when asked for in a direct and systemic manner. The difference of 74% impotence in routine against 53% in subtle estimation can be understood to be part of a greater gray area, in this case dependent on the doctor's input as well as the patients' degree of complaint.

What is the main reason for diabetic impotence, its central etiology, assuming it is a somatic one? Up to now the question – formulated as an *overall* attempt at clarification – has been unresolved, unless one accepts the answers that there are several reasons or diabetes as such is *the* reason. For a diabetologist, this answer might not be surprising because diabetes itself represents a divergent kaleidoscope of events and sequences of the underlying shortage of insulin or insulin action.

Here it could be worthwhile remembering the steps in the history of diabetes: failure of or resistance to insulin – the most remarkable endocrine agent – with anabolic effects in all areas of metabolism (carbohydrates, protein, or fat) – establishes the primary event of the disease, which is marked by hyperglycemia and glucosuria, or by symptoms such as weakness, weight loss, polydipsia, or polyuria, demonstrating the catabolism in insulin deficiency.

Not surprisingly this metabolic derangement of untreated diabetics may rapidly cause impaired sexual function in man, resembling events during other acute illnesses. This impotence is reversible with treatment, e.g., with insulin insofar more owing to energy deficit and general weakness than specially to the diabetes: that is the temporary (early) form of impotence in diabetics showing both loss of libido and potency.

Insulin deficiency via hyperglycemia with time initiates specific functional and/or morphological changes in certain susceptible tissues and compartments of the organism, leading to the late complication syndrome.

Several mechanisms are under discussion concerning the way this disaster takes place: by favoring the so-called sorbitol pathway, hyperglycemia can establish – perhaps by lowering the myoinositol content and Na/K-ATPase activity, pathobiochemical derangements intracellularly or situated in the membrane. Hyperglycemia too is the condition which accelerates the nonenzymatic glycolysation of protein (and nucleic acid) substrates, thus leading to glycosylated adducts such as glycohemoglobin (HbA) to mention the best known. The glycosylation of nearly all protein moieties so far studied has been elucidated today, as shown by Vogt et al. 1982 in autopsy material.

The glycosylation-induced alteration of the physicochemical properties of substrates produces the multi-coloured detailed picture of the morphological and functional sequelae of diabetes, such as thickening of basal membrane protein in capillary blood vessels or glomerulae, loss of transparency of lens crystalline, forming diabetic cataracts, and altered myelin structure in nervous tissue. Carrier proteins, structure proteins, enzymes, hormones, nothing escapes this disastrous sugar impregnation. Only biological repair-mechanisms, measured as protein turnover rates, are able to restore the original state when further glycosylation is stopped by appropriate therapy, leading to normoglycemia. Prominent targets of glycosylation (and the exciting events of *advanced* glycosylation coming into attention recently) are vascular as well as neuronal structures. Additionally the glycosylate extracellular collagen matrix comes into consideration. From a clinical point of view the three pathobiochemically defined areas establish the battle fields of late diabetic complications: microangiopathy, polyneuropathy, and the steadily emergent diabetic collagen – a syndrome with certain links also to the macrovascular disease. These areas are therefore prime candidates when looking for the etiology of diabetic impotence once the temporary form has gone and the permanent or chronic version has appeared.

A number of clinical studies have been dedicated to describing one specific etiology: Do the results clarify the point? No, my understanding is that they induce another looking at.

The neat study of Lehmann and Jacobs in Philadelphia (1983) is a suitable example to demonstrate the situation: The authors evaluated 31 male diabetics for sexual dysfunction. Patients were examined by an endocrinologist, psychologist or psychiatrist, urologist, and neurophysiologist. They measured penile blood pressure and pudendal nerve latency and performed psychological and laboratory tests. The overall finding was that "68% of the patients had evidence of vascular occlusion, 26% had neurological abnormalities, 19% had low plasma testosterone levels, and 38% had relevant psychological problems; also the condition was considered primarily psychogenic in only 19%." The authors themselves interpret their observations to suggest that "vascular occlusion is the most prevalent abnormality in impotent diabetics and may predate neurological abnormalities" correlated to the severity of diabetes.

A multifactorial etiology would be a concurrent or better interpretation and could best fit with the above-developed understanding of late diabetes. In our small number of patients, for instance, we found more cases of concomitant neuropathy than microangiopathy. There is good evidence for more than one reason in favor of *neuropathy*. Ellenberg (1980) claims autonomic neuropathy to be a reason. Tegada et al. (1984) were able to demonstrate thickening of basement membranes of perineural cells as well as of Schwann's cells with electron microscopic investigation of penile tissue, thus underlining neurological causation. Blacklay et al. (1984) measured reduced levels of VIP vasointestinal polypeptide noradrenaline, and to a smaller extent further neurotransmitters in peniles of diabetic rats and men. Similar findings were reported by Melman et al. (1980). We understand these findings to be in accordance with demonstration of prolonged latency periods in bulbocavernosus reflex as a measure of the somatosensitive innervation.

In favor of *vascular etiology* are, e.g., the findings by Herman et al. (1978) in angiographic studies in impotent men. Similarly Jevtich et al. (1982, 1985) found arterial penile obstruction to be the cause of insufficiency.

In contrast to the vascular and neurological findings, which have been more or less accepted, the hypothesis of an *endocrine* imbalance or dysfunction leading to impotence – primary or secondary hypogonadism or prolactin disorders – until now has had a lack of convincing evidence in diabetics – at least to explain the major cause of insufficiency. This latter statement is corroborated by the demonstration of impotence in men with a normal endocrine status and by the lack of convincing evidence when hormonal therapy is used in an attempt to overcome the dysfunction.

Phenomenologically or naively diabetic impotence represents the disturbance of blood conservation under pressure within the corpora cavernosa and spongiosa as a combined result of illness-derived vascular (micro- and macroangiopathic) and neurological dysfunction, a concept which can explain clinical correlations with both vascular and neurological complications, shown by McCulloch et al. (1980) e.g. for retinopathy, neuropathy or nephropathy. Nevertheless the scientific game – vascular against neurological arguments – may go on: The clinical sence might be the translation of findings in therapeutic strategies: revascularization-oriented surgery on one hand and attempts at neurostimulatory intervention on the other.

Since papaverine and phentolamine have been found to be effective, an injection trial should be tried in all causes. The results of doing so will be the beginning of permanent treatment (CAT = cavernosal autoinjection therapy) or a further clue to understanding the underlying cause: insufficient erection after drug injection into the corpora cavernosa may be of vascular origin or due to venous leakage or aterial stenoses, thus further clarifying the etiology of somatic diabetic erectile dysfunction in the individual case.

The question of whether erectile impotence is psychogenic or somatic (Bancroft 1982), although of the utmost diagnostic and therapeutic value, in general seems to be answered easily, although it may present difficulties in individual cases. Nocturnal penile tumescence (NPT) measurements may be helpful in differential diagnosis. Kolodny et al. (1974) calculated 10% of impotence in diabetics to be psychogenic, lower than previously much greater calculations. Bearing in mind that both soma and psyche represent a biological unit, an absolute separation is neither possible nor desirable.

Which symptoms are typical of diabetic impotence? Chronic diabetic impotence establishes itself as an isolated erectile dysfunction, which develops in a slow progression from erectile weakness to inability, while libido (and ejaculation) may be preserved until finally weakened in reaction to reality.

By analysis of 18 questions answered by 257 patients, Rouleau et al. (1984) achieved 80% accuracy in discrimination of diabetic versus nondiabetic impotence, thus emphasizing the special entity of this condition. Eleven symptoms were significantly different: (1) Achieving only partial erection had the highest weight, followed by (2) not being able to climax under any circumstances, (3) a slow rather than sudden onset of the problem, (4) sustained sex drive, (5) no climax during intercourse, (6) decreased testicular pain sensation, (7) impotence not specific to partner, (8) loss of erection, (9) retarded ejaculation, (10) not being able to obtain a full erection and, lastly, (11) impotence present during nonintercourse sexual activities. Nevertheless, Fairburn et al. (1982) caution against oversimplification of the concept of diabetic impotence to a stereotyped picture. In Fairburn et al.'s cohort of impotent diabetics, morning erections were at least preserved in over 50% of cases, 30% having intact spontaneous erections, but sexual interest being reduced in 44%.

The practical consequences of looking for symptoms therefore only reduce diagnostic expenditure, but lead to the risk of misinterpretation. As a diagnostic arsenal for better differentiation, the specialists recommend: *angiology*, Doppler measurements of penile blood pressure, nocturnal tumescence tests, (digital substraction angiography), cavernosography, and SKAT, i.e., injection of papaverine and phentolamine. The *neurological* arsenal consists of systemic neurophysiological status, bulbocavernosus reflex latency, autonomic nervous function tests of bladder, and gastrointestinal and cardiovascular functions.

Treatment may be unspecific or specific: *Basic or specific therapy* or better *prevention* is identical to the best possible treatment of the diabetic state itself, e.g., intensified insulin treatment (CSII or intermittent following the basis-bolus-concept) to achieve a near normal metabolic state. The Vienna group of Irsigler (Najemik et al. 1984) reported recovery from impotence during insulin pump treatment for 1 year in a small group of 6 out of 18 patients. All treatment results nevertheless have to be looked at with caution, since Jensen (1986) found recovery after 6 years from sexual problems even without therapeutic procedures and even without any changes in diabetic state (speculating from this that psychological factors are of major importance as previously thought).

Adjuvant or unspecific measures consist of normalization of diabetes-associated hypertension, while avoiding certain potency-weakening drugs especially antihypertensive drugs (particularly in combination), diuretics of the thiacid group, beta-blocking agents, vasodilatatory agents, central effective agents such as clonidine, methyldopa, and reserpine, and also psychopharmacological especially tricyclic antidepressive drugs, neuroleptics, or alcohol.

Finally all kinds of *unspecific* treatment [sex counseling, pharmacological agents, administered systemically (?) or better locally (papaverine and phentolamine), revascularization surgery, implantation of penile prostheses, or perhaps neurostimulation techniques] have to be discussed and may be applied according to the patient's or the couple's degree of complaint. Testosterone treatment, unless replacement is indicated, is unnecessary or even contraindicated because it stimulates libido without enhancing potency. Both diagnosis and therapy may be carried out in "staircase"-like strategies. Psychological approaches aiming either to cure or to help at coping with an otherwise incurable problem are often indispensable too.

At the very end of my lecture it is to conclude:

1. The occurrence of impotence among diabetic men has got into interest in scientific, medical and public thinking as well.
2. We have to distinguish different kinds of appearance:
   2.1 Early transient forms, which belong to acute metabolic, catabolic derangement and are reversible with metabolic recovery.
   2.2 As a chronic illness diabetes may induce a certain amount of impotence from primary psychogen origin: expression of impaired selfesteem and reduced wellbeing.
   2.3 The intrinsic form nevertheless represents impotence in form of an isolated erectile dysfunction which – with good reasons – may be embedded in the late diabetes syndrom – a multi-coloured combination of vascular, neurological and collagen sited disturbance.
3. The modern diagnostic arsenal is suited to differentiate in specific cases the dominating etiology, a part of which already is to achieve by subtle analysis of symptoms and signs.

4. Therapeutic measures ranging from psychologic to surgical techniques have been enriched by the phentolamin-papaverin injection procedure. Together with the establishment of normoglycemia or near normal metabolic state we now therefore have to our disposal a realistic therapeutic arsenal, too: perhaps the turning-point of my theme, the sexual disturbances in male patients with diabetes mellitus.

References

Bancroft I (1982) Sexuality of diabetic women. Clinics in Endocrinology and Metabolism 11:785–789
Blacklay P, Crow R, Lincoln J, Pryor J, Lumley J, Burnstock G (1984) Vasoactive intestinal peptide and other neurotransmitter agents in the diabetic penis, pp 205–209
Ellenberg M (1980) Sexual function in diabetic patients. Ann Intern Med 92:311–333
Fairburn CG, Wu FCW, Mc Culloch DK, Borsey DQ, Ewing DJ, Clarke BF, Bancroft JHJ (1982) The clinical features of diabetic impotence: a preliminary study. Brit J Psychiat 140:447–452
Henrichs HR (1985) Störung der Potenz als Folge des Diabetes mellitus. Teil I: Versuch einer klinischen Übersicht. Teil II: Therapeutisches Vorgehen nach einem Fünf-Stufen-Schema. Sexualmedizin 14:266–272, 325–330
Herman A, Adar R, Rubinstein Z (1978) Vascular lesions associated with impotence in diabetic and nondiabetic arterial occlusive disease. Diabetes 27:975
Jensen SB (1985) Sexual dysfunction in younger insulin-treated diabetic females. Diabète Métab 11:278–282
Jensen SB (1986) Sexual dysfunction in insulin-treated diabetic. A six-year follow-up study of 101 patients. Arch Sex Behav 15:271–283
Jevtich MJ, Edson M, Jarman WD, Harrera HH (1982) Vascular factor in erectile failure among diabetics. Urology 19:163–168
Kolodny RC, Kahen CB, Goldstein HH, Barnett DM (1974) Sexual dysfunction in diabetic men. Diabetes 23:306–309
Lehmann TP, Jacobs JA (1983) Etiology of diabetic impotence. J Urol 129:291–294
Melmann A, Henry DP, Felten DL, O'Connor B (1980) Effects of diabetes upon sympathetic nerves in impotent patients. South Med J 307–309
Mc Culloch DK, Campbell IW, Wu FC, Prescott RI, Clarke BF (1980) The prevalence of diabetic impotence. Diabetologia 18:279–283
Najemnik C, Kritz H, Irsigler K (1984) Impotenz bei Typ I (Diabetikern). Verhalten nach 12 Monaten verbesserter metabolischer Kontrolle, 19. Jahrestagg. Dtsch. Diab. Ges. München 1984. Akt Endokrin 5:110
Podolsky S (1982) Diagnosis and treatment of sexual dysfunction in the male diabetic. Med Clin North Am 66:1389–1396
Rollo J (1798) John Rollo's Book. Cases of diabetes mellitus. Dilly, London. Zit. nach Reichel G (1987) Vegetative Symptome bei diabetischen Polyneuropathien. Fortschr Neurol Psychiat 55:107–129
Rouleau JL, Abel GG, Mittelman MS, White RDV, Becker JV, Cunningham-Rathner J (1984) Sexual symptoms specific to diabetes. Diabetes and Impotence, pp 215–219
Tejada JSM, Andry C, Blanco R, Goldstein I, Krane RJ (1984) Ultrastructural studies of autonomic nerves within the corpus cavernosum of impotent diabetic patients. Diabetes and Impotence, pp 210–214
Vogt BW, Schleicher ED, Wieland OH (1982) γ-Amino-lysine bound glucose in human tissues obtained at autopsy: increase in diabetes mellitus. Diabetes 31:1123–1127

Sexual Dysfunction in Epileptic Patients: A Preliminary Report

S. B. Jensen, P. Jensen, P. S. Sørensen

From Rigshospitalet University Hospital, Dept N, DK 2100 Copenhagen Ø, Denmark

From the Myth of Epilepsy and Sexuality to a Biopsychosocial Approach

Epilepsy has a prevalence of 1% in most Western societies. It is mostly accepted as a chronic disease related to cerebral dysfunction and the treatment is primarily the administration of medications, some of which are known to have an impact on hormonal balance. Epileptics share in common with other chronic diseases that the patients will live in a chronically ill role. The epileptic patient and the couple where one partner has an epileptic symptomatology are at risk of developing sexual dysfunction as part of this general role as chronically ill – from epilepsy-specific factors and from the same factors as individuals without any chronic disease.

A critical review of the literature reveals considerable methodological concerns and may question many of the conclusions drawn from these studies. It is obvious that myths of epilepsy and sexuality may range from witchcraft to comparisons of epileptic convulsions and sexual orgasm. The reported frequencies of sexual problems among epileptics are considerable. Most studies report that more than one-half of male epileptic patients and 60%–70% of epileptic women have sexual problems. The main flaws of previous studies concern the skewed patient-material, where the patient may often have many associated medical and neurological complications or may live in institutions. The different subgroups of epileptic patients and the different treatment programs in different clinics will further complicate the picture.

Although some biological explanations have been offered, mostly of a hormonal nature or as a direct central cerebrotemporal factor, it would be reasonable to state that we are without a simple explanation of sexual dysfunction in epileptic patients. The complicated nature of the symptom picture, and the psychosocial aspects which are known to be of influence on the epileptic patient, makes it more natural to see the sexual symptom from a biopsychosocial approach.

This approach has been elaborated in our recent textbook *Sexuality and Chronic Illness. A Comprehensive Approach* (Schover and Jensen 1987). From this perspective the sexual symptom is seen as a result of the interaction of biological, psychological, and social factors in a time perspective. In the book criteria for studying sexual dysfunction in chronic disease are discussed, and this comprehensive approach is chosen in the study of epileptic outpatients we have performed in the past months. We are able to present some of our preliminary results here.

Sexology
Eds.: W. Eicher, G. Kockott

Preliminary Results of the Study

During a period of 6 months 244 epileptic patients were seen in the epilepsy clinic in a neurological department at the University Hospital in Copenhagen. Included in the study were patients 21–55 years of age and patients with detailed specified epileptic syndromes with focus on cryptogenic epileptics, while other convulsive conditions, for example, alcohol- or medication-induced convulsions, were excluded. Patients with a severe psychopathology, severe mental retardation, and associated chronic somatic disease (like diabetes, hypertension, and sclerosis) were excluded.

Seventy-five patients (30%) did not meet the age criteria and 69 patients were excluded because of associated medical disease ($n=20$), severe mental retardation ($n=18$), and other exclusion criteria, leaving 100 patients who were asked to participate. Eighty-six patients, 38 men and 48 women, agreed to participate and were evaluated by questionnaire, clinical interview, and hormonal tests. The neurological data were systematically drawn from the files. The mean age was 38 years (21–55 years) and 75% of the patients were married or were living with a steady sexual partner.

Most patients were in good control based on values of antiepileptic drugs in the blood and the reports of number of convulsions inside the past month and the past year. Fifty percent had no attack inside the past year and only five patients, all having psychomotorical epilepsy, had more than five attacks inside the past month. Seventy-five percent were on monotherapy, with carbamazepine as the most common drug. Disease acceptance was evaluated clinically and by questionnaire and classified into three groups, based on a previous study, as good, medium, or bad, Nearly 80% of the patients had a good disease acceptance with an adequate coping behavior and treatment compliance. All patients had a test of their hormonal status, including androgenic status, estrogenic status, FSH, LH, prolactin, thyroid hormones, and electrolytes. The level of antiepileptic medicine in the blood was controlled as well.

Results concerning sexual dysfunction were compared with results from a control group from a previous study of diabetics and controls (Jensen 1981) – a study carried out in the same research group with similar methodology. Sexual dysfunction was not seen with any higher frequency among epileptics compared with the nonpatient control group. Seventeen percent of the men and 27% of the women reported at least one sexual dysfunctional symptom:

In men: erectile dysfunction, 3%; reduced sexual desire, 3%; retarded ejaculation, 8%; and premature ejaculation, 3%.

In women: reduced sexual desire, 19%; orgasmic dysfunction, 19%; and vaginismus, 0%. Hormonal tests showed no significant differences on any parameter studied comparing epileptics with and without sexual dysfunction. As a group epileptic males had a slightly decreased level of free testosterone compared with the normal range, but still inside the normal limits. These results in epileptic men were significantly different from results from the percentages of sexual dysfunction in diabetic males, while similar for epileptic women compared with diabetics.

The preliminary conclusion from this study is that sexual dysfunction in this group of epileptic patients is not different from results in studies of a nonpatient population – and none of the hormonal factors measured could offer a single factor explanation for the sexual symptoms. This difference compared with the literature may be explained by the fact that this patient group did not include epileptic patients with complicating diseases and included only outpatients, where most of them were occupationally active (87%). This offers the perspective that epileptic patients in good medical control and with a good disease acceptance may have a sexual life which is not necessarily influenced by the disease or the treatment of the disease. This perspective does not call for a neglect of the sexual life and problems of epileptics, which is common in most textbooks and patients' guides. It presents the importance of combining an optimal medical treatment with an optimal caretaking of the psychosocial aspects of the disease to avoid unnecessary sexual suffering among these patients and their partners.

Reference

Schover LR, Jensen SB (1987) Sexuality and chronic illness. A comprehensive approach. Guilford, New York

Cancer and Sexuality in Women

C. Buddeberg

Abteilung für Psychosoziale Medizin, Universitätsspital Zürich,
8091 Zürich/Switzerland

The opinion that sexuality is for healthy people only, that sick people should abstain from sexual intercourse, is widespread: Not only healthy people and physicians, but often also sick people themselves are convinced that when they are sick they do not need sexual activity. How important is sexuality in the life of women that have cancer? Is it, as a disease that threatens life, only an unimportant matter, in which, as the case may be, sexologists are interested, or is it of some importance in the life of a woman with cancer? In the past few years the question concerning the quality of life in the treatment of cancer patients has been increasingly observed. Very different aspects, such as time of life, psychic and physical condition, interpersonal relations, material resources, use of leisure time, meaning of life and goals of life, and, not least of all, the experience of the own body and sexual satisfaction have meaning for the quality of life of the woman with cancer.

Within a prospective study to examine the problem of coping in the course of a malignant disease, we asked 107 newly afflicted women with breast cancer about their quality of life. Sexual dissatisfaction was given first, followed by dissatisfaction with the altered own body as the second most important problem. Especially in the case of a gynecologically malignant disease, the woman feels herself deeply unsure in her female identity, the image of her body, and her sexuality. Yet it is often the question of sexuality that is strictly avoided by both the patient and her partner and also by the physician. Sexuality is regarded as relatively unimportant and is therefore neglected frequently in the treatment of cancer patients. What are the reasons for the neglect and slighting of sexual matters in the treatment of these patients? It seems that our attitude toward persons suffering from cancer is allied with a widespread and more or less unconscious belief *that sexuality itself is a disease, which only healthy people can endure*. For the ill, as is often argued, sexual activity, primarily orgasm, is something which they should avoid. What fears are there behind the prejudice that is deeply rooted among both the healthy and the sick that disease and sexuality are not to be combined? In the counselling of women with cancer and their partners certain motives for fears appear over again in the reference to sexual questions; I list them here:

- One fear is that sexual activity is too strongly demanding and contains the danger of a sudden "love-death", that is death during sexual intercourse. In the widest sense this has to do with fear of death, for the defence against which general caution, not least in sexual activities, is recommended to the sick person.
- There is a fear of the healthy person that by sexual intercourse with a patient he or she might become infected with the disease. This fear one finds, e.g.,

Sexology
Eds.: W. Eicher, G. Kockott

among men whose wives have undergone surgery and irradiation because of genital cancer, and who then no longer engage in sexual relations with their wives.

- There is a fear that the sick person, especially after mutilating surgery, will shock their partner by the sight of their injured body and that they will be left as a consequence of the shock, by the partner; it is a fear of loss.
- Finally there are the fears of insufficiency, which arise foremost among those woman patients whose disease has led to an impairment of the capacity for sexual function. This is the case primarily after genital surgery and irradiation of the genital organs.

The fears mentioned are not at all specific for cancer patients and their partners. One finds them among other sick people, too, and among bodily healthy persons who are insecure in their competence for sexual reaction and experience. Just as there is no typical person with cancer and no typical characteristics of women suffering from cancer, there are no typical sexual problems of these women.

Sexual Difficulties of Women with Cancer

In my work as a psychosomatic consulting physician at the Gynecological Clinic of the University Hospital of Zurich, I repeatedly experience that sexual difficulties of tumor patients are frequently not noticed, are slighted, and are not treated at all or in a doubtful way. Sexual problems are mostly signals of difficulties not only of the cancer patient, but as often of difficulties of the partner, too, in coping with the psychosocial consequences of cancerous disease.

The effects of cancer upon the sexuality of the afflicted person have so far been investigated most profoundly among women with breast cancer (Buddeberg 1985, 1987; Frank et al. 1978; Spengler and Wickert 1981). The results of various studies may be summarized in the following conclusions:

The sexuality of women suffering from breast cancer is determined strongly by the age of the individual woman. Younger women are more active at all levels of sexual interaction and rather able to reintegrate sexuality soon after mastectomy. Conversely women who are more than 55 years old frequently develop a behavior of sexual avoidance that is determined by complete lack of sexual desire. Disturbances of sexual function in the proper sense as a consequence of mastectomy are relatively infrequent. Among many healthy women, too, the biological and psychosocial changes in the phase from the 50th to the 60th year of life lead to a lessening of sexual wishes and sexual activities. Conversely, however, sexual inappetence and behavior of sexual avoidance can also be symptoms of an unsuccessful adaptation to the new life situation. In the sexuality of couples in which women have undergone mastectomy, many fears and conflicts of coping with the disease can be shown symbolically.

Also among women with a genital carcinoma the reduction of sexual desires and behavior of sexual avoidance are frequent problems (Spengler and Schneidermann 1981; Raboch et al. 1985) which can disturb the rehabilitation of these women. Besides, as a sequel of radiotherapy, lubrication can be impaired and with it to various degrees the ability for sexual function.

How much may these findings that were obtained from women suffering from cancer be generalized? Since the adaption to a serious disease is influenced not only by its nature and seriousness, but also through intrapsychic factors of the sick person as well as environmental factors (Lazarus and Launier 1978; Lipowski 1970), the influences of a malignant disease on the sexuality of the individual patient are multiple and rather different. There are woman cancer patients whose sexual life is not deranged by the disease or only slightly, and equally women for whose sexual life the disease has profound consequences. The sexuality of woman cancer patients should therefore not be seen separately from the way in which they cope with the disease. Still, according to my experience, there are some aspects which are of special importance for the sexuality of women sick with cancer:

In the first months after the diagnosis and if the disease is progressing, sexual wishes and activities have a subordinate role; in these periods there is, however, a great need for bodily closeness and a feeling of "homeness," which only few cancer patients can express. Since their partners, because of their own fears regarding the disease, do not perceive these needs, frequently an emotional and bodily separation arises between the two. Some couples succeed, after the stabilization of the physical course of the disease, in removing this separation without help from outside; yet others are not able to overcome again the emotional distance that has been caused by the illness. In such cases, in the presence of a somatically favorable course of the illness, a situation that is increasingly onerous for both partners may occur, which they cannot overcome without help from outside. The sexual difficulties of which woman cancer patients complain most frequently are deficiency of libido, and, when libido is present, a behavior of sexual avoidance. Disorders of sexual desire as a whole are, together with other symptoms, a reference to a depressive syndrome that is caused by the disease. The avoidance of sexual contacts in the presence of sexual desires can indicate that the woman has not yet succeeded in identifying herself with that image of her own body that has been altered by the cancerous disease.

Sexual reserve and passive behavior become reinforced additionally by the sexual patterns of roles that are as effective now as they have been in the past. If it is valid that even the healthy woman should react sexually, as the occasion may occur, to the initiatives of her male partner, but not act of her own volition, then this is valid in a special way for sick women. I have repeatedly heard from women with breast cancer that their male partners receive very poorly from them their cautious indications of erotic wishes. More important though than general determination seems to me to be the understanding of the individual coping processes and those of the dynamics of the couple; I mean those processes that make understandable the sexual difficulties of a pair in consequence of cancer. Two brief case reports may exemplify and clarify this:

Case 1, Behavior of Sexual Avoidance

A 36-year-old woman reported 6 months after undergoing mastectomy that since then she had neither shown her scar to her husband nor had sexual relations with him. She wanted to know from me how long her husband could endure this without taking up sexual relations with another woman. Before the operation on the breast her sexual life had been very intensive and satisfying for both partners. In the discussion the patient frankly expressed her feelings of shame because of her mutilation and her fear of losing her husband. Before I invited the husband to a joint consultation, I discussed with the wife concrete possibilities leading to a gradual removal of her behavior of sexual avoidance. It seemed possible to her while wearing at first a brassiere and a T-shirt to begin sexual relations with her husband; the husband, too, agreed. After some weeks the woman was able to exchange with her spouse intense caressing over the whole body except the mastectomy scar.

Case 2, Intensified Sexual Activity

As a consequence of a carcinoma of the cervix uteri with two local recidivations, a woman of 48 years of age had a vagina that is only 5 cm long. She reported that since the last operation her husband wished daily sexual intercourse, which she allowed unwillingly, that otherwise her spouse was very loving and considerate of her, and that, however, his sexual drive had increased since her cancer operation to such a degree that it was no longer tolerable for her. She felt nothing at all during sexual intercourse, yet was fearful of rejecting her husband. In a joint consultation with her husband, it was found that his increased sexual activity was the expression of his fears of losing his wife. He sensed the daily execution of sexual union as the proof that his wife was still healthy and had overcome her illness. The wife had quite strong fears of injury and the idea that too frequent intercourse could lead to a recidivation of her cancerous disease. For this couple the sex counselling had as its purpose, besides reducing the fears of loss and of injury, discussing with both partners possibilities of a nongenital sexual practice.

As was mentioned initially, sexual satisfaction plays a not unimportant role in the quality of life of women with cancer. Therefore, sexual counselling should be a fixed part in the aftercare of women who have or have had cancer. Their own inhibitions and inadequate sexual medical knowledge prevent, however, now as in the past, many physicians from discussing sexual questions with their patients. Sexual difficulties as a result of mutual behavior of avoidance of both partners can often be removed with an advisory talk or can at least be lessened. The transmission of information about the interaction of somatic and psychic factors for the attainment of a satisfactory sexual life, the diminution of false conceptions and inhibitions, and the discussion of possible behavioral changes for overcoming the behavior of mutual avoidance are the most important tasks of such counselling. The ability to experience sexual activity and satisfaction despite limited physical health, which is threatened moreover by the disease, for many people suffering from cancer is an aid to accepting the disease and living with it.

References

Buddeberg C (1985) Ehen krebskranker Frauen. Urban & Schwarzenberg, München
Buddeberg C (1987) Sexualberatung – Eine Einführung für Ärzte, Psychotherapeuten und Familienberater, 2nd edn. Enke, Stuttgart
Frank D, Dornbush RL, Webster SK, Kolodny RC (1978) Mastectomy and sexual behavior: a pilot study. Sexuality and Disability 1:16–26
Lazarus RS, Launier R (1978) Stress-related transactions between person and environment. In: Pervin LA, Lewis M (eds) Perspectives in interactional psychology. Plenum, New York, pp 287–327
Lipowski ZJ (1970) Physical illness, the individual and the coping process. Int J Psychiatr Med 1:91–102
Raboch J, Boudnik V, Raboch J Jr (1985) Das Geschlechtsleben nach der Hysterektomie. Geburtsh Frauenheilk 45:48–50
Spengler A, Schneidermann S (1981) Abdominale Hysterektomie und Sexualität. In: Schorsch E, Spengler A (eds) Zur psychischen und sexuellen Situation von Patienten nach Genitaloperationen. Forschungsbericht, Hamburg, pp 21–66
Spengler A, Wickert J (1981) Mastektomie und Sexualität. In: Schorsch E, Spengler A (eds) Zur psychischen und sexuellen Situation von Patienten nach Genitaloperationen. Forschungsbericht, Hamburg, pp 67–126

Gynecological Cancer and Sexual Disturbances

D. Richter

District Hospital, Department of Obstetrics and Gynecology, Meisenhartweg, 7880 Bad Säckingen, FRG

Treatment of gynecological carcinomas has progressed enormously, achieving considerable cure and survival rates. Nevertheless, the prejudice of being incurable continues to be held against this disease, and it also continues to be closely associated with the attributes of sinister, treacherous, and incalculable. In an unrestrained consumer society in which youth and beauty, health, and vitality are glorified above all else, the notions of physical invalidism and incurable disease are pushed into the background, and the problem of death is taboo. These social conditions promote fear of cancer as well as it is fatalistically regarded as a disease with a fatal outcome. Neither extensive preventive medical programs nor health education campaigns have changed this very much. Far-reaching therapeutic measures such as surgery, radiotherapy, and chemotherapy change and deform the body and lead to serious damage of self-esteem. Female cancer patients feel devalued, socially and emotionally no longer capable of communication, socially isolated, and sexually unattractive. In fact, even though they are pitied to a certain extent, they are often shunned at work, by friends, yes even by their own family and beloved partner. Thus, to have cancer not only means fear of being in the hands of a treacherous disease, but especially fear of social isolation and of losing recognition and affection. Beyond the individual psychological disorder of the female patient, the diagnosis of cancer leads to damage in the family and environmental situation.

The idea must be discarded that everything has been done by initiating surgery, radiotherapy, or chemotherapy. The reality we must face is the individual woman who has fallen ill with cancer. Besides her cancer disease, she has many further qualities. She has her family, her profession, her position in society, her character, her convictions, her love, and her sexuality. To begin with, a female patient's quality of life largely depends on the success of surgery, radiotherapy, or chemotherapy. In this case, scientific interest with regard to assessment of treatment success centers on cancer cure rates. Until now, the question of "how" the female cancer patient has lived between discovery of the disease and cure or death has scarcely or insufficiently been asked. In spite of the fact that, recently, attention has also been given to problems of a female patient's quality of life, an objective estimation of the intensity and duration of the annoyances and strain, of the pain and misery, and of the fears and needs a woman with cancer may experience is still lacking. Care of cancer patients must take more and more into account the need to define goals of special importance for the lives of these women; tumor aftercare will have to develop concepts which give substance to the idea of quality of life.

Sexology
Eds.: W. Eicher, G. Kockott

Table 1. Sexual dysfunction of gynecological cancer patients

Author	*n*	Carcinoma	Frequency (%)
Froewis, Picha (1955)		Endometrial	30
Erkrath, Randow (1967)		Cervical	50
Henning, Schulz (1975)	201	Cervical	50
Maguire (1978)		Breast	33
Eicher, Herms (1979)		Breast	50
Pfleiderer, Richter (1979)	100	Cervical, endometrial	22
Herschbach et al. (1985)	95	Cervical	18
Herschbach et al. (1985)	385	Breast	14

Psychosexual disturbances constitute a special problem during or after cancer treatment. Yet, sexual problems are all too frequently, if not altogether, ignored by doctors and nurses. However, especially patients with breast and genital carcinomas have a strong desire to talk about these problems. For many women, sexuality, as a closely ego related way of making experience, is a sphere of conflict even when in a healthy condition; this holds true much more for female patients who have gone through drastic carcinoma therapy affecting their genital organs. For instance, carcinosis of the genital organs may elicit numerous feelings of guilt.

According to Eicher and Herms (1979), e.g., half the number of female patients who have had mastectomy anticipate a disturbance of the relationship with their partner and, consequently, react with enormous sexual disorders. All investigators have unanimously arrived at the result that the sexual life of female carcinoma patients degenerates. In spite of the fact that the various studies applied very different methods, it can be stated in general that the most obvious results are a decrease in libido, a decrease in coitus frequency, an increase in orgasm disturbance, and an increase in pain during sexual intercourse (dyspareunia).

Table 1 lists studies carried out in the past 30 years which investigated sexual life after genital cancer. Striking is the fact that, lately, sexual disturbances seem to appear less frequently than in the past. With 62% of our patients treated for a uterus carcinoma between 1974 and 1976 we found sufficient libido, and this at an average age of more than 50 years. Sexual intercourse, still achieved by 78% of the couples before the onset of the disease, continued with 65% of the couples after the disease was diagnosed. Ability to experience orgasm, testified by 79% of women before, continued in 57% of cases after onset of the disease. We agree with Herschbach et al. (1985) that these more favorable results in recent time have to do with better information and psychosomatically oriented care given to the female cancer patient. As early as in the course of preparatory talks before surgery or radiotherapy, the attempt must be made to evaluate the patient's psychosexual situation. In order to be able to detect possible irrational fears and apprehensions, it has proven advantageous to question the patient in a direct manner – after the reasons for surgery or radiotherapy have been explained to her by the doctor – whether or not and, if yes, which physical, mental, and sexual changes she expects. On one hand, this method reveals the patient's level of information, and false ideas can be corrected. On the other hand, the psychosomatically oriented gynecologist can find out whether innermost fears and apprehensions exist which might increase after surgery.

Directly after surgical treatment, however far-reaching or even mutilating it has been, the attempt is made, following a reactive phase of shock or sorrow varying in length, to reconcile the patient with her body, to help her accept her modified body once again. Doctors, nurses, or physiotherapists can contribute substantially to this process of reconciliation by providing emphatic, unreserved, and loving care. As early as during the stay in hospital, sexual life after cancer treatment is made a topic of detailed conversation, if possible together with the partner. If necessary, exploration of the partner alone can take place. In this case, widespread prejudices, such as men's fear of infection by sexual intercourse with their cancer-affected wife, may arise. Furthermore, as a prophylactic measure aiming at mental hygiene, we try to make partners of cancer patients understand that it is favorable for the course of the disease and for the final recovery from carcinoma if they are able to give their wife the feeling that she continues to be erotically attracting and sexually desirable. As far as necessary, the direct effects cancer treatment might possibly have on the genital organs are discussed, such as disturbance of vaginal lubrication, fibrosis of the vaginal tube after radiotherapy, vaginal atrophy, stenosis, or conglutination. We have experienced that the best prophylactic measure against coition inability is for the woman to resume sexual intercourse in due time, 2–6 weeks after the end of hospital treatment, of course with adequate care taken by the partner. The couple's attention is also drawn to the fact that a bloody vaginal discharge after coitus can be caused by reopening conglutination, which is not harmful, but, on the contrary, favorable to the improvement of sexual intercourse.

The woman undergoing therapy against cancer suffers from a feeling of sexual insufficiency toward her partner. This is where our help must begin. The confidential talk with her doctor – during the examination before discharge from hospital, at the latest – and, if possible, with the partner's participation, is an important aspect of medical aftercare of cancer patients, helps diminish anticipation anxiety, and prevents secondary psychosexual problems in many cases.

In addition, long-term psychosomatically oriented care of female cancer patients should include the following aspects: after individual information about the nature of the disease, removal of fear, depression, and guilt from the patient; learning to cope with physical changes caused by therapy in order to strengthen self-esteem and a positive body image; immediate inclusion of the partner and family when given a diagnosis and planning treatment; communication and encouraging support when it is time to resume the sexual relationship; and improvement of social contacts.

Despite the fact that psychosomatically oriented guidance of female cancer patients within a comprehensive treatment plan is still in its swaddling clothes, its necessity must be underlined.

References

Eicher W, Herms V (1979) Zur Epidemiologie des Mamma-Carcinoms. Fortschr Med 97(38):1638

Erkrath FA, Randow H (1967) Vita Sexualis nach Karzinombehandlung im Vergleich zu nicht krebskranken berufstätigen Frauen. Zbl Gynäk 89:1210–1216

Froewis J, Picha E (1955) Der Einfluß der Radikaloperationen bei Carcinoma colli uteri auf das Sexualleben der Frau mit besonderer Berücksichtigung der Wertheimschen Operation. Geburts Frauenheilk 15:806–810

Herschbach P, Rosbund AM, Brengelmann JC (1985) Probleme von Krebspatientinnen und Formen ihrer Bewältigung. Onkologie 8:219–231

Henning G, Schulz St (1975) Sexualverhalten von Patientinnen nach der Therapie von Zervixkarzinomen. Zbl Gynäk 97:1562–1570

Maguire GP (1978) Psychiatry problems in the first year after mastectomy. Br Med J 1:963

Pfleiderer A, Richter D, Thiessen P, Kissel U, Tibi P, Nowara P (1979) Aktuelle Probleme bei der Nachsorge von Patientinnen mit Carcinomen der Cervix und des Corpus uteri. Onkologie 2:62–69

Male Sexuality and Cancer

M. Beutel

Institut und Poliklinik für Psychosomatische Medizin,
Psychotherapie und Med. Psychologie der Technischen Universität München,
Langerstraße 3, 8000 München 80, FRG

Suffering from a chronic disease like cancer causes a disruption in a person's life, necessitating readaptation not only in daily living activities, but also in self-concept and relationships to others. How patients handle manifold stresses of cancer is explored under the *stress-coping paradigm*. This implies that patients are not seen as passive victims of a hardly bearable illness, but as active constructors of a reality which is at least tolerable. Affective state, social functioning, etc., in this perspective depend not so much on objective stresses, but on *how* these are appraised and dealt with. Coping strategies are highly individually variable and aim either instrumentally at changing the aversive situation or at dealing with painful emotions when the problem itself cannot be modified (Beutel 1987).

Especially for male cancer patients sexuality is one important area of adaptation distinguished from others by its special features of shame and speechlessness. It is striking that sexual problems are rarely expressed spontaneously. Occasional remarks are made incidentally in a joking or even obscene manner. This should not obscure the amount of suffering behind sexual problems.

A 74-year-old former test pilot with tonsillar cancer is referred to consultation because of "lack of social support." The depressive and mistrustful patient emphasizes there is nothing wrong with him. He would be only concerned because of the impending sale of his house. As the reason for this he claims that neigbors would make up to his wife during his hospitalization. During the consultation, anxieties of losing his 10-year-younger wife, disfigurement, and losing his potency become clear. The discussion of these issues provides a marked relief for the patient.

The wife the same age as her husband, a 54-year-old engineer with inoperable pancreatic cancer, complains incidentally about the complete lack of sexual interest of her husband during a phone call for arranging an appointment. When the topic is brought up in the joint conversation by the therapist, the patient reveals that he feels the disease and the loss of vocational activity and physical ability is a "demascularization," toward which he reacts deeply depressively, and for the first time since the diagnosis the couple resumes sexual contact.

On behalf of the – in the majority also male – *physicians* there is often little inclination to address sexual concerns or refer to specialized treatment when needed. Causes for this reservation are certainly manifold. Investigations of general physicians (e.g., Pacharzina 1979) demonstrate significant lack of sexological knowledge. In addition to language barriers and untested beliefs according to which sexuality has only minor importance in the face of the vital threat of cancer,

Sexology
Eds.: W. Eicher, G. Kockott

Table 1. Sexual problems in patients with testicular cancer

Ejaculatory dysfunction	35%–80%	Bracken and Johnson (1976)
	81%	Klippel and Weisbach (1976)
	45%	Narayan et al. (1982)
	37%	Rieker et al. (1985)
	57%	Schover and von Eschenbach (1985)
Reduced orgasmic intensity	38%	Schover and von Eschenbach (1985)
Erectile dysfunction	25%	Klippel and Weissbach (1976)
	10%[a]	Schover and von Eschenbach (1985)
Fears of infertility	21%	Schover and von Eschenbach (1985)
	31%	Rieker et al. (1985)
Strains by mutilation	44%	Klippel and Weissbach (1976)
Relationship problems	25%	Schover and von Eschenbach (1985)
	32%	Married couples, Rieker et al. (1985)
	74%	Unmarried couples, Rieker et al. (1985)

[a] ≥50% of the tima: lymphadenectomy, 6.5%; plus chemotherapy 2.6%; +radiotherapy ±chemotherapy 23.5%.

concerns of inducing sexual dysfunctions by preparatory information, etc., are further reasons.

As recent research (e.g., Verres 1986) has shown, cancer still carries the stigmata of immoral conduct, just punishment, and contagion in the healthy population. This is also expressed by comparisons with plague, cholera, and venereal diseases. Over 40% of the healthy sample studied by Verres (1986) voiced strong resentment toward close physical contact with cancer victims.

The speechlessness mentioned initially has been reflected in a lack of *studies* on sexual problems of male cancer patients, while the sexual consequences of cancer of the breast or gynecological cancer have been the subject of many investigations.

I wish to give an overview over some more recent studies on sexual problems of male cancer patients, exemplified by testicular and prostatic cancer, and I wish to conclude with some remarks on coping and counselling issues.

1. Sexual problems in patients with testicular cancer. Hardly any other cancer has been subject to such a decisive progress in treatment which raises longterm survival even for metastatic disease (from about 10% to 70%–80%) so drastically (Dold and Sack 1985). The disease strikes mostly young patients in their 2nd and 3rd decades. Therapeutically mostly a unilateral orchiectomy is performed, seminoma being treated by irradiation, other cancers by resection of paraaortal lymph nodes, in the case of systemic spread by chemotherapy. Table 1 presents an overview of sexual problems.

In the foreground of sexual problems of mostly curatively treated testicular cancer patients (studied betwen 2 and 10 years after treatment) are *ejaculatory dysfunctions* (between 35% and 81%) with reduced semen volume. This is often accompanied by reduced orgasmic intensity (38%). An important organic cause is retrograde ejaculation due to a lesion of the sympathic nerve plexus by retroperitoneal lymphadenectomy. According to Narayan et al. (1982), however, there

Table 2. Sexual problems in patients with prostatic cancer

Erectile dysfunction	75% 79%	Bergman et al. (1984) Goldstein et al. (1984)
Discontinued coital activity	41% 39%	Bagshaw et al. (1975) Bergman et al. (1984)
Ejaculatory/orgasmic dysfunction	20%	Bergman et al. (1984)
Maintenance of sexual desire	70% 88% 42%	Spengler and Kleber (1982) Goldstein et al. (1984) Bergman et al. (1984)

is a tendency toward recovery of anterograde ejaculation within 2–3 years after treatment. In general, *erectile dysfunction* is rarely observed, but may increase with the progression of the tumor stage and intensity of therapy, according to Schover and von Eschenbach (1985) from an average of 4% after lymphadenectomy (without chemotherapy) to about 25% after lymphadenectomy plus radiotherapy plus chemotherapy.

Fears of infertility are common, raised either by the ejaculatory disorder or fears to transmit the disease to the offspring. Important measures like sperm cryoconservation (if possible) or attempts at treating the ejaculation disorder by sympathomimetic substances are by themselves insufficient without detailed counselling.

The few studies exploring *subjective meaning* or phantasies of losing one testicle show strains by mutilation for almost half the patients. While *problems* in the *partner relationship* are reported by 25% in one study (Schover and von Eschenbach 1985), Rieker et al. (1985) found problems in 32% of those married and even in 74% of unmarried patients.

2. Sexual problems in patients with prostatic cancer. Distinct from testicular cancer, prostatic cancer is a very frequent disease in a much older population. When the cancer is confined to the prostate, radical operation or radiation are mostly performed. Estrogen treatment and bilateral orchiectomy, respectively, or radiation are employed in the metastatic stage. In general previously sexually active patients are studied (e.g., Bergman et al. 1984), whose mean age is about 70 years. Table 2 presents an overview.

Partial or total *erectile dysfunctions* are observed in about 80% of the patients, organically caused by neurological lesions of the parasympathic nervi erigentes or a radiation-induced vasculitis. Total erectile dysfunction means discontinuation of coital activity, and often sexual partner contact is totally relinquished. In contrast to the deleterious somatic consequences of radical perineal or abdominal operation, transurethral resection (mostly performed for benign tumors) is followed by *ejaculation disorders*.

Quite in contrast to prevailing stereotypes of a "natural" decrease of sexuality with age, up to 80% of patients report the *maintenance of sexual desire*. Among the patients who reported preoperative coital activity, at least between 40% (Bagshaw et al. 1975) and 50% (Spengler and Kleber 1982) maintained this activity, although with reduced frequency.

Table 3. Determinants of sexual functioning in male cancer patients

Individual
– Age
– Information and attitude
– Affective state
– Sexual fears/concerns
Disease/medical treatment
– Stage/site of disease
– Extent of treatment
– Time elapsed since therapy
– Communication with physician
Partner relationship
– Previous sexual relationship
– Communication and mutual affection
– Stigmatizing misconceptions

3. Conclusions. Although some of the data cited have to be considered cautiously for methodological reasons, it is shown that testicular cancer is associated with a high frequency of ejaculation disorders which often concur with a decrease in orgastic satisfaction. More deleterious erectile dysfunctions are common in the much older group of prostatic cancer patients. The considerable discrepancy of maintained sexual desire and the high rate of erectile dysfunctions points to a high measure of subjective suffering in many cases. Comparatively serious debilitating effects are described for the radical therapy of bladder and rectum cancer (MacDonald and Anderson 1985).

Special attention is required by the following risk groups for sexual readaption:

- Young, unmarried patients who are still insecure in their sexual identity
- Older patients who are handicapped by misconceptions about "natural" sexual decrease in old age
- Patients lacking the ability to communicate about sexuality and disease problems
- Patients with sequelae of radical and combined treatment

To summarize, a number of determinants of sexual functions for male cancer patients can be discerned (Table 3):

On behalf of the *patient*, sexuality is influenced by many variables, especially age, information, attitude, and affective state. Depression and anxiety are well known to inhibit sexual desire and functioning.

While a number of specific and unspecific organic determinants have been cited (e.g., severity of disease and extent of treatment, neurological and vasculogenic impairment), psychogenic and organic factors are closely interwoven as recent studies (e.g., Buvat et al. 1983) suggest. One connecting link is the often-described *self-enhancing mechanism* (Fig. 1), which illustrates how even mild or transient (cf. Narayan et al. 1982) dysfunctions can initiate a cycle of critical self-monitoring, fear of failure, threat to self-esteem and narcissistic insult, negative partner response, and avoidance behavior.

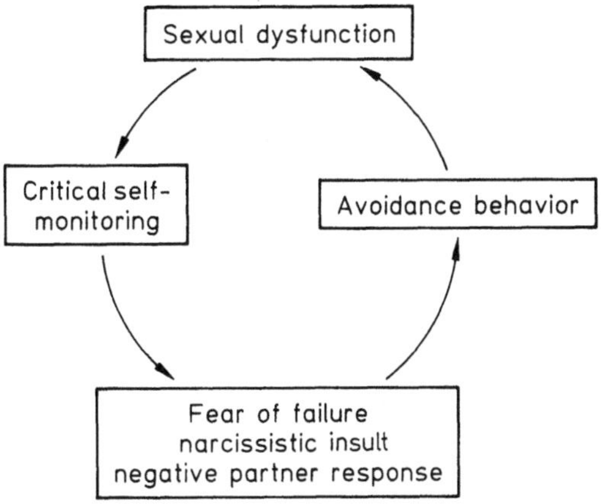

Fig. 1. Self-enhancing mechanisms of sexual dysfunctions

The literature cited mostly portrays a narrow understanding of human sexuality, reducing it to coital activity. Accordingly, treatment suggestions refer mainly to restoration of coital functions (e.g., penis protheses; cf. Rieber 1979).

While it is mostly acknowledged that male cancer patients' sexual problems go along with strains in the *partner relationship*, little is known about sexual readaptation of patients and their partners.

In the study by Leiber and collegues (1976), as an exception, patients with progressed disease and their partners reported an increase of the need for physical closeness (nearly 50% versus 6% decrease), while 50% reported a decrease of the need for coital activity.

Reestablishing sexual contact after cancer therapy can be taken both as an indicator and as a strategy for coping with the disease, treatment sequelae, and their impacts on a patient and his/her partner relationship.

Respecting research has shown that men are especially vulnerable to a decline in active, assertive, and achievment-oriented aspects in their lives, while women may be more capable of maintaining self-esteem in the face of these threats and rely more easily on social resources for that purpose (Mages and Mendelsohn 1979). As sexual functioning has strong achievement-oriented implications for men in our society, their sexual failure may constitute just that kind of threat to male self-esteem.

Total avoidance of sexual contact has been described as a strategy of defending an already fragile self-esteem, or of not exposing a physical disfigurement or painful dysfunction. On the other hand, maintaining or resuming sexual contact may be an important coping strategy to restore physical closeness and intimacy and mobilize emotional support (e.g., Tausch and Tausch 1985). Regaining sexual functioning may be an important device for restoring a sense of completeness and mastery (cf. Spengler and Kleber 1982). This need may be expressed by an *increase* of sexual activity reported by some cancer patients.

Stigmatizing misconceptions of sexual needs of the chronically ill, the common speechlessness and shame of male patients require active communication and information about sexuality by the physician. This is stressed by research reports which show that between 48% and 98% of cancer patients wish to be completely informed about the sexual sequelae of the disease, while only one-fourth actually felt sufficiently informed. While these numbers may be spuriously high for male cancer patients (mostly women investigated in Bullard 1980; mixed sample of stoma patients in Gloeckner and Starling 1982), the tendency is clear. Leaving sexual issues totally aside from the interaction between physician and male cancer patient easily transmits the feeling to the patient that it is an illegitimate or taboo topic. Especially since sexual functioning is so importantly connected with self-esteem, male identity, etc., it is difficult for many patients to express sexual problems actively. This necessitates a tactful initiative on behalf of the physician, who helps the patient to alleviate feelings of failure and stress of performance (cf. Kochenstein 1987). This need for counseling should be satisfied by the primary care physician as this is desired by most patients and is often easier in an already existing trustful relationship which would have to be built up in psychiatric or psychotherapeutic consultations.

Furthermore, information should be presented sufficiently and in a preventive manner.

Zohar et al. (1976) showed in a quasiprospective study that patients who had been informed *before* transurethral prostatic resection (prostatic adenoma) about the sexual consequences had much lower rates of total erectile failure than an uninformed group. In the last group misconceptions prevailed that prostatic operation inevitably means "impotency." Another study (Gloeckner and Sterling 1982) showed that erectile failure in preoperatively insufficiently informed patients placed great strain on the patient-physician relationship.

Models of sexual counselling and therapy have been described by many authors in recent years (cf. Buddeberg 1987; Loewit 1986, etc.). Most of these also apply for cancer patients.

Whatever counselling or therapeutic strategy is applied, it is desirable to include the partner with his own anxieties, considerations, or frustrations as a reaction to the sexual handicap in sexual counselling and to address sexual readaptation as a conjoint task of the couple. Sexual information and counselling presupposes sufficient sexological knowledge and unprejudiced readiness for self-reflection. When it is understood in this way it may help the patient to reduce unnecessary strains and satisfy elementary needs for closeness, intimacy, and valuation in the partner relationship even when confronted with continuing or debilitating effects of the disease.

References

Bagshaw MA, Ray GR, Pistenma DA, Castellino RA, Meares EM (1975) External beam radiation therapy of primary carcinoma of the prostate. Cancer 36:723–728

Bergman B, Damber JE, Littbrand B, Sjoegren K, Tomic R (1984) Sexual function in prostatic cancer patients treated with radiotherapy, orchiectomy or oestrogens. Br J Urol 56:64–69

Beutel M (1987) Verarbeitung chronischer Krankheit. Edition Medizin, Weinheim

Bracken RB, Johnson DE (1976) Sexual function and fecundity after treatment for testicular tumors. Urology 7:35–38

Buddeberg C (1987) Sexualberatung. Eine Einführung für Ärzte, Psychotherapeuten und Familienberater. Enke, Stuttgart

Bullard DG (1980) Discussing sexual concerns with cancer patients. Sexuality and Disability 3:68–70
Buvat J, Dehaene L, Lemaire A, Buvat-Herbaut M (1983) Arteriell bedingte erektile Impotenz. Sexualmedizin 12:248–251
Dold U, Sack H (1985) Praktische Tumortherapie. Thieme, Stuttgart
Gloeckner ML, Starling JR (1982) Providing sexual information to ostomy patients. Dis Col Rect 25:575–579
Goldstein I, Feldman MI, Deckers PJ, Babayan RK, Krane RJ (1984) Radiation-associated impotence. A clinical study of its mechanism. JAMA 251:903–910
Klippel KF, Weißbach L (1976) Sexualleben semikastrierter Hodentumorpatienten. Sexualmedizin 5:331–333
Kochenstein P (1987) Sexualtherapie: Strategien für die tägliche Praxis. Sexualmedizin 16:60–65
Leiber L, Plumb MM, Gerstenzang ML, Holland J (1976) The communication of affection between cancer patients and their spouses. Psychosom Med 38:379–388
Loewit K (1986) Zur Psychosomatik der sexuellen Störungen. In: von Uexküll Th (ed) Psychosomatische Medizin. Urban and Schwarzenberg, Munich, pp 641–649
Mac Donald LD, Anderson HR (1985) The health of rectal cancer patients in the community. Europ J Surg Oncol 11:235–241
Mages NL, Mendelsohn GA (1979) Effects of cancer on patients' lives: a personological approach. In: Stone GC, Cohen F, Adler NE et al. (eds) Health psychology – a handbook. Jossey-Bass, San Francisco, pp 255–284
Narayan P, Lange PH, Fraley EE (1982) Ejaculation and fertility after extended retroperitoneal lymph node dissection for testicular cancer. J Urol 127:685
Pacharzina K (1979) Der Arzt und die Sexualität seines Patienten. In: Sigusch V (ed) Sexualität und Medizin. Kiepenheuer und Witsch, Köln, pp 17–40
Rieber I (1979) Die operative Implantation von Penisprothesen bei Erektionsstörungen des Mannes. In: Sigusch V (ed) Sexualität und Medizin. Kiepenheuer und Witsch, Köln, pp 177–201
Rieker PP, Edbril SD, Garnick MB (1985) Curative testis cancer therapy: psychosocial sequelae. J Clin Oncol 3:1117–1126
Schover LE, von Eschenbach AC (1985) Sexual and marital relationships after treatment for nonseminomatous testicular cancer. Urology 25:251–255
Spengler M, Kleber R (1982) Psychische und sexuelle Situation von Patienten nach radikaler Prostatektomie. Münchn Med Wochenschr 124:221–225
Tausch AM, Tausch R (1985) Sanftes Sterben. Rowohlt, Reinbek
Verres R (1986) Krebs und Angst. Springer, Berlin Heidelberg New York
Zohar J, Meiraz D, Maoz B, Durst N (1976) Factors influencing sexual activity after prostatectomy: a prospective study. J Urol 116:332–334

Sexuality and Antihormonal Therapy in Prostate Cancer

L. Rousseau [1], A. Dupont [2], F. Labrie [2], and M. Couture [3]

[1] Department of Psychiatry, Laval Hospital, 2725 Chemin Ste-Foy, Québec, GIV 4G5, Canada
[2] Department of Molecular Endocrinology, Laval University Medical Center, 2705, Laurier Blvd, Quebec, GIV 4G2, Canada
[3] Private Practice in Sexology, 120 Montmorency Street, Boischâtel, Quebec, GOA 1HO, Canada

Introduction

Cancer of the prostate is the second most frequent cause of death due to cancer in man. So far surgical castration and the administration of high doses of estrogens have been the two most commonly used forms of treatment. Although significant clinical improvement in 60%–80% of patients has been associated with these two forms of treatment, this was for limited time intervals (Resnick and Grayhack 1975). Orchiectomy has psychological limitations and estrogens have serious cardiovascular side effects (Nesbit and Baumm 1950; Vacurg 1967; Resnik and Grayhack 1975; Murphy and Slack 1980). Chemical castration has been proposed as an alternative to these two treatments. It can now be achieved by the chronic administration of LHRH agonists with no side effects other than those due to hypoandrogenicity (Labrie et al. 1980, 1982).

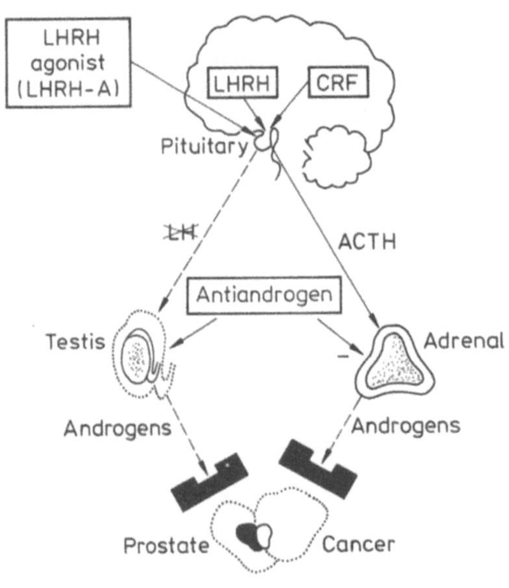

Fig. 1. Schematic representation of the combined action of an LHRH agonist and a pure antiandrogen in the treatment of prostate cancer. The LHRH agonist blocks testicular androgen formation, thus achieving medical castration, while the pure antiandrogen neutralizes the action of the remaining male hormones, especially those produced in the prostate cancer from precursors secreted by the adrenal cortex.

Sexology
Eds.: W. Eicher, G. Kockott

Recently our group has developed a new method of treatment aimed at a more complete blockade of androgens of both testicular and adrenal origin (Labrie et al. 1982, 1984, 1985 a). In order to inhibit the androgenic influence of extratesticular origin (arising from adrenal secretion and peripheral conversion), we have combined the administration of an LHRH agonist with an antiandrogen (Fig. 1). This new combined treatment brings a complete deprivation of male hormones which was not the case with previous treatments that left the adrenal sex steroids free to stimulate the cancer. In addition, the combined treatment decreases by approximately 50% the serum levels of the four adrenal precursors, thus further depriving the cancer from male hormones and decreasing the amount of male hormones to be neutralized by the antiandrogen in the cancer tissue.

Hot flashes and the lowering of sexual drive and performance are the side effects observed with this treatment (Labrie et al. 1986). In order to measure more precisely the changes in sexual activity accompanying the combined antiandrogen treatment, we have submitted 128 patients to a retrospective questionnaire on their sexual life in the 5 years prior to the diagnosis and since the diagnosis. We also have obtained data on the sexual attitudes and behavior of 44 of those 128 patients who completed a 6-month follow-up period.

Method

Subjects

One hundred and sixty-three new consecutive patients admitted to the prostate cancer clinic were asked to answer the retrospective questionnaire at the moment of the medical workup preceding the start of the antihormonal therapy. Thirty-three patients were excluded for the following reasons: bad general condition and/or too much in pain (24), did not speak either French or English (4), lack of time (3), uneducated (1), and suffering from a second cancer (1). Two patients were eliminated because of inconsistencies in their answers to the questionnaire. Thus 128 patients were kept in the study. Their age, civil status, presence of a regular sex partner, and attendance at religious services are illustrated in Table 1. Their academic level, occupation, and income level are illustrated in Table 2.

Table 1. Our population ($N=128$, values in percent)

Age (years)	<50 6	50–60 14	61–70 54	>71 26		% 100
Civil status	Single 6	Married 83	Divorced 6	Widowed 3	Separated 2	% 100
Regular sex partner	Yes 77	No 23				% 100
Attendance at religious services	Once a week or more 42	Once a month or less 45	Never 13			% 100

Table 2. Our population ($N = 128$)

Academic level	Grade school	High school	College	Uni-versity				%
	7	26	30	37				100
Occupation	Manual	Profes-sional	Business-man	Civil servant	Farmer	Pen-sioned	Unem-ployed	%
	2	26	21	2	45	45	2	100
Income level (thousands Canad. $)	<20	20–50	50–75	>75				%
	20	52	12	16				100

Table 3. Cancer stage (Whitmore 1973)

	N	%
A_2	1	1
B_2	2	2
C	13	10
D_1	4	3
D_2	108	84
	128	100

Sixteen patients had a prostate cancer stage A_2, B_2, or C (limited to the prostate) and 112 patients had prostate cancer stage D (metastatic) (Table 3, Fig. 2) proven by histology and all the clinical and laboratory tests as described (Labrie et al. 1983). Aside from the good general condition, the inclusion criteria were a normal hypothalamohypophysogonadic and adrenal axis and absence of other cancer.

Eighty-three percent of the patients were married, although only 77% of them claimed to have a regular sex partner. We must understand that 6% of them did not have an active sexual life with their spouse, and consequently did not consider their spouse as a regular sex partner.

Fifty-nine percent of the patients had been submitted to previous transurethral resection of the prostate for diagnostic purposes or for the treatment of benign prostatic hyperplasia (Table 4). In addition a large number of patients had received, prior to the beginning of the combined treatment, other forms of therapeutic regimen, as illustrated in Table 4.

The questions in our retrospective study referred to the 5 years before the discovery of their prostate cancer, and since the diagnosis.

Forty-four among those *128 patients* did complete a follow-up questionnaire 6 months after the beginning of the antihormonal therapy combining the antiandrogen flutamide with medical (LHRH agonist) or surgical castration (Tables 8–19). These data are also presented since they indicate the evolution of the sexual desire and activity of 44 patients after 6 months of treatment with flutamide (antiandrogen) and medical (LHRH-A) or surgical castration.

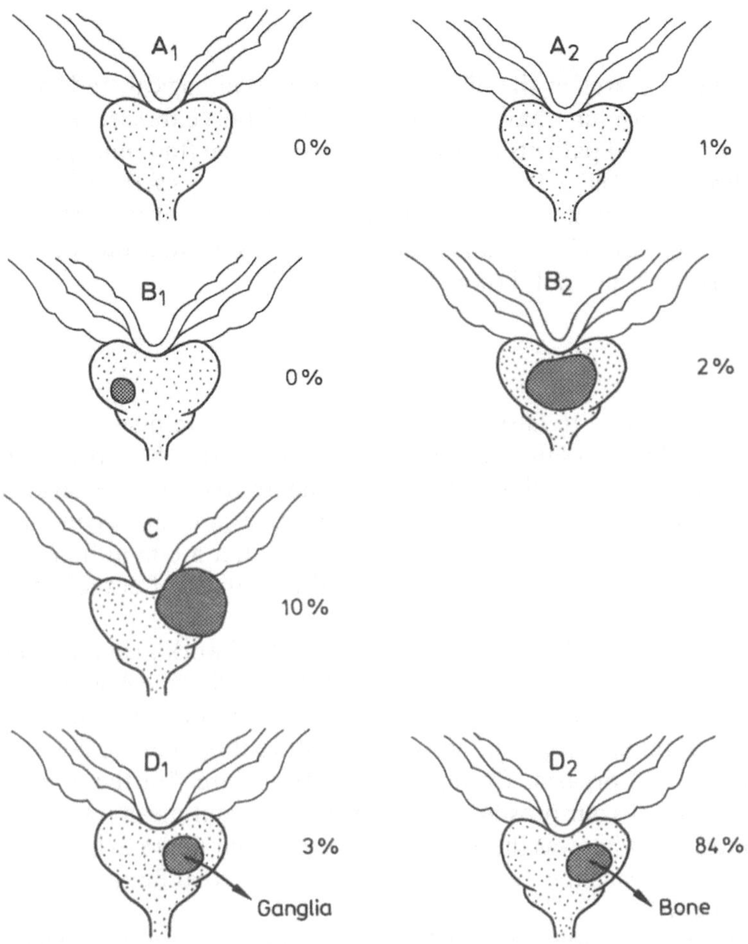

Fig. 2. Cancer stage ($N = 128$). (See Table 3.) (Whitmore 1973)

Table 4. Previous treatment profile (before the antihormonal therapy) ($N = 128$) (one more treatments)

Treatment	Yes	%
Prostatic surgery (TUR)	75	59
Estrogens	50	39
Surgical castration (orchiectomy)	46	36
Radiation therapy	39	31
Antiandrogen (Androcour-Euflex)	6	5
Corticosteroids	6	5
Aminoglutethimide (Citadren)	2	2
LHRH (analog)	7	06

Protocol

The patient population as well as the clinical, urological, radiological, and endocrinological tests and procedures have been described in detail (Labrie et al. 1984, 1985 a). Surgically castrated patients received the antiandrogen (flutamide) at the dose of 250 mg three times daily. Patients from the nonsurgically castrated group received the same dose (250 mg) of the antiandrogen in association with the LHRH agonist (D-Trp^7) LHRH ethylamide administrated subcutaneously at the dose of 500 μg daily for 1 month followed by 250 μg daily.

Procedure

Each of the *128 patients* had to answer a 100-item retrospective questionnaire. The patients were divided into small groups of four to five under the supervision of a research assistant. The "Sexual Attitudes and Behavior Inventory" is divided into two parts, one addressing the 5 years before diagnosis and the second addressing the period since diagnosis. The *44 patients* seen after a 6-month period provided answers to 30 more questions addressed to the 6 months after the beginning of the antihormonal therapy.

Patients were told by their physicians during their medical workup at the clinic that the chemical castration proposed might or might not have some negative influence on their sexual life. The research assistant provided answers to questions pertaining to the definition of certain terms like masturbation, coitus, fantasy, erection, ejaculation, and orgasm. Examples of questions are: "in the 5 years preceding the diagnosis of your prostatic cancer, what was your mean frequency of sexual intercourse,..., what was the mean frequency of your desire to have sexual intercourse,..., what was the mean frequency of your sexual fantasy (erotic thoughts) during the week?"

The 44 patients seen at follow-up were asked questions like: "since the beginning of your treatment at this clinic, what is your mean frequency of intercourse,..., what is the mean frequency of your desire for intercourse,..., what is the mean frequency of your sexual fantasies (erotic thoughts) during the week?"

We used the Wilcoxon matched-pairs signed-ranks test to analyze our data. Since we compare individual differences in sexual functionning at various periods, this test was chosen because it can tell the sign of the difference between any pair of patients and rank the differences in order of absolute sign. The *P* value was established at <0.05.

Results

Before moving on to our results, we must caution the reader about the possible influence of some factors on the level of sexual desire and activity of our patients. Age, the silent evolution and the unknown presence of a prostate cancer, the availability of a sex partner, and the medication (Table 5) taken by some patients are important factors to take into acount. Moreover we shall not forget that many patients have received one or more treatments for their cancer (Table 4) between the moment of diagnosis and the start of the antihormonal treatment.

Table 5. Medications taken by patients

None	42	33
Diabetes	7	5
Cardiac condition	17	13
Lung problem	0	0
High pressure	24	19
Nervousness	5	4
Depressive condition	1	1
Sleep disorder	6	5
Other	26	20
	128	100

Serum Androgens

As illustrated in one patient serving as his own control (Fig. 3), the treatment decreases the serum testosterone concentration from pretreatment levels of 4.7 ± 0.3 to 0.26 ± 0.08 ng/ml. Dihydrotestosterone, similarly, decreases from 0.54 ± 0.07 to 0.06 ± 0.021 ng/ml, while serum 17β-estradiol is reduced to approximately 30% of control. The serum concentration of testosterone is thus decreased to approximately 5% of pretreatment values, this inhibition remaining constant for as long as treatment continues (Labrie et al. 1985 b). There has been no difference found in serum androgens between orchiectomy and treatment with LHRH agonists except for the 2- to 3-week delay before castration levels of serum androgens are achieved with the LHRH agonist. An immediate blockade of androgen action is, however, obtained with the antiandrogen administrated 1 day before orchiectomy or administration of the LHRH agonist (D-Trp[7]) LHRH ethylamide.

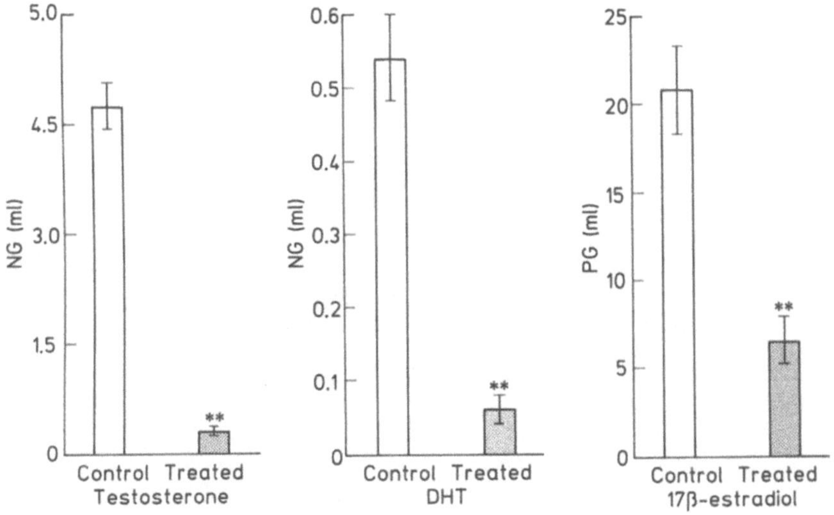

Fig. 3. Effect of combined treatment with an LHRH agonist or surgical castration with the antiandrogen flutamide on the serum levels of T, DHT, and 17-β-estradiol after 1–2 months of treatment

Level of Sexual Fantasies and Desire

In the group of *128* patients, only 45% had one or more sexual fantasy a week since their diagnosis, as opposed to 78% ($P=0.0000$) of them in the 5 years before diagnosis (Table 6). The frequency of their desire for intercourse (once every 2 weeks or more) dropped significantly ($P=0.0000$), from 78% before diagnosis to 31% after diagnosis (Table 7).

Table 6. Frequency of sexual fantasies ($N=128$)

Frequency	In the 5 years before diagnosis (%)	Since diagnosis (%)
<once a month	22	55
1–2/week	49	33
3–5/week	17	7
6–10/week	10	3
>11/week	2	2
	100	100

$P=0.0000$.

Table 7. Frequency of desire for intercourse

Frequency	In the 5 years before diagnosis % ($N=125$)	Since diagnosis % ($N=124$)
Never	5	37
<once a month	17	32
Once every 2 weeks	12	7
1/week	31	15
2–3/week	26	7
>4/week	9	2
	100	100

P: 0.0000.

Table 8. Frequency of sexual fantasies

Frequency	Since diagnosis % ($N=44$)	Six months after beginning of antihormonal therapy % ($N=44$)
<once a month	43	73
1–2/week	41	25
3–5/week	9	0
6–10/week	5	0
>11/week	2	2
	100	100

P: 0.0010.

Table 9. Frequency of desire for intercourse

Frequency	Since diagnosis % (N=44)	Six months after beginning of antihormonal therapy % (N=44)
Never	34	68
<once a month	32	20
1/2 weeks	7	5
1/week	16	7
2–3/week	7	0
>4/week	4	0
	100	100

P: 0.0016.

In the follow-up group of 44 patients, although 57% of them had maintained a level of at least one sexual fantasy a week, only 27% (P=0.001) of them still had that level of sexual fantasy 6 months after the beginning of the antihormonal therapy (Table 8). The frequency of desire for intercourse also shows a dramatic decline, since 88% (P=0.0016) of patients seldom or never desire intercourse 6 months after the beginning of the antihormonal therapy, from the 66% they were at the moment or shortly after diagnosis (Table 9).

Level of Sexual Functioning

The actual frequency of intercourse shows an even sharper decline than the level of sexual fantasies, as only 21% (P=0.0000) of the patients acknowledged having intercourse once every 2 weeks or more since diagnosis, as compared with 73% in the 5 years before diagnosis (*group of 128 patients*) (Table 10). The quality of erectile capacity also decreases significantly, going from 72% of patients who declare 51% to 100% rigidity during intercourse before diagnosis to only 20% (P= 0.0000) of them after diagnosis (Table 11). The level of 51%–100% of intercourse with orgasm drops by half (P=0.0000) between these two periods (Table 12). Fi-

Table 10. Frequency of intercourse

Frequency	In the 5 years before diagnosis % (N=125)	Since diagnosis % (N=123)
Never	9	58
<once a month	18	21
1/2 weeks	17	7
1/week	33	11
2–3/week	17	3
>4/week	6	0
	100	100

P: 0.0000.

Table 11. Penile rigidity during intercourse

Degree of rigidity	In the 5 years before diagnosis % (N=118)	Since diagnosis % (N=92)
No degree of rigidity	4	41
1%–50% of rigidity	24	39
51%–100% of rigidity	72	20
	100	100

P: 0.0000.

Table 12. Percentage off intercourse with orgasm

Percentage	In the 5 years before diagnosis % (N=117)	Since diagnosis % (N=75)
Never	4	41
1%–50% of intercourse	18	23
51%–100% of intercourse	78	36
	100	100

P: 0.0000.

Table 13. Frequency of masturbatory activities

Frequency	In the 5 years before diagnosis % (N=128)	Since diagnosis % (N=128)
>4/week	2	0
2–3/week	2	2
1/week	8	3
1/2 weeks	9	3
1/month or less	42	16
Never	37	76

P: 0.0000.

nally 21% of patients used to masturbate once every 2 weeks or more before diagnosis, and only 8% (P=0.0000) of them did so after diagnosis (Table 13).

In the group of 44 patients, 77% of patients had intercourse never or less than once a month since diagnosis (Table 14). This figure increases to 95% (P=0.0008) after 6 months of antihormonal therapy. The penile rigidity of this group of patients decreases sharply, although these data are not significant (P=0.1614) (Table 15). The percentage of *no* intercourse with orgasm rises from 31% to 79% 6 months after the beginning of the antihormonal therapy (Table 16). The P value (P=0.0431) of these data suggests caution. Finally we find, 6 months after the beginning of the antihormonal therapy, absolutely no patient maintaining masturbatory activities (P=0.0077), as compared with 20% of patients who had at

Table 14. Frequency of intercourse

Frequency	Since diagnosis % (N=44)	Six months after beginning of antihormonal therapy % (N=41)
Never	52	85
<once a month	25	10
1–2 weeks	7	3
1/week	14	2
2–3/week	2	0
>4/week	0	0
	100	100

P: 0.0008.

Table 15. Penile rigidity during intercourse

Degree of rigidity	Since diagnosis % (N=28)	Six months after beginning of antihormonal therapy % (N=18)
No degree of rigidity	32	67
1%–50% of rigidity	50	16
51%–100% of rigidity	18	17
	100	100

P: 0.1614.

Table 16. Percentage of intercourse with orgasm

Percentage	Since diagnosis % (N=23)	Six months after beginning of antihormonal therapy % (N=19)
Never	31	79
1%–50% of intercourse	17	11
51%–100% of intercourse	52	10
	100	100

P: 0.0431

least some such activity at the moment of diagnosis or shortly thereafter (Table 17).

Nocturnal or Morning Erections

Sixty-seven percent of the *128 patients* admitted having at least one nocturnal or morning erection every 2 weeks or more before diagnosis as opposed to only 18% (P=0.0000) after diagnosis (Table 18).

Twenty-five percent *of the 44 patients* reported having at least one nocturnal or morning erection every 2 weeks or more at the moment of diagnosis compared

Table 17. Frequency of masturbatory activities

Frequency	Since diagnosis % (N=44)	Six months after beginning of antihormonal therapy % (N=44)
>4/week	0	0
2–3/week	0	0
1/week	2	0
1/2 weeks	2	0
1/month or less	16	0
Never	80	100
	100	100

P: 0.0077.

Table 18. Frequency of nocturnal or morning erections

Frequency	In the 5 years before diagnosis % (N=128)	Since diagnosis % (N=128)
Never	13	56
1/month or less	20	26
1/2 weeks	11	6
1/week	36	4
2–4/week	20	8
	100	100

P: 0.0000.

Table 19. Frequency of nocturnal or morning erections

Frequency	Since diagnosis % (N=44)	Six months after beginning of antihormonal therapy % (N=44)
Never	43	84
1/month or less	32	9
1/2 weeks	11	2
1/week	5	3
2–4/week	9	2
	100	100

P: 0.0006.

with 7% (P=0.0006) of them after 6 months of antihormonal therapy (Table 19).

Discussion

Retrospective questionnaires are known to have limited validity. Moreover going as far back as 5 years before the diagnosis of a disease is a fairly long period during which sexual activity may decrease progressively. Other methodological difficulties in our study include the fact that we do not have a control group, that the patients were not blind to their own treatment and had to deal with the information physicians gave them about the possibly negative effects of these substances on their sexual drive and performance. The survival preoccupation of our patients confronted with a life-threatening disease should also be taken into account. All the above do limit somewhat the validity of our results. However, these results may shed some light on the sexuality of patients treated for prostatic cancer with antihormonal therapy.

Sexuality changes with aging. Many authors (Freeman 1961; Rubin 1965; Weinberg 1975; Weizman and Hart 1987) have studied healthy elderly males. Among the 52 potent patients of their cohort of 81 aged 60–70 years, *Weizman and Hart* reported 54% of patients having sexual intercourse more than four times a month. We obtain similar results, as 56% of 128 patients report having sexual intercourse once a week or more before diagnosis. The age span of our population is different, running from 45 to 80 years of age. However, 54% of the 128 patients are between 61 and 70 years of age. We must consider though that they report on their sexual activity in the 5 years prior to diagnosis, which is referring to a period of their lives when they were younger than 61–70. The frequency of one masturbatory activity a week or more is reported by 12% of our patients, as compared with 19% in the Weizman and Hart study. A more striking difference between their and our data concerns the frequency of nocturnal or morning erections. Whereas 28% of their 81 patients reported an unchanged frequency of spontaneous day or night erections, 67% of our 128 patients reported one nocturnal or morning erection every 2 weeks or more. The difference in these results may partly be explained by the fact that 20% of our population is of a younger age group and that even the patients between 61 and 70 years of age reported on a 5-year retrospective period.

Disease and its corresponding medical treatment (medications) is well known to affect sexual functioning. Forty-two percent of our patients were taking medications for diabetes, a cardiac problem, high pressure, nervousness, or depression. An even more important factor affecting sexual functioning is the presence of a slowly evolving prostate cancer. This condition, even if unknown to the patient, may affect his general wellbeing and consequently his sexual functioning. This is a highly important consideration for our patient population since 87% of them had a metastatic carcinoma at the moment of diagnosis. This means that this cancer was evolving for months, possibly years.

Among the 44 follow-up patients, 57% had transurethral resection of the prostate, 36% received estrogens, 21% were surgically castrated, 27% received radiation therapy, 11% received antiandrogen, and 5% received LHRH-A. All these treatments, aside from the anxiety of having a cancer, certainly affected the level of sexual desire and activity of these patients since diagnosis, even before the beginning of the antihormonal therapy. It is then easy to explain why, in adding the antiandrogen flutamide and the LHRH-A (for the nonsurgically castrated patients), only 27% still have sexual fantasies, 32% maintain some level of desire for intercourse, 15% effectively have intercourse (of which 10% less than once a month), 33% maintain some level of penile rigidity, 21% occasionally have an orgasm, 0% masturbate, and only 7% have one nocturnal or morning erection every 2 weeks or more.

The issue of surgical castration, antiandrogen medication, androgen withdrawal, or replacement therapy is well documented in the literature (Skakkebaek et al. 1981; Salmimies et al. 1982; Bancroft et al. 1974; Bancroft and Wu 1983; Cooper et al. 1972; Berlin and Meinschke 1981; Heim and Hursch 1979; Gagné 1981). These authors studied the effects of the presence or absence of male hormones on the level of sexual fantasies, quality of erections, and frequency of sexual activity. Our results from the 44 follow-up patients surprisingly show a greater decline in sexual activity than in sexual fantasies and desire. Such a small amount of serum androgens should affect desire more than activity. We must, however, put this in the context of patients and spouses struggling with the anxiety of having cancer.

We are convinced that the present treatment using the pure anti-androgen flutamide in association with an LHRH agonist or surgical castration achieves a more complete blockade of androgen action and that it could be used more effectively than cyproterone acetate or medroxy progesterone acetate in the treatment of sexual offenders. This is confirmed in our population of 44 patients by the sharp decline in the frequency of sexual fantasies, intercourse, masturbatory activities, and reported frequency of nocturnal or morning erections. Our data need to be extended to more than 44 patients and to be objectivated by appropriate means, like nocturnal penile tumescence, before we use this new antihormonal therapy with sex offenders. This is, however, a highly promising way of future research.

References

Bancroft J, Wu FCW (1983) Changes in erectile responsiveness during androgen replacement therapy. Arch Sex Behav 12:1

Bartsh W, Voigt KD (1984) Endocrine aspects of aging in the male. Maturitas 6:243–251

Berlin FS, Meinschke CF (1981) Treatment of sex offenders with antiandrogenic medication: conceptualization, review of treatment modalities and preliminary findings. Am J Psych 138:5

Cooper AJ, Ismail AA, Phanjoo AL et al. (1972) Antiandrogen (cyproterone acetate) therapy in deviant hypersexuality. Br J Psych 120:59–63

Davidson JM, Chen JJ, Crapo L, Gray GD, Greenlaf W, Catania JA (1983) Hormonal changes and sexual function in aging men. J Clin Endocrinol Metab 57:1

Freeman JT (1961) Sexual capacities in the aging male. Geriatrics 16:37–40

Gagné P (1981) Treatment of sex offenders with medroxyprogesterone acetate. Am J Psych 138:644–646

Heim N, Hursch CJ (1979) Castration for sex offenders: treatment or punishment. A review and critique of recent European literature. Arch Sex Behav 8:281–304

Huggins C, Hodges W (1941) Studies of prostatic cancer. I. Effect of castration, estrogens and androgen injections on serum phosphatases in metastatic carcinoma of the prostate. Cancer Res 1:293–295

Huggins C, Stevens RE, Hodges CW (1941) Studies on prostatic carcinoma. II. The effect of castration on advanced carcinoma of the prostate gland. Arch Surg 43:209–211

Labrie F, Bélanger A, Cusan L, Séguin C, Pelletier G, Kelly PA, Lefebvre FA, Lemay A, Raynaud JP (1980) Antifertility effects of LHRH agonists in the male. J Androl 1:209–228

Labrie F, Dupont A, Bélanger A, Cusan L, Lacourcière Y, Monfette G, Laberge JG, Emond JP, Fazekas ATA, Raynaud JP, Husson JM (1982) New hormonal therapy in prostatic carcinoma: combined treatment with an LHRH agonist and an antiandrogen. Clin Invest Med 5:267–275

Labrie F, Bélanger A, Dupont A, Emond J, Lacourcière Y, Monfette G (1984) Combined treatment with an LHRH agonist and a pure antiandrogen in advanced carcinoma of the prostate. Lancet:1090

Labrie F, Dupont A, Bélanger A (1985 a) Complete androgen blockade for the treatment of prostate cancer. In: De Vita VT, Hellman S, Rosenberg SA (eds) Important advances in oncology. Lippincott, Philadelphia, pp 193–217

Labrie F, Dupont A, Bélanger A, Lachance R, Giguère M (1985 b) Long-term treatment with luteinizing hormone releasing hormone agonists and maintenance of serum testosterone to castration concentrations. Br Med J 291:369–370

Labrie F, Dupont A, Bélanger A, St-Arnaud R, Giguère M, Lacourcière Y, Emond J, Monfette G (1986) Treatment of prostate cancer with gonadotropin-releasing hormone agonists. Endocr Rev 7:67–74

Martin CE (1981) Factors affecting sexual functioning in 60–79 year-old married males. Arch Sex Beh 10:5

Murphy GP, Slack NH (1980) The questionable use of hormone therapy in advanced carcinoma of the prostate. Urol Clin North Am 7:631–638

Nesbit RM, Baum WC (1950) Endocrine control of prostatic carcinoma: clinical and statistical survey of 1818 cases. JAMA 143:1317–1320

Resnick MI, Grayhack JT (1975) Treatment of stage IV carcinoma of the prostate. Urol Clin North Am 2(1):141–161

Rubin I (1965) Sexual life after sixty. Basic, New York

Rousseau L, Dupont A, Labrie F, Couture M (to be published) Changes in sexuality in prostate cancer patients receiving the antihormonal therapy combining the antiandrogen flutamide with medical (LHRH agonist) or surgical castration: a pilot study. Arch Sex Behav

Salmimies P, Kockott G, Pirke KM, Vogt HJ, Schill WB (1982) Androgen replacement with oral testosterone undecanoate in hypogonadal men: a double blind controlled study. Clin Endocrinol 14:49–61

Skakkebaek NE, Bancroft J, Davidson DW, Warner P (1981) Androgen replacement with oral testosterone undecanoate in hypogonadal men: a double blind controlled study. Clin Endocrinol 14:49–61

Toradello P, Boscia FM (1985) Sexuality in aging: a study of a group of 300 elderly men and women. J Endocrinol Invest 8: suppl 2

Tsitouras PD, Martin CE, Harman SM (1982) Relationship of serum testosterone to sexual activity in healthy elderly men. J Gerontol 37:288–293

Veterans Administration Cooperative Urological Research Group (1967) Carcinoma of the prostate: treatment comparisons. J Urol 98:516–522

Weinberg J (1975) Geriatric psychiatry. In: Freedman AM, Kaplan HI, Sadock BJ (eds) Comprehensive textbook of psychiatry, 2nd edn. William and Wilkins, Baltimore, p 2405

Weizman R, Hart J (1987) Sexual behavior in healthy married elderly men. Arch Sex Behav 16:39–44

Whitmore WF Jr (1973) The natural history of prostate cancer. Cancer 32:1104

VIII. Sexuality and the Handicapped

Team Approach to Sexual Counseling in Patients with Spinal Cord Injuries

H. J. Hachen

Medical Director, Spinal Injuries Centre, Geneva University Hospital, 1211 Geneva 4, Switzerland

The comprehensive management and medical rehabilitation of patients with spinal cord lesions is presently based on internationally defined and accepted guidelines. In recent years the quality of monitoring and nursing in the acute, post-traumatic stage and the techniques of functional rehabilitation have continuously improved. In spite of severe polytrauma, more than 90% of these patients survive and eventually return to their home, their families, and society at large. According to statistics compiled at our center in Geneva, there are in Switzerland approximately 26 new cases with spinal cord lesions per million inhabitants per year. The average age of these patients is the mid-twenties. Before becoming paralyzed they belonged to a highly active part of society. As there exist, at present, no ways and means of restoring neurological function in patients with complete spinal cord lesions, our therapeutic efforts aim at restoring the highest level possible of independence in daily life.

Comprehensive management requires close collaboration, professional expertise, and good interdisciplinary team-spirit. Survival in the acute stage depends on the combined efforts of rescue workers, specialists in cardiovascular and respiratory intensive care, neurosurgeons, and traumatologists. Subsequent medical rehabilitation relies on a team of physicians, nurses, physiotherapists, occupational therapists, social workers, and psychologists (Fig. 1), all specially trained in the field of spinal cord injury. Early emphasis lies on bladder and bowel training. Subsequently the rehabilitation program encompasses wheelchair indepen-

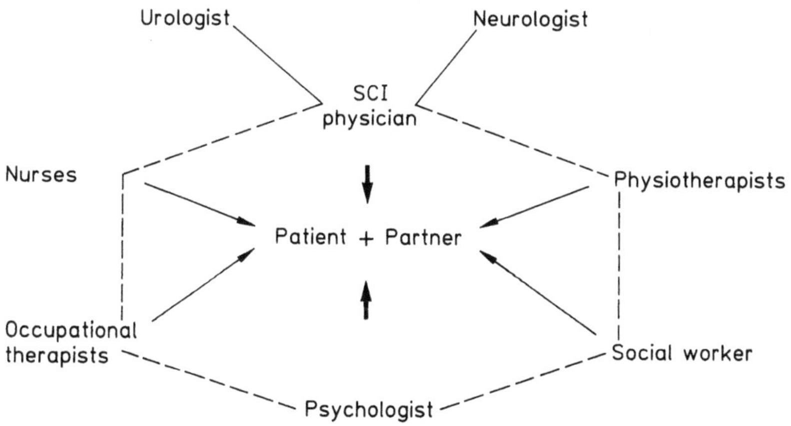

Fig. 1. Team approach in sexual counseling

Sexology
Eds.: W. Eicher, G. Kockott

dence and, in patients with lower dorsal or dorsolumbar fractures, walking exercises with orthotic devices. All necessary adaptations at the patient's home should be completed within 3–4 months postinjury, so as to allow early reintegration of the patient in his or her community; optimal solutions for vocational training should be worked out concomitantly.

During the early stage of functional rehabilitation emphasis quite naturally lies upon medical aspects – on repeated neurological assessment of the patient's functional deficit, on neurourological studies, and on comprehensive management of such complications as severe spasticity and chronic pain. Both physicians and the nursing staff are well aware of the many somatic implications of acute spinal cord trauma. The patient's psychological needs, on the other hand, are often underestimated and possibly neglected. This is particularly the case in large centers where an individualized patient approach is more difficult, due to frequent changes within the nursing staff.

There are considerable differences among patient's attitudes toward physical handicap. Depending on age, creed, education, family background, professional status, level and type of injury, a paralyzed person is more or less well prepared to cope with future life in a wheelchair. Twenty-five years of daily contacts with spinally injured persons have taught us a great deal about the profound psychoaffective impact of paralysis and the need for efficient long-term psychological support.

Some decades ago the sexual needs of physically handicapped persons were clearly underestimated. A pilot study on sexual readjustment and modified sexual behavior was initiated at our center in 1968. The essential driving force for this program came from the patients themselves, who felt a growing need to discuss their sexual problems with a competent medical professional. The aim of this program was to offer all patients the opportunity to discuss sexual problems freely, whenever they wish to do so, with a therapist of their choice, to provide a comfortable and private setting for these discussions, to analyze and understand sexual needs, to provide expert professional guidance and advice in order to render sexual activities as enjoyable and pleasurable as possible, to promote the gradual adoption of a new range of sexual attitudes and behaviors that are compatible with a person's degree of physical impairment, and, last but not least, to foster the recognition that all of us, rehabilitation specialists, nurses, physiotherapists, etc., must give due consideration to all needs of our patients, and this definitely includes their sexuality.

In 1973, we published our preliminary findings based on questionnaires answered by a series of 214 patients. With this experience in mind we established a more detailed protocol for a second study, which covered the 5-year period between 1974 and 1979 and included 172 spinal cord injured (SCI) patients. Their level and type of lesion are indicated in Table 1. Their marital status at admission and 5 years postinjury is shown in Table 2. The large majority of these patients, both para- and tetraplegics, were in their early twenties when they became paralyzed (Tables 3, 4). Eighty-four percent completed the full course of sexual counseling, 7% only wanted precise answers to a few specific questions, and 9% felt no need or wish to talk about sexual readjustment. The degree of sexual activity, evaluated 2 years postinjury, indicates major differences between the subgroups

Table 1. Neurological level ($N = 172$)

Tetraplegia	67 (39%)	Complete	38 (57%)
		Incomplete	29 (43%)
Paraplegia	105 (61%)	Complete	44 (42%)
		Incomplete	61 (58%)

Table 2. Marital status in 172 male SCI patients

	Paraplegia ($N = 105$)		Tetraplegia ($N = 67$)	
	At time of injury	5 years postinjury	At time of injury	5 years postinjury
Single	58	36	47	43
Married	37	49	19	12
Separated/divorced	8	9	1	5
Separated + remarried	–	2	–	–
Widowed	2	1	–	1
Widowed + remarried	–	1	–	–
Unknown		7		6

Table 3. Age distribution of patients with paraplegia

Type of lesion	15–20 (years)	20–30 (years)	30–50 (years)	>50 (years)	Total
Complete	11 (18.3)	19 (24.8)	9 (39.5)	5 (54.7)	44 (29.6)
Incomplete	7 (19.1)	17 (26.5)	3 (37.6)	2 (56)	29 (27.9)

Table 4. Age distribution of patients with tetraplegia

Type of lesion	15–20 (years)	20–30 (years)	30–50 (years)	>50 (years)	Total
Complete	14 (18.7)	9 (25.2)	9 (42.6)	6 (61.3)	38 (31.4)
Incomplete	19 (19.4)	17 (24.5)	16 (37.4)	9 (63.5)	61 (32.0)

Table 5. Sexual functions in male SCI patients with incomplete lesions (2 years postinjury)

Number cases	Type of lesion	Libido < = >			Erection	Ejaculation	Orgasm	Coitus
57	Central	5	41	11	55	51	51	39
33	Peripheral	0	29	4	26	21	19	19

Table 6. Sexual functions in male SCI patients with complete lesions (2 years postinjury)

Number cases	Type of lesion	Libido < = >			Erection	Ejaculation	Orgasm	Coitus
58	Central	14	34	10	52	4 (retrograde = 8)	0	22
24	Peripheral	2	18	4	0	0	0	2 (penile prosthesis)

with complete and incomplete lesions and also between central and peripheral types of injury. The highest level of performance was achieved by patients with incomplete central lesions (Table 5); the poorest results were seen in subjects with complete peripheral lesions (Table 6).

Our program of sexual counseling addresses three specific subgroups of patients:

1. Teenagers and single adults below the age of 20 years.
2. Adults having reached a certain degree of sexual maturity and having had experience with various forms of sexual behaviors. Approximately two-thirds of the patients in this group were already married or had a steady relationship before getting paralyzed.
3. Elderly patients who had already somewhat limited their sexual activities prior to their injury.

In our experience this approach greatly facilitates the dialogue between patient and therapist, as each subgroup is inclined to adopt a distinct generation-related vocabulary and attitude. In fact, at each age sex has different meanings and is described and analyzed in different terms.

For the teenager and young adult, sex frequently is a means to boast his ego, to raise his self-esteem, and prove to others and himself that he has success in social life. Sex identifies with pleasure and provides a chance to get rid of worries and tension.

Paraplegic youngsters start to ask questions very early, sometimes as soon as 2 weeks after admission. At this moment bladder training requires intermittent catheterization, urodynamic investigations, etc., and the patient becomes intensely aware of the complete loss of sensation in his genitalia. A syndrome of "castration" may cause severe frustration, feelings of inadequacy, and inferiority and be viewed as the major component of the handicap – more important even than the paralysis of both legs.

At this stage of the rehabilitation program each patient should be instructed, in practical, explicit terms, about the complex neurological disorders brought about by spinal cord injury. In general the functional disturbances of the bladder and bowel are closely intricated with functional disorders in the sexual sphere. The voluntary control of the anal and urethral sphincter is lost. Most male patients carry a condom urinal; in some cases it is necessary to place an indwelling catheter. Urethral sphincter spasticity may justify the administration of spasmolytic agents that adversely affect erectile strength. Medical rehabilitation of the spinally injured patients encompasses a multitude of specific areas that are closely linked and have to be dealt with concomitantly. Medication that is clearly indicated and beneficial in some areas may, at times, be detrimental in others. With regard to sexual activity this is particularly the case for alpha-adrenergic inhibitors, anticholinergic agents, and tranquilizers.

Guidelines for Sexual Counseling

From a general viewpoint it is highly important to choose the appropriate time and setting for sexual counseling and to tailor the techniques and modalities to each patient's individual needs. It takes time for a patient to make initial adjustments to his or her disability. Table 7 shows the sequence of psychological reactions to acute physical impairment and loss of body functions as seen in spinal cord injury. The five stages are shock, denial, anger, depression, and adjustment. The time interval between subsequent behaviors varies greatly from patient to patient. The capacity to solve sexual problems may be jeopardized by previously established personal taboos, religious considerations, and overreaction to sexual items and documentation used in counseling. It is important regularly to inform all members of the paramedical staff about the degree of understanding reached by every single patient during subsequent sessions, so as to avoid confusion and misinterpretation.

Our program comprises four 2-h sessions at 1-week intervals.

Session 1 deals with normal sexual function, reproduction, and anatomy in both the male and female (ovulation, menstruation, spermatogenesis, erection and ejaculation, pregnancy, etc.). Following this basic introduction the patient receives information on all possible modes of contraception. Audiovisual material

Table 7. Sequence of psychological reactions to acute spinal cord injury

Shock	Anxiety Cognitive disorganization
Denial	Defensive retreat
Anger	Hostility
Depression	Feelings of guilt Loss of hope
Adjustment	Progressive adaptation

is used to illustrate the practical meaning of complicated medical terminology. The patient is made aware of the large scope of sexual activities. He or she learns about the importance of foreplay and the changes that take place during the four successive stages of arousal, plateau, orgasm, and resolution. The therapist then describes the many causes of sexual dysfunction, both organic (neurogenic, vascular, endocrine) and psychic (failure to communicate, performance anxiety, premature ejaculation, etc.). The therapist then goes on to describe the effects of certain drugs which activate or impair sexual functions and analyzes with the patient the age-related changes that determine male and female sexual attitudes. Particular emphasis is put on the importance of fantasy and exploring and stimulating the many erogenous zones. The patient is told that each human being must make his or her own free choice of what is acceptable, pleasing, and gratifying to him- or herself and his or her partner.

During the 2nd h of the session the patient is encouraged to express freely what sex means to him or her. The type of response obtained reflects particular personality traits and enables the therapist to optimize the program and adapt it to individual requirements. The patient soon realizes that sexual counseling is just one facet of a comprehensive rehabilitation program that will eventually enable a new positive life-style to be adapted to. Before attending the following session the patient is encouraged to consult books and journals on sexual functions both valid for the physically handicapped.

Session 2 is centered on the leitmotiv: "sexuality, an essential part of the human relationship." It focuses on sex as a strong binding force between individuals. The patient who previously identified sex with intercourse must learn that there are many more ways to express sexual feelings in interpersonal relationships. We must teach our patients about the large variety of activities that culminate in joy, happiness, and sexual fulfillment. Whenever possible, the patient's partner should actively participate in these discussions.

Session 3 centers on specific problems encountered by spinally injured men and women when they engage in sexual activities with an able-bodied partner. Most paralyzed persons in a wheelchair expect to be rejected, as if there were something dirty or contagious attached to paraplegia. In our center the incontinent paraplegic woman is taught to practise self-catheterization prior to intercourse. Regular bowel emptying prevents embarrassing fecal incontinence. Adequate, comfortable positioning of the body is important to prevent pressure sores. In patients with severe flexor-adductor spasms in both legs it is sometimes necessary to destroy some motor end-plates by chemical coagulation after careful identification by electrostimulation. Capsular and ligamentous retractions of the hip joints and severe limitation of joint mobility by para-articular ectopic bone formation also require surgery. When tetraplegic persons are aroused sexually they may experience acute autonomous dysreflexia accompanied by systemic hypertension, bradycardia, and cluster headache.

Session 4 deals with procreation. The mechanisms of reflexogenic and psychogenic erection are explained again. The patient learns about the structural and functional changes that occur in the testicle and affect spermatogenesis. Subcutaneous eserine (physostigmine salicylate) is administered at regular intervals in order to improve the quality and quantity of semen. The possibility of sperm banking is discussed. In vitro fertilization offers new possibilities to hitherto infertile couples.

The paraplegic woman receives detailed instruction about contraception. If she has a spastic lesion and does not smoke we let her use oral contraception. If the paralysis is of the flaccid type, oral contraceptives are contraindicated as they significantly enhance the risk of venous thrombosis. These women should request their partner to wear a condom and in addition use a local spermicidal foam. We are rather reluctant to allow the use of intrauterine devices. Due to total lack of sensation, local intolerance and infection may not be diagnosed until expulsion occurs, with a risk of septicemia.

In our own experience one of the major problems that arises when one wishes to put theoretical sexual counseling into practice is the total lack of privacy in most rehabilitation units. SCI patients who are hospitalized for many months often lack the psychological support of their families, friends, and lovers because there simply is no opportunity for privacy and intimate relationship. Hospital administrators should be made aware of this situation and accept the idea of a specially designed private room for physically handicapped persons.

References

Cole TM, Chilgren R, Rosenberg P (1973) A new programme of sex education and counseling for spinal cord injured adults and health care professionals. Paraplegia 11:111–124

Comarr AE, Vigue M (1978) Sexual counseling among male and female patients with spinal cord and/or cauda equina injury. Am J Phys Med 57:215–227

Eisenberg MG, Rustad LC (1976) Sex education and counseling program on a spinal cord injury service. Arch Phys Med Rehabil 57:135–140

Evans RL, Halar EN, Defreece AE (1976) Multidisciplinary approach to sex education of spinal cord injured patients. Phys Ther 56:541–545

Fitzpatrick WF (1974) Sexual function in paraplegic patient. Arch Phys Med Rehabil 55:221–227

Hachen HJ (1973) Paraplégie et fonction sexuelle. Med Hyg 31:1753–1755

Hanson RW, Franklin MR (1976) Sexual loss in relation to other functional losses for spinal cord injured males. Arch Phys Med Rehabil 57:291–293

Held JP, Cole TM, Held CA et al. (1975) Sexual attitude reassessment workshops: effect on spinal cord injured adults, their partners and rehabilitation professionals. Arch Phys Med Rehabil 56:14–18

Hohmann GW (1972) Considerations in management of psychosexual readjustment in the cord injured male. Rehab Psychol 19:50–58

Jackson RW (1972) Sexual rehabilitation after cord injury. Paraplegia 10:50–55

Romano MD, Lassiter RE (1972) Sexual counseling with spinal-cord injured. Arch Phys Med Rehabil 53:568–572

Siller J (1969) Psychological situation of the disabled with spinal cord injuries. Rehab Lit 30:290–296

Singh SP, Magner T (1975) Sex and self; the spinal cord injured. Rehab Lit 36:2–10

Tarabulcy E (1972) Sexual function in the normal and in paraplegia. Paraplegia 10:201–208

Weber DD, Wessman HC (1971) A review of sexual function following spinal cord trauma. Phys Ther 51:290–295

Weiss AJ, Diamond MD (1966) Sexual adjustment, identification, and attitudes of patients with myelopathy. Arch Phys Med Rehabil 47:245–250

Sexuality in Spinal Cord Injured Women

V. Banthien

Keplerstraße 22, 6900 Heidelberg, FRG

Studying the literature about the sexuality of the spinal cord injured, I found that there was very much written about the sexual problems of male patients, but very little about women except for the fact that their ability to have sexual intercourse, to get pregnant, and to deliver is maintained. Being a woman myself I thought that sexuality surely is more than sexual intercourse and pregnancy, but as Romano (1978) states:

> It can be agreed that for women sexuality is more than the act of sexual intercourse. It involves for most women the whole business of relating to another person: the tenderness, the desire to give as well as take, the compliments, casual caresses, reciprocal concerns, tolerance, the forms of communication that both include and go beyond words. For women, sexuality includes a range of behaviors from smiling through orgasm; it is not just what happens between two people in bed.

So I was curious to find out what sexuality is to spinal cord injured women. A questionnaire was developed for semistructured interviews consisting of 81 questions concerning the meaning of, the experiences in, and the attitudes toward sexuality of spinal cord injured women. The questions related to the time before the injury, during medical rehabilitation, and after it.

Forty women with a spinal cord lesion were interviewed, 30 paraplegics and 10 quadriplegics; 33 were in a wheelchair. The disability was caused by accidents in 35 cases (87.5%), 4 (10%) had had a disease, and 1 (2.5%) was the consequence of a suicide attempt. The interviews were performed individually in the department of treatment and rehabilitation of spinal cord injured patients in the Orthopädische Universitätsklinik Heidelberg, where the subjects were seen as out- or inpatients. The subjects' age ranged from 18 to 47 years, the disability existed for at least 1 year, and primary rehabilitation was finished at least 6 months previously. The average age was 31 years; the average time since injury was 8 ½ years. All but one woman lived and cared for themselves without professional help and only assisted by their partners or relatives. Sixteen lived with a partner, ten lived alone in apartments, seven lived with their parents, five shared an apartment with roommates, one was undergoing vocational rehabilitation in a boarding school, and one lived in an apartment with a professional helper. The subjects' marital status was as follows: 23 unmarried, 11 married, 2 living with a partner without being married, 2 widows, and 1 divorced. Ten, that is 25% of the interviewed women, had children at the time of the injury. One of them had another child after her spinal cord lesion, and the other 7 (17.5%) had their first child after they had been handicapped. Altogether 17 (42.5%) brought up children as a spinal cord injured mother. While before the injury 37 (92.5%) of the subjects had a pro-

Sexology
Eds.: W. Eicher, G. Kockott

fession or were still at school, after the injury only 23 (57.5%) worked or continued with their education. The percentage of housewives rose from 5% before to 32.5% after injury. Regarding the financial situation the number of women earning their living decreased from 22 to 14 after rehabilitation, while 10 (40%) lived on a pension afterwards.

In the following I will sum up some of the results of the study, concentrating on the most important ones: The subjects were asked whether the spinal cord injury had had an impact on their sexuality, and 32 (80%) felt so. Twenty-one (52.5%) even reported that the sexual impairment was a very weighty restriction caused by the handicap. Many subjects stressed the loss of sensitivity as the most important loss in sexuality.

We tried to find out how important sexuality was to the women before the spinal cord injury, during rehabilitation, and after it. The subjects marked their statements on a seven-step scale: one meaning "not important at all," seven meaning "most important." The means of the data thus achieved show that sexuality grew less important during hospitalization and then grew in significance after rehabilitation. The contentment with their sexual life was rated even higher on the same scale: The means were 5.0 before and 5.1 after injury.

In order to understand these results a little better we had to obtain more detailed information. Romano states that for disabled women it is difficult to become a "sexual object," that is to be regarded as a sexual being to find a partner. The women of our sample stated that 29 (72.5%) had a partner at the time of the interview. Before the injury 34 had a partner (85%), and two-thirds of these relationships were changed considerably during the time in hospital. Fifteen of 31 (48.4%) lost their partner as a consequence of the injury. That means, they were left by the partner, they decided to separate, or the partner died. At the time of the study, five of the women still had the partner they had before. Of the remaining 35, 33 had fallen in love after the injury, 28 of them starting a love affair at least once since then. Among the interviewed women we found only 6 (15%) who had not had any sexual experience since injury. The reasons for their abstinence may be found in the fact that the time since injury was too short or that the gravity of their disability made them dependent on living with their parents' assistance, so they did not have a chance to find a partner or to meet him in intimacy. More than half of those who had had sexual intercourse since injury reported their first experience as positive, about 30% described it as difficult or even negative, but at the time of the interview, 73% stated that their experience with intercourse had become better and more satisfying than at the beginning. Twenty-four percent reported disappointing experience or total loss of interest in coital activities.

We tried to find out what could be the factors that help women with a spinal cord injury to enjoy sexual encounters. Our first hypothesis was that satisfaction in sexual activity depends very much on the level of lesion in the spinal cord: women with no sensitivity in the genital area and with no control of the bowel and bladder should enjoy sex less than those with an incomplete injury.

According to the information we obtained from the interviews, this is not necessarily true. Many women with a complete lesion and consequently no sensation in the genital area reported that they enjoy intercourse and even stated that they had orgasms at least sometimes. Some even said that their orgasm felt better than before the injury, while others, whose sensitivity was fully functioning, enjoyed sex much less and had problems with their orgasm. This information seems most important to me, because it shows that other than the sheer medical facts play an important role in the enjoyment of sexual activity.

One determining factor for sexual satisfaction seems to be age: Those women who say they enjoy sex are on average 9 years younger than those who report to have very little sexual satisfaction. The subjects that regarded themselves as sexually attractive tended to be more satisfied with their sexual activities. Perhaps further investigation might find some more factors that are relevant for sexual counseling and therapy in order to help handicapped women to enjoy life more.

As we wanted to know how spinal cord injured women arrange their sexual activities, we asked many questions about preparatory and logistic issues. Thirty-four of the 40 women had sexual experience and helped us by speaking frankly about the intimate details. Two of our sample were lesbian, one of them deciding to prefer female lovers only after the injury. While before the accident 23 (57.5%) reported to have masturbated, only 7 (17.5%) practiced masturbation after injury. This might be a matter of age, but loss of sensation in the genital area seems to be at least partially the reason for this change of habit.

We asked the subjects about the worries and concerns they experienced the first time they had intercourse after the injury: Most of them were about the partner's reaction about their ability to move adequately and to enjoy sex, and about an impending leak of the bladder. With growing experience most women were less concerned about these things and they learned how to handle the actual problems by preparatory activities. So 18 (52.5%) preferred to go to the toilet before intercourse in order not to risk a leak. Eleven (32%) still had problems with bladder incontinence, only one (3%) reporting bowel incontinence during intercourse. All partners tolerated this according to the subjects. Increased spasticity during sexual activity was noted by 5 (14.7%); one of them felt this was a handicap for sexual satisfaction and decided to take antispastic medication before intercourse. Three women (8.8%) complained about lack of lubrication during intercourse, but 10 (31.1%) of the subjects who also had a complete lesion had no problems with lubrication. Six (17.6%) women were helped in their bowel and bladder routine by their sexual partners. Only one regarded this as a handicap in their sexual relationship. One subject had an indwelling catheter. She reported that her partner felt disturbed by it in sexual contacts. During intercourse 13 (38.2%) could feel movements in the vagina, and 23 (67.6%) had marked vaginal sensations in this situation. Asked about the possible positions for sexual intercourse 67.7% (22) reported that they had found different acceptable positions. Ten (29.4%) said that the only possible position was lying on their back, with their partner on top of them. Another preferred position was lying sideways facing the partner or being on top of the partner. The reasons given for the preferred positions were better mobility, better respiration, less spasticity, more comfort, etc. Other sexual activities like caressing one another, kissing, and petting were reported to be as important as or even more important than intercourse to the majority of the interviewed women.

According to Romano, handicapped women need more open and intense communication about sexual activities and desires with their partners. In our study we found that 30 of 34 women (88.2%) were talking frequently or occasionally with their partners about sexual topics and about what aroused them most. One important issue we tried to explore in our interviews was how much information the spinal cord injured women remembered to be given about sexuality during their rehabilitation. More than 50% of them stated that they had not been given any information, 80% felt they had not received enough information about changes in sexuality, and only 17.5% believed they had had the right amount of information at the right time in hospital. It seems, that – whatever information the patients had really been given during primary rehabilitation – most of them had not been impressed by it, or the information did not meet their needs at that period (for example the fact that they are able to bear children and that their menstruation would be regular after some time). Besides physicians and nurses, female copatients seem to play a very important role as informants and models for newly injured women. The exchange of experience and opinions also about sexuality and partnership seems to have great impact on the newly developing self-image as a handicapped woman.

At the end of the interview the women were asked about their attitude toward men and their own sexuality. About half of the subjects indicated that they were afraid of taking the initiative when meeting a man. The male reactions to a disabled woman in a wheelchair were estimated as negative, i..e, frigthened and helpless, by 24 (64.8%) and positive, i.e., helpful and careful, by 8 (21.6%), while the others did not note any difference to the male reactions before the injury.

The last question, and probably one of the most important ones, was whether the spinal cord injured women regarded themselves as sexually superior, equal, or inferior compared with nondisabled women. None of them valued themselves as superior, about half of them regarded themselves as inferior, and the other half thought they were equal.

Looking at the results of this study the following can be drawn:

- Sexuality is – also to disabled women – much more than intercourse and pregnancy, it is both a very important factor for self-esteem and self-confidence and a kind of social interaction that makes it possible to share intimacy and deep feelings with a partner.
- Spinal cord injured women tend not to become neuter but most of them try to find a partner and sexual fulfilment. As this is a way of coping well with a disability it should be supported by the rehabilitation team.
- Sexuality should be a more important issue in the rehabilitation of spinal cord injured women. This means that sexual information and counseling should be offered to the patients and their partners in hospital and rehabilitation centers. In order to fulfil this demand, the staff – doctors, nurses, and other therapists – have to be trained in dealing with sexual questions.
- Sexual fulfilment of a spinal cord injured woman does not depend only on the level of lesion and the preserved sensitivity or motor function, it also depends on the psychological situation and the attitude of the patients. Further research and therapeutic concepts are necessary in order to help handicapped women to activate their sexual potential and thus make them feel more satisfied and self-confident.

References

Friedmann BE (1978) Female sexuality following spinal cord injury. Cheever Publishing, Bloomington

Paeslack V (1984) Sexualität der querschnittgelähmten Frau. In: Stöhrer, Palmtag, Madersbacher (eds) Blasenlähmung. Thieme, Stuttgart

Romano MD (1978) Sexuality and the disabled female. Sexuality and disability, vol 1, No 1

Trieschmann RB (1980) Sexuality and spinal cord injury. In: Trieschmann (ed) Spinal cord injuries: psychological, social and vocational adjustment. Pergamon, New York

Fertility in Male Paraplegia

C. Pons

Rehabilitation Cent, Zandbergsweg 111, NL 6432 CC Hoensbroek, Netherlands

Introduction

Fertility is an important part in the sexuality of handicapped people. For society in general, the handicapped person is someone who, by definition, is without sexuality. There is a very clear literary example: 50 years ago D. H. Lawrence wrote Lady Chatterley's Lover. Lawrence describes Chatterley, a paraplegic invalid of the First World War, as being impotent, making Lady Chatterley's extramarital affairs a natural consequence. The image of the impotent paraplegic is matter of factly accepted not only in the literature, but also by the professional healthcare worker. Certainly in the initial phase of their handicap, but often later as well, handicapped people also see sexuality as something that is definitively past; something that cannot longer fit in with such a seriously damaged physical image. It is difficult for nonhandicapped people to imagine what it is like to have a spinal cord lesion. Cole (1975) attempts to resolve some of the difficulty by means of a realistic description.

It would be helpful if the reader would imagine that he has become suddenly paraplegic. He is totally paralysed and has lost all ability to feel bodily sensations from the midchest down. He is a head and shoulders floating in space. He can still feel normally above the mid-chest area. Automatic bodily functions have been altered and bladder and bowel control has been lost. The bladder may empty itself spontaneously into diapers or clothing, or it may be continually drained off by a tube in the bladder which passes out of the urethra and travels down to a plastic bag strapped to the leg and filled full of urine.

Because bowel control has also been lost, faecal incontinence can occur at any time. There is no superficial or deep sensation in the genitals, and one would have to be watching to know that the genitals were being touched or manipulated. The physical experience of orgasm no longer can occur. In the case of the male, erotic stimulation which previously produced erections no longer does. The body has become abruptly altered and its normal contours have been changed. Areas of looseness and sagging may appear together with other areas of atrophy and loss of muscle mass. The individual can no longer stand or walk. He moves about seated in a wheelchair, causing him to converse with erect people by looking upward. Everyone is taller than he. It is not difficult to imagine that this altered body condition could lead to self consciousness and feeling of inadequacy which may cause the individual to actively avoid sexual encounter.

An intensive and all-questioning learning process will be necessary in order to reach any level of acceptance of such a violated body; an acceptance based on

Sexology
Eds.: W. Eicher, G. Kockott

those possibilities which remain, including those in the sexual areas. These possibilities may not be rejected or negated. Specific examination and knowledge of these possibilities is the primary pre-condition for learning to cope. It is important to realise that the sexual act is only a part of the vast problem and possibility of sexuality. Any sexuality has more aspects than the genital aspects. The neuromuscular aspect, the body as instrument and the psycho-social aspect are just as important as the genital aspect. In this short paper only some genital aspects are considered.

What is a Paraplegia?

A transverse lesion can be defined as damage to the spinal cord and/or to the nerves running through the spinal canal, resulting in an interruption in the continuity of the ascending and descending nerve fibres.

Resulting in a trias of symptoms:
- motor disturbances
- sensory disturbances and
- vegetative disturbances.

Three simple words: motor, sensory and vegetative, but placed in the description of Cole, it becomes more realistic but still hardly understandable. In the United States, spinal cord injury occurs most frequently in young persons with a mean age of 29.7 years, the most frequent age at injury of 19 years, with a 4:1 ratio of males:females (Stover 1987). The picture as described by Cole becomes more accurate: The young male paraplegic with all his expectations for life, including sexuality and fertility.

Neurophysiology of Male Sexual Functioning

The course of sexual activity comprises four phases:
- erection of the penis,
- emission of semen: internal transport,
- ejaculation in the narrowest sense (expulsion), and
- orgasm.

Erection

An erection is caused by a swelling of the corpora cavernosa and spongiosa as the result of a hyperaemia which is due to arterial dilatation. The erection is maintained by the pinching of the vein between the swollen corpora and the stiff tunica albuginea. Neural influence originates from sacral segments S2–4, via efferent parasympathetic fibres (nervi erigentes). An erection can also be brought about by impulses from the sympathetic centres (Th11–L2), efferent via the hypogastric nerves, and it is of a cholinergic character. Visual, aural, olfactory or tactile external stimuli can cause an erection, as can fantasies. Such stimulation leads to an erection via the spinal cord and peripheral nerves; the sympathetic centres also play a role in this type of psychogenic erection. It is possible too to produce an erection by directly stimulating the external sexual organs.

Direct tactile stimulation results in a reflexive erection. Psychogenic erection requires proper brain functioning, long pathways in the spine and the sympathetic reflex centre (centrally and psychogenically activated centre). Reflexive erection requires that the sacral reflex centre and reflex arc are intact. Specific receptores, e.g. those sensitive to vibration, play a significant role in the genital area.

Seminal Emission

This is defined as the emission of the secreted products from the seminal vesicles and prostate, plus the spermatozoa from the testicles via the vasa deferentia in the proximal portion of the urethra. Just prior to this emission, the neck of the bladder is closed, thereby preventing a retrograde ejaculation. Neural influence is sympathetic, arising from the sympathetic reflex centre Th11–L2, efferent via the hypogastric nerves.

Ejaculation (Expulsion)

An ejaculation is brought about by clonic contractions of the bulbocavernosus and ischiocarvenosus muscles. These are striped muscles with somatic innervation. Neural control is from segments S2–4, efferent via the pudendic nerve. A very precise interplay between sympathetic, parasympathetic, and somatic influences is required for an ejaculation. In practice, ejaculation is clearly more vulnerable than the erection.

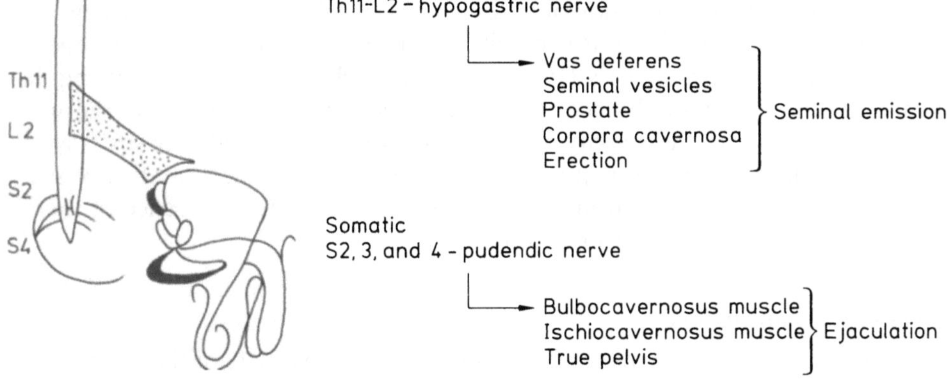

Fig. 1. Mechanism of ejaculation

Orgasm

Orgasm is difficult to define. Neurophysiologically, orgasm and ejaculation are seen as being the same thing, aslong as further reactions are also included, such as changes in respiration, circulation and muscle tone. Orgasm during masturbation will be experienced differently from an orgasm experienced during a valued act of love. Psychological and social factors, as well as physiological factors, certainly play a role in experiencing orgasm (Masters and Johnson 1966).

Disturbances in Male Sexual Function as a Result of a Spinal Cord Lesion

The medical examination. In addition to the general anamnesis, it is necessary to ask specific and detailed questions concerning the sexual behaviour of the patient before and after the lesion. The partner, if there is one, can provide important information. It is essential to use simple terminology during this conversation. The medical examination includes a general internal examination, and the neurological examination of active motor abilities, sensitivity, and reflexes, which will determine the location of the lesion, the type of spinal cord lesion, and whether or not damage to the myelum is complete. The level of the lesion is determined for all functions and is expressed in terms of the segmental myelum level; identifying the cord lesion by its spinal level is not a reliable indicator. The examination of sacral functions is extremely important. The examination of sensitivity often reveals the existence of some residual sacral function. Finding this is of great significance for further classification and for patient counselling. An examination of the ability to voluntarily tense the anal sphincter and the levator ani provides information about voluntary motor abilities at the sacral level. Examination of the superficial anal reflex, the bulbocavernosus reflex and cremasteric reflex provides information on sacral reflex activity. The Achilles reflex provides information about the somatic reflex activity S2–4. A urodynamic examination (including an electro-myelographic examination – EMG – of the pelvic musculature), carried out when regulating a neurogenic bladder, provides important details about the functioning of the sacral myelum.

Classification

With the aid of this examination of reflex activities, voluntary motor activity, and sensitivity at the sacral level, it is possible to determine the type of "neurogenic sexuality" following Comarr's (1978) very useful classification. The typing depends on the presence or absence of reflex activities via segments S2–4 of the myelum. The presence of the activity indicates the existence of "reflexive sex" (synonym: upper motor neuron sex); when it is absent, this is called "areflexive sex" (synonym: lower motor neuron sex). Complete means a total absence of sacral sensitivity and voluntary motor control.

Reflexive Complete Sex

The reflex activity via segments S2–4 is intact, while sensitivity of the penis, scrotum and perineal tissue is lacking, as too is voluntary motor control of the pelvic musculature. A reflexive erection can be expected by 90% or more of these patients. This erection will be useful for coitus for 70% of these patients. The majority are not capable of ejaculation (1%–5% successful ejaculation).

Reflexive Incomplete Sex

Reflex activity via the sacral segments is present. Sensitivity is lacking and voluntary motor control of the pelvic muscles is present, or vice versa: sensitivity is partially present in combination with a partial or complete lack of voluntary motor control. Generally, 98% of this group can achieve an erection (reflex), while 83% can use this erection for coitus. About 45% can be expected to be able to achieve a psychogenic erection, as well as a reflexive erection. Of this group capable of successful coitus, thirty-five per cent can achieve ejaculation.

Areflexive Complete Sex

Reflex activity via the sacral segments is lacking. There is a total loss of sensitivity in the sacral tissue, and a complete lack of voluntary muscle control of the pelvic musculature (analogous to the lower motor neuron lesion in the classification of neurogenic bladders). Although patients in this group are incapable of a reflexive erection, 25% can generally achieve psychogenic erection. Of these patients, approximately 25 per cent can have successful coitus. Ejaculation occurs in 20%–35% of these cases, which almost exclusively includes those patients whose lesion is located below Th12.

Areflexive Incomplete Sex

There is no reflex activity via the sacral segments. There is a complete loss of sensitivity in the sacral tissue, while voluntary motor control of the pelvic muscles is present, or vice versa: sensitivity is partially present in combination with a partial or complete lack of voluntary motor control. The majority of these patients (83%) have psychogenic erections. 75 per cent achieve successful coitus and 50% achieve ejaculation. Sometimes "psychogenic" emissions are seen.

This classification must be seen as a framework, into which each individual patient must be fitted. Too many exceptions prove the rule of the categorization. Differentiating between a complete and an incomplete lesion can sometimes be very difficult.

Statements concerning the sexual function to be expected can be made only after the neurological picture had stabilised: statements in the initial phase are valueless. Anamnesis is not always very reliable. A role is played by secondary factors, such as medication, infection and urological and neurosurgical measures.

Reviewing these groups, we find psychogenic erection varying between 90% in the areflexive incomplete sex group and 0% in cases of reflexive complete sex. Ejaculation occurs significantly more in the areflexive sex group than in the reflexive sex group.

Treatment

The relativity of the term treatment must be emphasized. Treatment can only be partly effective, and is sensible only when it is a part of a total program of adaptation and guidance.

Erection: How to Improve?

- masturbation
- vibratory stimulation as a starter
- endoprosthesis: such as a fixed permanent form and the inflatable form
- exoprosthesis: an exoprosthesis is an artificial penis, consisting of a thick-walled, stiff condom which is worn over the unaroused penis. A new erection assistence device is the correct aid.

Erection can be improved or prolonged by the use of a condom, fixed with tape at the base of the penis, creating a tourniquet effect, which can help sustain the erection. The same effect is achieved by sexual technique of the partner, the "stuffing" technique.

Chemically Induced Erection by Local Injections:

- phenoxybenzamine (Brindley 1986)
- phentolamine
- papaverine (Wyndaele et al. 1986)

Brindley does not combine drugs. Their secondary side effects must be considered (e.g. priapism, hypotension).

As Brindley stated at the workshop: "sexual aspects of spinal cord injury," held at Stoke-Mandeville in May 1987: "the prosthesis is the main line to come."

Experimental is the sacral arterial root-stimulation, on the level of S1–S2, as developed for management of the neurogenic bladder (still experimentally).

Disturbances in Ejaculation

As stated before, ejaculation in the spinal paralyzed man is rarely obtained spontaneously, as reported by all authors: less than 10% (Francois 1986).

Disturbances in ejaculation must more often be seen within the framework of fertility and procreative functions, and less in the light of an erotic sexual relationship.

Provoking ejaculations is done by manual methods, mechanical methods, and electroejaculation and pharmacological stimulation. The manual method is masturbation, either by the handicapped or by the partner, for example in cases of cervical lesion accompanied by disturbances of hand function.

Vibration

The condition is that the reflex arc exists, and that the appropriate technique is used. Frequency of 40–120 Hz and lower frequencies of 30–60 Hz will provoke erection; higher frequencies (80–100 Hz) are used to induce an ejaculation. A high amplitude is necessary. The site of application is the ventral surface of the glans. The Wahl-2 speed vibrator is a good example. A very expensive one is the VIBRECTOR. In a high lesion vibration can be more dangerous than electrostimulation by provoking autonomic dysreflexia, which will continue even if the vibration is stopped. With electroejaculation it has been seen many times that the blood pressure begins to fall as soon as stimulation is stopped; with the vibrator it seems that this is not so (Brindley 1981).

Electroejaculation

The advantage is that it is the only technique acting by direct stimulation on the sympathic pathways. "Electroejaculation" is the word generally used to denote the collection of semen by electrical stimulation with electrodes in the rectum (Brindley 1981). In 84 patients with spinal injuries, Brindley (1981) described 36 patients with external success and 14 patients with retrograde success. Side effects were: intolerable pain (incomplete in L4–5 and sacral), aftereffects on spasms, micturation, erection, rise in blood pressure (above Th5).

Drug-Induced Ejaculation

The use of intrathecal Prostigmine (neostigmine) as described by Guttmann has been abandoned because of severe autonomic dysreflexias. Physostigmine (parasympathomimetic agent) by subcutaneous injection was described by Chapelle (1983). If the lesion affected Th12, L1, and L2 the test failed. No autonomic dysreflexia was observed; the side effects were: An orthostatic hypotension and nausea and vomiting.

The following schedule is used: The patient is lying down, having fasted for 6–8 h and not having received any ganglioplegic therapy. Injection of 40 mg of Hyoscine-*N*-butylbromide (Buscopan®) is given followed 20 min later by 2 mg of physostigmine. Masturbation is carried out 10 min later. If ejaculation does not occur within 30 min a supplementary injection of 1 mg physostigmine is given.

Chapelle has recently reported 27 pregnancies for 80 paraplegics using this technique (Francois 1987).

Brindley and Francois tend more and more to use a combination of vibrator application or electroejaculation with a drug such as: idazoxan (alpha$_2$-adrenoceptor block), 40–60 mg, orally; bromocriptine (dopamine-antagonist) 2.5, or 5 mg orally; physostigmine subcutaneously.

The first choice is masturbation, then vibrator application, if necessary combined with a drug. If results are negative, electroejaculation or subcutaneous physostigmine must be performed. One can only consider the term "non-fertility" if all these methods are used and several trials have been performed.

New techniques are: implanted stimulation of the anterior sacral root direct collection of semen from the vasa deferentia and seminal vesicles, and in vitro fertilization when one or two spermatozoa are brought into the oocyte.

A Few Remarks About Retrograde Ejaculation

If retrograde ejaculation occurs due to sphincter dyssynergia, pudendal block can be considered.

If retrograde ejaculation occurs, in the literature the use of desipramine (50, 75, or 100 mg, given 3 to 24 h before ejaculation) is recommended.

Retrograde ejaculation is more often seen using the technique of electrostimulation than in reflex ejaculation.

Bladder neck incision is often the cause of retrograde ejaculation in reflex ejaculation.

If retrograde ejaculation occurs: the bladder must be empty, catheterization is necessary, and concentration of urine with the right pH with isotonic or hypertonic urine must be performed.

The Sperm

The volume and percentage of spermatozoa in spinal men are very diminished, although the technique used influences the volume: vibration gives better results than electroejaculation. The quality of the sperm increases with regular ejaculation, either by vibration or by electroejaculation, even if the spinal cord has been damaged for many years. The damage is done in the first 6 weeks, mostly by urogenic complications (Bakker 1985). Even if the quantity is poor (less than 10^6 spermatozoa/ml), the quality is more important. The low motility percentage is the dominant characteristic and also the most important factor in achieving fertility. Deep scrotal temperature is an important factor (higher in spinal man than in normal man); when above 36.4 °C, there is a very low motility. Freezing of semen in sperm banks causes a decrease in quality of the sperm. The best way of improvement of the sperm in terms of removal of seminal plasma, selection of spermatozoa, and enhancement of motility means direct application to the cervix.

As stated by Francois (1987) in the jubilee issue of the *International Journal of the Spinal Cord* in 1987:

"In spite of numerous factors, it is possible to be relatively optimistic" ... "If one takes into account all the factors which come into play, as well as the gynaecological status of the women and the couple's perseverence, this result corresponds to 38% of pregnancies by those really wanting a child."

We have reached the post-Chatterley era.

References

Bakker H (1985) Ejaculatie bij mannen met een ruggemergletsel. Ned Tijdschr Geneesk 129:1931–1933

Brindley GS (1981) Electro ejaculation: its technique, neurological implications and uses. J Neurol Neurosurg Psychiatr 44:9–18

Brindley GS (1981) Reflex ejaculation under vibratory stimulation in paraplegic man. Paraplegia 19:229–302

Chapelle PA (1983) Treatment of an ejaculation in the total paraplegic by subcutaneous injection of physiostigmine. Paraplegia 21:30–36
Cole TM (1975) Sexuality and physical disabilities. Arch Sex Behav 4:389–403
Comarr AE (1978) Sex classification and expectations among quadriplegics and tetraplegics. Sexuality and Disability 1:252–259
Francois N, Maury M (1987) Sexual aspects in paraplegic patients. Paraplegia 25:289–292
Pons C (1985) Sexual aspects and neurological injuries in cases of transverse lesions. In: Dechesne BHH, Pons C, Schellen AMCM (eds) Sexuality and handicap, problems of motor handicapped people. Woodhead-Faulkner, Cambridge, pp 49–93
Stover SL, Fine PR (1987) The epidemiology and economics of spinal cord injury. Paraplegia 25:225–228
Tarabulcy E (1972) Sexual function in the normal and paraplegic. Paraplegia 10:201–208
Wyndaele JJ, de Meyer JM, de Sy WA, Claessens H (1986) Intracavernous injection of vasoactive drugs, an alternative for treating impotence in spinal cord injury patients. Paraplegia 24:271:275

Pregnancy and Labor in the Paraplegic

V. Paeslack

Abteilung für Behandlung und Rehabilitation Querschnittsgelähmter
Schlierbacher Landstraße 200a, 6900 Heidelberg, FRG

The ability of paraplegic women to conceive has to be considered normal. Spinal cord injured women ought to be informed in good time about the chances and risks of pregnancy and parturition. Experience proves that as a rule this information may have a positive psychological effect on therapy and rehabilitation. The formerly held opinion that paraplegia and pregnancy have to exclude one another, and moreover that pregnancy may cause an additional danger for the paraplegic woman, cannot be confirmed. So the physician should emphatically contradict such views.

Experience shows that there is no medical or social contraindication of pregnancy if the paraplegic woman is in good physical and psychological health. Pregnancy in paraplegics or tetraplegics, however, requires careful supervision by cooperating gynecologists and specialists in spinal cord injury. Risks of congenital malformations particularly of the spine and spinal cord should be considered not increased in comparison with nondisabled women. Regarding the course of gravidity certain medical aspects must be considered. The frequency of urinary tract infections may be increased during the first trimenon. Women suffering from renal complications before the onset of pregnancy should be carefully supervised for gestosis during the full term of gravidity. Frequently there will be manifestations of iron deficiency anemia observed. Prophylactic ferrotherapy may lead to nausea and gastrointestinal incompatibility. In pronounced cases, blood transfusions may become necessary.

In women suffering from paraplegia above T5/6 in particular in cases of tetraplegia the risk of paroxysmal hyperreflexia with sudden hypertension should be considered. This syndrome will be provoked by an acute rise in intraabdominal pressure mainly caused by disturbances voiding the bladder or by insufficient evacuation of the rectal ampulla.

Acute infections of kidneys or bladder have to be treated carefully by antibiotics, avoiding drugs, which may have an embryotoxic effect. During the final phase of pregnancy, disturbances of the micturition will frequently be found as result of the enlargement and displacement of the uterus. Bladder training is no longer successful; insertion of an indwelling catheter connected to a closed bag system may be unavoidable. As a rule such disturbances will be normalized after delivery, and former reflex bladder function will return within some weeks.

Severe problems may appear in cases of pregnant women sustaining a spinal cord injury with paraplegia or tetraplegia as a consequence. On the one hand a concomitant traumatic lesion of the uterus and embryo should be considered. In 1971 we published two cases of congenital brain damage caused presumably by

Sexology
Eds.: W. Eicher, G. Kockott

the trauma which struck the pregnant mothers during the first trimenon and left them paraplegic. On the other hand, hazards should be considered resulting from drugs – anticoagulants, antibiotics, ganglioblockers – from X-ray examinations, anesthesia, or unavoidable surgical interventions, administered to the pregnant paraplegic mother.

There seems to exist no detailed knowledge as to whether the embryo may suffer damages, caused by spinal shock. At any rate in the case that spinal cord injury hits a woman in the first stage of pregnancy advantages and dangers of an interruption need to be discussed carefully.

Labor and Delivery

If the traumatic paraplegic suffers from a lesion above T10, the risk of premature labor onset is higher than in nondisabled women. For this reason it is recommended that these patients be taken under clinical surveillance 3–4 weeks prior to the term of birth. Rupture of the membranes may occur unnoticed, and loss of amniotic liquor may be misinterpreted as reflex micturition.

Paraplegics suffering from lesions above T8 as a result of analgesia frequently do not recognize the onset of labor. Sometimes signs of paroxysmal hyperreflexia are the only and most important indications of the onset of birth. The activity of labor is independent of spinal regulations and will not be influenced by paraplegia.

„Silent partus" may happen through lack of any sensory feeling for labor and parturition, possibly in connection with evacuation of the bowels. Because of paresis of the abdominal muscles, paraplegic parturients are unable actively to support bearing down effects.

Delivery may be facilitated in flaccid paralysis of the pelvic floor but made more difficult under conditions of intense spasticity. The view that every paraplegic parturient should be deliverd by cesarean section is apparently no longer tenable nowadays. Indications for delivery by operation are the same as those for nonparalyzed women. Exceptions for this rule are paraplegias above T4 and tetraplegias. In such cases of high-level spinal cord injury an early planned operative delivery may help to prevent complications.

Special attention should be given to autonomous dysregulations, arising during bearing down efforts and delivery. This hyperreflex syndrome is characterized by severe headache, profuse hyperhidrosis, bradycardia, sometimes unconsciousness, convulsions, and in rare cases retinal and cerebral hemorrhage. Under such conditions delivery must be completed in the quickest way. Treatment with ganglioblockers may be helpful in such urgent situations but does carry the risk of excessive hypotonic depression. Some authors recommend delivery under peridural anesthesia.

During 15 years – between 1971 and 1986 – we observed 75 pregnancies in 45 spinal cord injured patients. The group of patients consisted of 32 paraplegics and 13 tetraplegics. Six times pregnancy was interrupted by abortion at an early point. In five cases the interruption was made during the first trimenon. In about 40% of cases delivery was performed by cesarean section. Serious complications were observed in three women. Twice we observed massive hemorrhages after laceration of the cervix. One tetraplegic parturient suffered from convulsions in connection with autonomous hyperreflexia. There were no congenital injuries in the newborn except the above-mentioned two cases.

During the postpartum period as a rule there are no paraplegia-specific complications. Breast-feeding is possible without any particular problems. If the spinal cord injury level is above Th5 the region of the nipples is anesthetic. In this case lactation may be reduced or totally absent. Tetraplegic mothers will be unable to look after their babies and to handle them. These connected social and psychological problems need to be dealt with. Solutions should be discussed and found before delivery takes place.

To conclude it can be emphasized that for a well-rehabilitated paraplegic woman no additional dangers and complications are to be expected concerning pregnancy and labor. The birth of a healthy baby is an important positive event for the vast majority of spinal cord injured women. This is particularly true regarding their efforts for the beginning of a new and active life after the cruel experience of their handicap.

XI. AIDS

Sexual Behavior and AIDS

E. J. Haeberle

1100 Gongh Street 7C, San Francisco, CA 94109, USA

Eros and Thanatos, love and death, have long been regarded as two very powerful deities fighting over our souls and shaping our lives, as the greatest conceivable opposites that are nevertheless mysteriously related.

Some romantic and symbolistic poets and artists have even tried to make this relationship manifest in works celebrating the fulfillment of love in death. Richard Wagner, the most sensuous of composers, gave this yearning its perfect expression in Isolde's *Liebestod.*

However, the fascination with love and death did not begin or end in the nineteenth century. As early as the writings of the Marquis de Sade, love and death appeared as conflicting, yet mutually reinforcing experiences, and for many writers who came after him, sexual desire expressed both a lust for life and a death wish. This century, Sigmund Freud came to the conclusion that all human striving could be traced, if not reduced, to Eros and Thanatos as the two ultimate drives.

In view of all this, it is rather peculiar that the exact relationship between sexual behavior and fatal illness has hardly ever been the subject of empirical research. There are a few recent studies of sexual concerns in cancer patients and the chronically ill, but, regrettably, the actual data base remains small (Fischer 1983; Ford and Orfirer 1967; Gideon and Taylor 1981; Goldberg and Cullen 1985; Golden 1983, 1986; Grinker 1976; Haswell 1978; Jacobson 1974; Leiber et al. 1976; Levitan 1978; Money 1967; Patterson 1980; Schon 1968; Taylor 1983; Vaeth 1986; Wasow 1977, 1982; Waxberg and Mostel 1980; Wise 1977, 1978a, b, c, 1983; Wood and Trombrick 1983; Woods 1975).

However, the subject has now gained importance with the arrival of the sexually transmissible human immunodeficiency virus (HIV) and the various diseases caused by it. The most serious possible consequence of an HIV infection, aquired immune deficiency syndrome (AIDS), is now killing tens of thousands of men and women in many countries and is frightening millions more. Indeed, several millions may already be infected, and hundreds of thousands are now suffering from AIDS-related conditions (ARCs).

Under these circumstances, it would seem more than justified to take another close look at human sexual behavior. The behavior of the infected before and after their diagnosis, especially, merits examination. Unfortunately, so far, only a few, perfunctory observations have been made. For the sake of organizing systematic research in this area, one could perhaps divide the general population into five groups:

Sexology
Eds.: W. Eicher, G. Kockott

1. The unconcerned – either uninfected or infected without knowing it
2. The concerned but uninfected
3. The concerned who have no symptoms, but know they are infected
4. Persons suffering from ARCs
5. Persons suffering from AIDS

At first, one might simplify the task somewhat by considering the last two of these groups together. Those infected who have become ill with various temporary or chronic, light or severe symptoms are obviously forced to face a very serious reality, and this, in turn, can be assumed to affect their sexual interests and actions.

However, before we can begin to examine any of this, we have to face a certain widely denied reality ourselves: Many chronically ill and even dying patients do have sexual interests and seek opportunities to follow them.

This tends to be denied by hospitals, official social services, and religious counselors, even by the family members of patients. After all, traditionally patients with serious diseases have always been treated as nonsexual beings. Few if any hospitals, for example, make provisions for sexual contacts between patients and visitors. In the case of AIDS patients, this reluctance is reinforced by the potential for virus transmission and the fact that, at present, most of the patients are still homosexual and bisexual men. Should hospitals be asked to provide opportunities for homosexual contact? Or should they, on the other hand, try to prevent such contact at all costs?

These questions are not frivolous. In San Francisco, a disgruntled nurse has already accused the city's General Hospital of providing sexual opportunities for its AIDS patients, a charge that has been vigorously denied. However, it is recognized hospital policy to allow visitors to stay overnight in the patient's room and to put up sleeping cots for this purpose. The visitor may be the patient's current lover or previous sexual partner. Should this policy be discontinued? Should the hospital at least insist on "safe sex" on its premises? How?

Should "sexual" contact be prohibited, but "affectionate" physical contact be allowed? Where should the line be drawn and by whom? Another issue is raised by the availability of video recorders inside the AIDS ward. Should the staff encourage or prohibit the use of "porno videos" by patients?

All of these questions remain relevant as long as AIDS patients are hospitalized for long periods of time. In San Francisco they are, by now, largely academic, because our reorganized health care system has allowed us to cut the average hospital stay of AIDS patients down to under 2 weeks. Most of the care is provided at home. Thus, AIDS patients are hospitalized only during certain life-threatening episodes and released as soon as they are out of immediate danger. As a result, the above questions are of greater concern to hospice and other home-care providers. In the home, on the other hand, the issue of sexuality, once faced, is much easier to address.

As mentioned above, not very much is known about the sexual behavior of AIDS patients, but here I can at least offer some preliminary findings. One of my students, Patrick Glasscock, has begun a project, conducting extensive, Kinsey-style interviews with homosexual and bisexual AIDS patients, asking them about their sexual behavior before and after diagnosis. The first 50 of these interviews already yield some interesting clues:

- All patients reported continued sexual desire, although it appeared sharply reduced during episodes of acute illness. After recovery, the desire usually returned.
- Many reported a negative effect on their body image and self-esteem, although this effect was often transitory.
- A few patients reported sexual dysfunctions which began only after the diagnosis of AIDS.
- Most of the patients had dramatically reduced the number of sexual partners.
- There was a sharp reduction in "unsafe" sexual practices, with masturbation being the most frequent sexual outlet (Glasscock 1988).

Obviously, these partial, preliminary findings are inconclusive. I am mentioning them here, not for the purpose of proving anything, but merely to underline the importance of addressing the issue of sex and AIDS. After all, it should not come as a surprise to any of us that even AIDS patients are sexual beings with sexual needs. These needs can and perhaps should be met as far as circumstances allow. They may vary from case to case, but we probably should also ask ourselves some general questions. For example:

- Should physicians, counselors, and other health-care workers, or simply friends and lovers of AIDS patients help them to restore or increase their sexual desire? Should they help them to find partners and to have "safe" sexual encounters? Could this strengthen their overall health and contribute to their relative well-being?
- Should therapists treat sexual dysfunctions in AIDS patients? How?

Such questions become relevant once we accept and support the sexual interests of AIDS patients. Should we as sexologists offer this acceptance and this support? If not, why not? In any case, one thing seems to me quite clear: Our stand on these issues will be a reflection of how we really feel about sex, even in healthy men and women. Thus AIDS becomes an acid test of our professional commitment and competence. Do we consider sexual activity as a concession to be made to human frailty or do we see it as having value in itself? Do we have a restricted, stereotypical view of what is sexually "natural" or correct? Or are we capable of differentiation? Do we truly accept a wide spectrum of human sexual possibilities?

The latter question indeed becomes crucial when we turn from AIDS and ARC patients to those that are infected but have no symptoms. Some of them know of their infection, know that they are infectious to their sexual partners, and therefore try to adopt "safe sex" practices. They may be homosexual men without a steady partner or they may be in an exclusive relationship. They may be husbands who acquired the virus through a casual extramarital affair or through a blood transfusion. They may be hemophiliacs who acquired it through untreated blood products. No matter how they became infected, they now need help in their efforts to find sexual fulfillment and to protect their partners at the same time. These partners, in turn, whether they are casual acquaintances, or lovers or spouses, need help in protecting themselves while entering or maintaining the sexual relationship.

There are, unfortunately, some medical and other professionals who do not want to face this problem. Their refusal amounts to a denial of reality and an abdication of responsibility. To the extent that they fail to deal with the options of "safe sex" they also betray a lack of professional knowledge.

I do not want to comment here on the embarrassing statements made by certain German sex researchers who have called "safe sex" an "expression of U.S. moral imperialism" and who congratulated themselves on "having utterly failed in matters of 'safe sex'" (Amendt and Sigusch 1986). Instead, I would like to discuss very briefly an American example of failure which forces us sexologists to take sides, indeed, to stand up and be counted.

In the fall of 1985, the otherwise respected Dr. Helen Singer Kaplan published an editorial "AIDS and the Sex Therapist" in her *Journal of Sex and Marital Therapy* (Kaplan et al. 1985), revealing an appalling ignorance of both AIDS and human sexual behavior. When the editorial was widely protested, she made a formal reply in the fall of 1986, repeating her major errors and adding a gratuitous homophobic insult to the very groups that had done most to reduce the level of infection (Kaplan et al. 1986). However, the issue here is not the apparently uninformed and confused person of Dr. Kaplan; it is rather our own willingness to prove ourselves competent where she failed. If we do not supply this proof – and fairly soon – the men and women at risk from AIDS, and eventually the entire population, will lose confidence in our ability to make any meaningful contribution at all. Thus, the entire field of sexology could suffer irreparable damage.

Time limitations do not allow me to quote and refute Dr. Kaplan's two editorials in detail. I will therefore discuss only three of her most outrageous statements:

1. "There is no such thing as 'safe sex'."
2. "Single persons ... should not have sex with individuals in the high-risk group, unless that person is willing to be tested and cleared" (Kaplan et al. 1985, pp 211–212).
3. "Gay activist groups seem to have little concern about preventing the spread of AIDS in their determination to protect their ... civil rights" (Kaplan et al. 1986, p 163).

I will pass over the faulty grammar of the second statement and directly address the content of all three in sequence:

1. The first statement "There is no such thing as 'safe sex'." is very obviously false. Indeed, Kaplan herself later mentions "Masturbation, parallel masturbation, and celibate, affectionate, romantic relationships" as safe. However, this by no means exhausts the possibilities which include "telephone sex," certain sadomasochistic practices, "sensate focus" exercises, erotic massages and frottage, consensual voyeurism, and exhibitionism. Many of these, however, are practices traditionally condemned by psychiatrists as "perversions" or at least as "immature" and undesirable. Such ideological blinders today prevent many, not only Dr. Kaplan, from perceiving the obvious: Many formerly denigrated forms of sexual expression can be life-saving alternatives to unprotected coitus. Those therapists who, like Kaplan, equate "sex" simply with vaginal intercourse and who fail to see the full range of available options reveal a curious tunnel vision which prevents them from entering any meaningful dialogue with their clients and patients. This is particularly disturbing in a profession that has worked long and hard at broadening the concept of sex.

2. The second statement making "sex" dependent on the willingness of high-risk partners to be tested and "cleared" is even more disturbing. I have already mentioned married men and women who know they are infected and who have told their spouses. Should we declare the sexual side of their marriage to be over? Are we to end their sexual relationship by therapeutic fiat without helping them to develop some practical options? However, the most unsettling aspect of Kaplan's statement is the naive reliance on testing and "clearance" as a means of stopping the epidemic. I won't even mention the occasional false-positive and frequent false-negative test results seen up to several months after infection. Let us also forget the fact that any "clearance," even if justified, is good only on the day issued and no longer – the real problem is Kaplan's failure to see the potential social implications of widespread testing.

3. This becomes all too clear in her third, inaccurate and insulting statement about gay activist groups which care mostly for their own civil rights and show little concern about preventing AIDS. In the meantime, this pernicious slander has indeed gained some acceptance in so-called conservative, but actually right-wing, nearly totalitarian political circles and threatens to undermine the enormous prevention efforts that have already been made. First, the statement creates a false dichotomy: minority civil rights versus public health. In fact, however, the latter cannot possibly be protected without first protecting the former. Where the civil rights of sexual minorities are trampled underfoot, where homosexuals, drug users, or prostitutes, for example, are subjected to forced testing, where their positive test results are not kept strictly confidential, where they suffer the slightest discrimination in employment, housing, or freedom to travel, the majority courts disaster. Not only will these groups cease to cooperate with the authorities who will thus unintentionally end up driving the epidemic underground – causing it to spread much faster through the rest of the population – but, most importantly: the first steps leading down a very slippery slope will have been taken. At the bottom of this slope we will all find ourselves in a two-class society: on the one hand a large, if slowly dwindling number of certified "test-negatives" enjoying all social privileges, and on the other hand a smaller, but steadily growing number of unemployed, unemployable, homeless "test-positives" with nothing left to lose. This is a prescription for national financial ruin and permanent social unrest; it is an invitation to terrorism of a new kind, compared to which all previous group violence will seem almost benign.

Fortunately, the American public health authorities responsible, from the Surgeon General on down, see this danger clearly. They have therefore always warned against sacrificing anyone's civil rights and have rejected the false dichotomy suggested by Dr. Kaplan. They also know very well who has initiated and maintained the most effective AIDS prevention programs – none other than the gay activist groups so unjustly maligned by Dr. Kaplan. It is the historical truth that AIDS prevention through behavior change was begun by gay activists in San Francisco, New York, and other American cities, especially the Bay Area Physicians for Human Rights, the Sexologists' Health Project at our institute, the San Francisco AIDS Foundation, and the New York Gay Men's Health Crisis.

They all became active and developed "safe sex" guidelines at a time when Dr. Kaplan and many other sex therapists had nothing concrete to offer but general calls for caution. Therefore, her attempt to rewrite history is deeply offensive to any true pioneer of AIDS prevention.

There are now numerous studies available demonstrating just how successful the gay AIDS prevention programs have been. In one group of gay men studied in San Francisco, the infection rate dropped from over 12% in 1982 to 1% in 1986 (*San Francisco Examiner* 1987). In fact, about 90% of the San Francisco gay population has now adopted either sexual abstinence, strict sexual exclusivity, or a safe-sex lifestyle (CDC 1985; McKusick et al. 1985; Research and Decisions Corporation 1986; Winkelstein et al. 1987). The drastic change in sexual behavior is convincingly demonstrated by the falling rate of rectal gonorrhea cases in the city – from an average of about 550 per month in 1980 to about 20 per month in late 1986 (Echenberg et al. 1986; Echenberg and Stoller 1986). Similar results have been reported in New York city. Unfortunately, because of the long incubation period of the disease, the number of AIDS cases among gay and bisexual men continues to rise as most of these were infected years ago, before the prevention programs were fully developed.

It remains a fact, however, that these programs have produced such a dramatic behavior change in so many people in such a short time as to be virtually without historical parallel in their effectiveness. They have reached many previously unconcerned, although infected, and uninfected individuals, and motivated them to avoid the risk of infection or additional infection without denying themselves sexual fulfillment. And finally, the programs have forestalled a dangerous social division into the infected and ill on the one hand and the rest of the population on the other.

Indeed, we are all in this together. In the end, even the strictly monogamous or completely asexual person will be touched by the spread of AIDS, if only as a voter or taxpayer. All others, however, must learn to adjust their sexual behavior to the new, dangerous situation. The gay self-help groups have shown them how.

Returning again to the sexual needs and options of AIDS patients, we see more clearly the direction in which we must go. We must free ourselves and help free others of preconceived, narrow notions of sex and now evaluate all sexual behavior according to a new criterion. We must ask: Does this behavior carry a risk of infection? If so, we should judge it bad, if not, we should consider it good. Accordingly, we should explore all "good" sexual possibilities and develop a wide spectrum of "safe sex," from which we ourselves, our clients, and patients can choose.

We will also have to consider sexual options that are only "conditionally safe," such as the use of a condom, perhaps in combination with spermicidal preparations. It is not helpful to dwell on the possible failure of condoms, as Dr. Kaplan does. An immediate, universal use of condoms would certainly slow down the epidemic to a remarkable extent. This is the very reason why the Surgeon General of the USA recommends condoms in his official report.

The same recommendation is part of all current AIDS prevention programs in Europe and indeed the rest of the world. Again, this idea was first developed by gay activists who, before AIDS, had hardly ever used condoms, but then took a new look at them, experimented with them, and promoted them in their own communities. This promotion also included explicit instructions for their correct application, because it is well known that the failure rate of condoms as contraceptives is largely due to incorrect and inconsistent use.

At the same time, the most successful prevention programs combined detailed medical information with positive erotic messages in group settings. A recent study of programs run by the Gay Men's Health Crisis in New York has now demonstrated that this approach is indeed the best (unpublished study, results reported by Helquist 1987 and Jacobs 1987). Frightening people with the dangers of AIDS only seems to have a temporary effect. In the long run, AIDS prevention requires new, safe, but satisfying sexual habits, and these habits must be supported by a strong group solidarity, indeed by peer group pressure. It will therefore become necessary to eroticize "safe sex" for whole populations.

Here, however, we finally come to the crux of the matter: The still underinformed general public is not yet prepared to accept unconventional sexual behavior as possibly healthy and does not want it promoted under any circumstances. Hence the resistance to condom commercials on television, explicit educational language, "safe sex" pornos, "telephone sex," and masturbation clubs. By and large, the American gay community has accepted all of these and more, and it has changed its behavior accordingly. How will the public react when all of these changes are increasingly carried into the "straight," i.e., heterosexual, community? Perhaps the necessary transformation of values will provoke new forms of resistance and intolerance on both the right and the left. What will we sexologists do? Are we afraid of this potential intolerance? Will we be found on the side of its victims? I do not predict a comfortable position for any of us in the future. At any rate, one thing is clear: So far, AIDS prevention has not been hampered by the protection of minority civil rights, but by the protection of majority sexual prejudices.

When certain politicians have demanded "drastic measures" in fighting AIDS, usually they have not referred to any explicit ways of promoting "safe sex" – the only strategy proven to be effective – but to compulsory testing, registration, travel restrictions, and "quarantine" measures that are not only ineffective, but actually counterproductive. It is our duty as sexologists to expose this kind of swindle for what it is – cowardice in the face of powerful pressure groups that are unwilling or unable to see the true dangers of AIDS. These groups value their sexual ideologies higher than human life. They have opted for Thanatos over Eros, for death rather than life.

Let us not allow their ideas to prevail! We can make a life-saving contribution in the fight against AIDS by reaffirming the sexual rights of all men and women – in sickness and in health. Today, more than ever, serving the cause of life should be our highest priority.

References

Amendt G, Sigusch V (1986) In: Operation AIDS. Konkret – Sexualität March:26, 72

CDC (1985) Self-reported behavioral change among gay and bisexual men – San Francisco. Morbidity Mortality Weekly Rep 34:613–615

Echenberg DF, Stoller E (1986) Rectal gonorrhea in San Francisco, October 1984–September 1986. San Francisco Epidemiol Bull 2(12)
Echenberg DF, Rutherford GW, Darrow WW et al. (1986) The incidence and prevalence of LAV/HTLV-III infection in the San Francisco city clinic cohort, 1985. Paper presented at the 2nd international conference on AIDS. Paris, June 1986
Fisher SG (1983) The psychosexual effects of cancer and cancer treatment. Oncology Nursing Forum 10:63–68
Ford AB, Orfirer AP (1967) Sexual behavior and the chronically ill patient. Med Aspects Hum Sexuality 1:51–61
Gideon MD, Taylor PB (1981) A sexual bill of rights for dying persons. Death Educ 4:303–314
Glasscock P (1988) Sexual behavior of gay and/or bisexual males with a diagnosis of AIDS: an investigative study. (to be published)
Goldberg RJ, Cullen JO (1985) Factors important to psychological adjustment to cancer: a review of the evidence. Soc Sci Med 20:803–807
Golden JS (1983) Sex and cancer. Dan Med Bull 3:4–6
Golden JS (1986) Sexual problems of cancer patients, special issue: the physician's guide to sexual counseling. Med Aspects Hum Sexuality 20:70–76
Grinker RR Jr (1976) Sex and cancer. Med Aspects Hum Sexuality 10:130–139
Haswell GL (1978) Chronic illness and sexuality. In: Barnard J, Clany J, Krantz E (eds) Hum Sexuality Health Professionals. Saunders, Philadelphia
Helquist M (1987) Evaluation of safe sex educational interventions. Focus, a guide to AIDS research. March
Jacobs R (1987) A model for AIDS prevention. Focus, a guide to AIDS research. May
Jacobson L (1974) Illness and human sexuality. Nurs Outlook 22:50–53
Kaplan HS, Sager C, Schiavi RC (1985) AIDS and the sex therapist (editorial). J Sex Marital Ther 11(4)
Kaplan, Editorial 1985 (see above) pp 211 and 212
Kaplan, Editorial 1986 (see above) p 163
Leiber L et al. (1976) The communication of affection between cancer patients and their spouses. Psychosom Med 38:379–389
Levitan D (1978) The intimacy/sexual needs of the terminally ill and the widowed. Death Educ 2:261–280
McKusick L, Wiley JA, Coates TJ et al. (1985) Reported changes in the sexual behavior of men at risk for AIDS, San Francisco, 1982–84 – the AIDS Behavioral Research Project. Public Health Rep 100:622–629
Money J (1967) Sexual problems of the chronically ill. In: Wahl CW (ed) Sexual problems, diagnosis and treatment in medical practice. Free Press, New York
Patterson PR (1980) The role of sexual feelings in the terminal patient. Arch Found Thanatol 8:13–15
Research and Decisions Corporation (1986) Designing an effective AIDS prevention campaign strategy for San Francisco: results from the third probability sample of an urban gay community. Research and Decisions Corporation, San Francisco
San Francisco Examiner (1987) Safe sex can thwart AIDS, study shows. 10 April (The study mentioned here was undertaken by George Lemp of the San Francisco Department of Public Health. It was formally presented at the Third International Conference on AIDS in Washington, DC in June 1987)
Schon M (1968) The meaning of death and sex to cancer patients. J Sex Res 4:288–302
Taylor PB (1983) Understanding sexuality in the dying patient. Nursing 13:54–55
Vaeth JM (ed) (1986) Body image, self-esteem, and sexuality in cancer patients, 2nd rev ed. Karger, New York
Wasow M (1977) Human sexuality and terminal illness. Health Soc Work 2:105–121
Wasow M (1982) Sexuality assessment as a tool for sexual rehabilitation in cancer patients. Sexuality Disability 5:28–37
Waxberg JD, Mostel S (1980) Sex and the terminally ill: overcoming obstacles to gratification. Sexual Med Today 4:25–40

Winkelstein W Jr, Lyman DM, Padian N et al. (1987) Sexual practices and risk of infection by the human immunodeficiency virus: the San Francisco men's health study. JAMA 257:321–325
Wise T (1977) Sexuality in chronic illness. Prim Care 4:199–208
Wise T (1978a) Sexual problems resulting from interactions between medical and psychologic conditions. Med Aspects Hum Sexuality 11:71–89
Wise T (1978b) Effects of cancer on sexual activity. Psychosomatics 19:769–775
Wise T (1978c) Sexual counseling of the chronically and terminally ill. Med Aspects Hum Sexuality 12:29–30
Wise T (1983) Sexual dysfunction in the medically ill. Psychosomatics 24:787–805
Wood JD, Tombrick J (1983) Impact of cancer on sexuality and self-image: a group program for patients and partners. Soc Work Health Care 8:45–54
Woods NF (1975) Human sexuality in health and illness. Mosby, St. Louis

AIDS – Perspectives of a Malignant Epidemic (On the Need to Avoid Surprises)

M. G. Koch [1] and J. L'age-Stehr [2]

[1] VaC, 54600 Karlsborg, Sweden
[2] Robert-Koch-Institut, 1000 Berlin 65, FRG

Good judgement comes from experience –
experience comes from bad judgement.

History

It was not easy to understand what was going on, when, in 1980, a patient in New York died after a long and frustrating time of puzzling, incurable infections caused by normally harmless pathogens – viruses, bacteria, fungi, and protozoans – in combination with a rare blood-vessel malignancy called Kaposi's sarcoma (KS).

We now know that we were witnessing the take-off of an epidemic, in reality a pandemic, that soon would reach the world's remotest countries, leading us into an era, the duration of which we are not yet able to determine. It was a moment in medical history with grave implications for us all, for patients and the health-care system, for relatives and friends, and, finally, for the public. As professionals, we must concern ourselves immediately with the emerging medical consequences of this dreaded new disease; it would, however, be unwise to lose sight of other implications of this unfolding epidemic, especially the future perspectives.

More cases like the one described soon appeared: four in the New York area, five in California, all of them young homosexual men. The existence of infectious agent was immediately suspected because some clusters of contacts between patients were not explainable by random events. Leaving aside some early and rather farfetched theories about this enigmatic illness, suffice it to say that from the end of 1982 a virus, a retrovirus, became the prime suspect as the cause of this disease. Because it involved a breakdown of the immune system, the disorder was named AIDS (acquired immune deficiency syndrome). The concept of a viral origin soon proved correct: in January 1983 a French team of scientists led by Luc Montagnier (Institut Pasteur, Paris) identified the virus. The group isolated and described the agent and grew it in tissue cultures, and even developed a test for the disease based on antibodies against certain viral proteins. In their first publication (May 1983) Montagnier's team named the virus LAV (lymphadenopathy-associated virus). When some months later similar viruses (called IDAV-1, -2, etc., immunodeficiency-associated virus) were isolated from AIDS patients and their relationship to AIDS was established, the other terms were dropped and all virus variants were from then on referred to as LAV.

The British virologist Abraham Karpas (University of Cambridge) made similar observations during the following summer and published his findings in December 1983. Paul Feorino at the Center for Disease Control (CDC) in Atlanta had also found such a virus, although his would not at first survive in cell cultures.

Sexology
Eds.: W. Eicher, G. Kockott

Table 1. Nomenclature of the AIDS virus

Date	Scientist	Location	Name for AIDS virus
May 1983	Barré-Sinoussi, Cherman, Montagnier	Paris	LAV
September 1983	Barré-Sinoussi, Cherman, Montagnier	Paris	IDAV
December 1983	Karpas	Cambridge	C-LAV
May 1984	Popovic, Sarngadharan, Gallo	Bethesda	HTLV-III
August 1984	Levy	San Francisco	ARV
1983–1985	Feorino	Atlanta	LAV/HTLV-III-CDC-151, -451
August 1985	Rübsamen-Waigmann	Frankfurt	AAV
May 1986	ICTV (International Committee on the Taxonomy of Viruses)		HIV

At the National Cancer Institute (NCI) in Bethesda, Robert Gallo, who at the outset sought to demonstrate that the oncovirus HTLV-I was the cause of AIDS, finally had to confirm these findings. However, Gallo renamed the virus HTLV-III because of his conviction that it belonged to the same oncovirus group as the known human T-cell lymphoma/leukemia-associated viruses HTLV-I and -II. (Oncoviruses form one of three subgroups of retroviruses: onco-, lenti-, and spumaviruses.) Shortly after this, Jay Levy in San Francisco also identified the virus, calling it ARV (AIDS-associated retrovirus). Other scientists followed, confirming the Paris group's early findings. The proliferating nomenclature was very confusing, as shown chronologically in Table 1. Today, by international consensus, the virus is known around the world as HIV (human immunodeficiency virus). Gallo's suggestion that the AIDS virus belonged to the oncovirus family was understandable, but optimistic. Oncoviruses can give rise to tumors and immune deficiency, but most of them cause clinical disease only in a small proportion (between 0.1% and 10%) of infected individuals. In contrast, some members of the lentivirus subgroup of retroviruses cause disease in nearly all infected individuals, often with a mortality of up to 100%; for mankind, these are new and ominous properties. The lentiviruses, moreover, show a very long incubation period ("lenti" means slow), generally extending to between $^1/_3$ and $^2/_3$ of the host's life span, and unusual capabilities such as "antigenic shift," "antigen shedding," and survival in macrophages.

These features pose multiple and severe obstacles to the development of a vaccine. Today, it is a tragic fact that the virus causing AIDS turned out to be, after all, a lentivirus, as suggested by Montagnier, and not an oncovirus, as assumed by Gallo. Like the known animal lentiviruses, HIV has an insidious affinity for brain tissue and lung macrophages. The tropism for macrophages raised the possibility that antibodies could actually have an adverse effect upon inhibiting HIV infection, as is known from other viruses with tropism to macrophages (e.g., dengue virus). This effect is known as antibody-dependent virus enhancement (ADE), and has recently been shown to occur with HIV; this is likely to seriously hamper all conventional vaccine approaches.

Veterinary scientists have fought lentiviruses in sheep, goats, and horses for many years, but in vain. They have had no success in finding a treatment and have failed to develop a vaccine; their vaccination attempts actually produced more adverse effects in livestock. In the absence of a cure, it has been necessary to slaughter the infected stock. Now we must face the fact that the AIDS epidemic, as far as we know, is the result of the first lentivirus infection ever to hit mankind.

Detailed studies of HIV morphology, molecular biology, genomic structure, and the regulation of replication have shown some peculiar features. Although these features may be insufficient to place the virus in a taxonomic group of its own, the specific characteristics of HIV clearly show it to be in the lentivirus subgroup of retroviruses.

The Virus

The term retrovirus identifies a type of virus that reverses the biologically normal direction of transcription (from DNA to RNA), in which the normal cellular chromosomal information is transcribed into messenger substances that direct all life processes in the host cell. Since it consists of RNA, a retrovirus converts (a form of mimicry) its own genomic information into DNA, thereby enabling it to "hide" itself as a provirus in the genetic material of the host cell. This ability to integrate, by several enzyme-dependent steps, into the host's genome allows permanent existence of the DNA provirus in the chromosome – thus causing persistent infection in the cell. It has been shown by very sophisticated methods (hybridizing gene probes following gene amplification) that for every obviously infected cell (e.g., cells expressing viral antigen or replicating the virus), there are hundreds of cells containing so-called dormant copies.

When it has invaded the cell by penetrating the outer cell membrane, by a rather complicated process of receptor-mediated endocytosis, the virus can (after "uncoating") do without its auxiliary equipment – those structures of the nucleocapsid and membranes (shell and coats) which protect it from damage in hostile surroundings. Outside a cell's cytoplasm the virus can spread, but not replicate. H.R. Gelderblom (Berlin), P.A. Marx (Davis, California), and A.F. Bykovsky (Moscow) have made the most progress in unveiling the structure of the virus.

Oncoviruses and lentiviruses have differently shaped cores, but all the important components are essentially the same. The outer membrane, with its envelope glycoproteins, gives each virus a specific selective preference for certain target cells (the virus' tropism) and the ability to invade those cells.

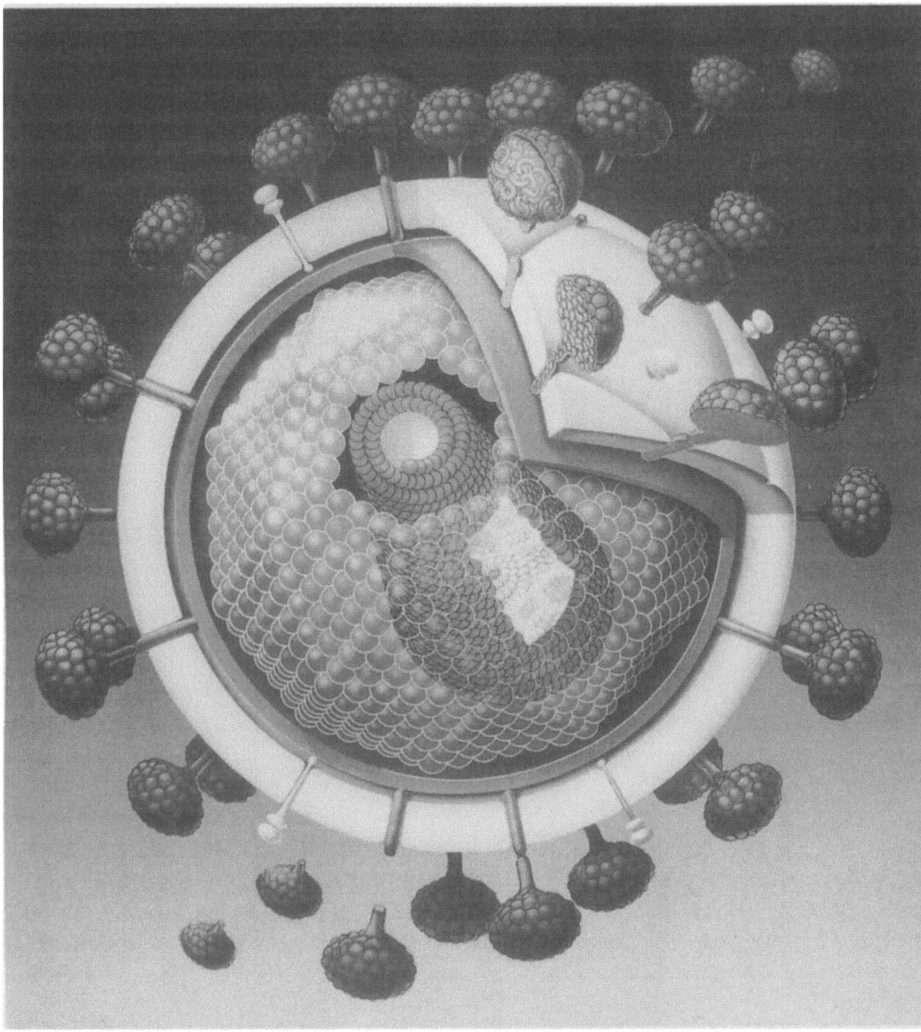

Fig. 1. Model of the HIV particle designed by us, based on hundreds of electron micrographs and especially on the ingenious studies on details of the virus structure by the groups of H. Frank (Tübingen; membranes), H. R. Gelderblom (Berlin; surface), P. A. Marx (Davis, California; core), and A. F. Bykovsky (Moscow; ribonucleoprotein complex) (Copyright 1987: M. G. Koch und GRAPHICO, Hamburg) (Michael G. Koch: Aids – Vom Molekül zur Pandemie. Spektrum der Wissenschaft, Heidelberg 1987)

The central ribonucleoprotein complex within the core contains the crucial viral information and the specific enzyme (reverse transcriptase) by which the viral RNA is converted (translated) into a DNA code indistinguishable from the host cell's own DNA. Whenever the proper conditions occur, this essential viral information is sufficient for replication at high rates. These copies can, on their own, by means of a complicated assembly process, reconstruct completely new virus particles capable of leaving the cell in order to look for new targets.

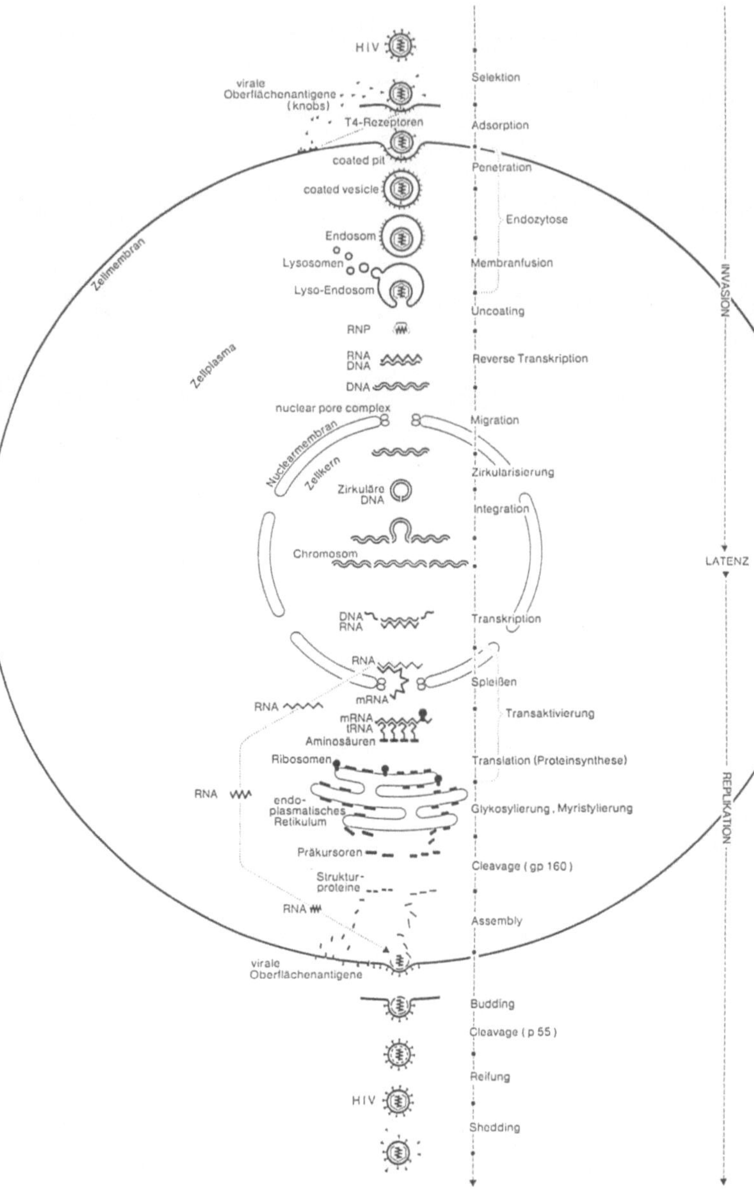

Fig. 2. The life cycle of HIV (Copyright: M. G. Koch und Spektrum der Wissenschaft, Heidelberg 1987) (Michael G. Koch: Aids – Vom Molekül zur Pandemie. Spektrum der Wissenschaft, Heidelberg 1987)

Viral information usually counteracts the cell's own metabolic instructions and thus subverts the internal life processes to the virus' own purposes and advantage – and to the cell's considerable disadvantage. Thus, through violent viral replication, the host cell is ultimately damaged or killed. This is the cause of the disturbed cell function and the accelerated death of those human cells – mainly part of the immune system – the virus has chosen to attack. Autoimmune antibodies seem to play an additional role in the destruction of T-helper cells and other cellular elements.

It is essential to understand that the integrated virus (not every HIV particle will necessarily integrate) will never again leave the safe position in the host's chromosome. Time and again it simply produces thousands of copies of itself to assure its survival and spread. This means that all conventional therapy is directed against the copies and cannot affect the integrated "original" provirus itself. It also explains why therapy has to be lifelong and may even have to be extended into the next generation.

Incubation time seems to be controlled by the virus' own sophisticated genetic code, even involving self-inhibitory action. Slowly accumulated viral precursors allow the host a long period of survival. In this way, the incubation period is prolonged by perhaps 5–15 years, thus optimizing the chances for intra- and interindividual virus spread. This suppression of reproduction seems to be most typical in immature macrophages (e.g., monocytes) and is possibly terminated by external stimulation. In the reproductive stage of its life cycle, HIV, mediated by the *tat* gene, can speed up its own reproduction in a way that very few other viruses can match.

Viruses are very tiny and structurally primitive. They have characteristics which may confer on them three essential advantages: the ability to hide, to replicate in tremendous numbers, and to adapt by rapid self-transformation to ever-changing living conditions.

Immunology

After leaving the host cell, the "newborn" HIV copies look for their specific targets: the T4 receptor (CD4 molecule) on T-helper cells, macrophages, and possibly certain cells in brain tissue. In order to understand what will happen if these cells are damaged, it is useful to become familiar with the normal function of those elements in the immune system that are the primary targets for HIV. The most obvious target is the T-helper cell, which interacts with most cells in the immune system. T-helper cells also activate B cells and macrophages and direct the T-killer cells towards pathogens and infected (or malign) cells that are to be destroyed by cytotoxic functions.

B cells are stimulated by T-helper cells to produce specific antibodies (immunoglobulins) that, by attachment to recognized surface antigens, label both the intruder's and infected cells' surfaces, thus activating the complement system, attracting killer cells, and opsonizing the marked target for macrophage action.

Killer cells also survey emerging abnormalities on cell surfaces (e.g., neoantigens in the course of carcinogenesis) and kill "irregularly" marked cells. This function plays an important role in the surveillance of malignancies in status nascendi.

Macrophages are part of a very effective system which is dispersed throughout the body and is represented in every organ by locally adapted phagocytotically active cells. These cells "clean up" whatever is recognized as alien and remove tissue destroyed by killer cells. It has been shown, with increasing evidence, that macrophages are likely to represent the primary target cell for virus invasion in mucosa and minor erosions. They even act as antigen-presenting cells (APCs), forming confluating giant cells and syncytia together with T-helper cells. The virus is shown to pass into uninfected cells through intercellular bridges, and is thus never exposed to circulating antibodies.

Cells in the colon, rectum, retina, cervix, and skin have been shown to be infected by HIV. The Langerhans cells in the skin and mucosa, especially, have proven to be easily infected. The presence of antibodies and complement seems to facilitate infection. Thus the chances of vaccine development are critically reduced.

In the brain there are both neuronal cells and macrophages (a locally adapted variant is called microglia) which are likely to bear the T4 receptor. These cells seem to be infected in HIV carriers, and the macrophages are seen as a possible "trojan horse" carrying the virus through the blood-brain barrier. The pathogenesis of the inflammatory and atrophic processes that lead to severe loss of brain tissue and to dementia are still to be elucidated in detail.

AIDS is the result of a systemic collapse and loss of function in all these cell types – a steadily increasing failure to survey and inhibit the development of malignancies and to fight different intruders such as viruses, bacteria, fungi, protozoans, and other parasites. Such pathogens include:

Viruses	herpes simplex virus (HSV), cytomegalovirus (CMV), varicella zoster virus (VZV), Epstein-Barr virus (EBV), human papilloma virus (HPV), Jacob Creutzfeldt virus (JC), molluscum contagiosum
Bacteria	*Mycobacterium tuberculosis,* Mycobacterium avium intracellulare (MAI), and other atypical mycobacteria, *Salmonella, Shigella, Nocardia, Rhodococcus, Actinomyces, Streptomyces, Calymmatobacterium, Spirochaeta, Chlamydia*
Fungi	*Candida, Cryptococcus, Histoplasma, Aspergillus, Blastomyces, Zygomycetes, Coccidioides, Petriellidium*
Protozoans	*Pneumocystis, Toxoplasma, Isospora, Eimeria, Cryptosporidium,* various *Microsporidia*
Parasites	*Strongyloides stercoralis, scabies*
Malignancies	Kaposi's sarcoma (KS), Burkitt's lymphoma (BL), B-lymphocytic lymphoma (BLL), Hodgkin's disease (HD), non-Hodgkin lymphoma (NHL), diffuse undifferentiated NHL (DUNHL), cerebral lymphomas, cancer of the oral and the rectal regions, certain small cell carcinomas and other malignancies

This great variety of diseases and symptoms following with the AIDS condition also includes inflammatory changes in the central and peripheral nervous system, rapidly developing brain atrophy, dementia, thymus atrophy, trophical and other disorders of the skin, thrombocytopenia, malabsorption and wasting, interstitial pneumonia, and other unusual and hidden inflammatory processes, including accelerated aging in general. The clinical spectrum seems to be ever widening. Lack of normal cutaneous reactions for common recall antigens (like tuberculin) is a strong indication of a severe defect in the cellular immune response; this defect seems to correlate with a decreased function of APCs (macrophages) and develops gradually over many years. This evolution gives rise to several stages or patterns of prodromal disease called pre-AIDS.

At the beginning of the course of the disease, we encounter very uncharacteristic complaints such as weight loss, fatigue, mental alterations, pyogenic skin infections, fever of unknown cause, shortness of breath, and a tendency to diarrhoea. There are unlimited variations and combinations of possible clinical features seen in this disease.

The CDC case definition of AIDS, including some recent adjustments, just outlines a late, sometimes semifinal or penultimate, stage of disease and not the disease itself. The disease itself, a contagious immunodeficiency, has no proper name. This reflects the initially incomplete understanding of the pathogenic processes that lead to AIDS. To maintain epidemiologically consistent reporting, this CDC definition – with repeated minor changes – is still adhered to all over the world. The essential text is the following:

(1) Presence of reliably diagnosed disease at least moderately indicative of cellular immune deficiency (e.g., Kaposi's sarcoma in a patient less than 60 years of age, pneumocystis pneumonia). (2) Absence of known underlying immune deficiency and of any other reduced resistance reported to be associated with the disease (e.g., immunosuppressive therapy, lymphoreticular malignancy).

Several typical and thus "qualifying" infections and malignancies are listed, and the symptoms are allowed to be less stringent in the presence of positive antibody-test results, of positive virus culture, or of other indicative laboratory findings (as of viral antigens or viral RNA). In simpler terms this means that the diagnosis of AIDS should be made only when there are typical laboratory findings and reliable indications of cellular immune deficiency without any other known underlying cause. This definition has been slightly adjusted to include specific pediatric features for children under 13 years of age.

Hitherto, most laboratory tests have been designed to show the existence of host antibodies against different protein components of the virus. Such antibodies can be found in the blood, saliva, urine, and spinal fluid of infected persons. Without doubt, there are virus carriers who do not produce specific antibodies at measurable titers. The latency period for seroconversion may be up to several years. These seronegative carriers are very difficult to detect and will remain a central point of concern for all screening procedures and prophylactic measures regarding blood transfusions, heterosexual contacts, occupational, and nosocomial risks. In the United States it has happened repeatedly that transfusion recipients have been infected by blood donors who had just had negative results on screening tests.

A very important question concerns the number of infected persons who will develop full-blown AIDS. This proportion is increasing continuously at an annual rate that seems to peak at about 8%–10%. The cumulative progression to AIDS is dependent upon the observation time (which seems to be the most important "cofactor"), and the annual progression rate has not yet been seen to decline. The longest follow-up studies (e.g., New York, Washington, Frankfurt) report a cumulative progression to AIDS of about 50%–65% and a deterioration in the clinical conditions in about 70%–100% of the observed cases (e.g., Washington, New York, San Francisco, Frankfurt). No final conclusion, however, can be drawn from these data because the incubation period is crucial for the final outcome and cannot yet be reliably defined. The largest follow-up studies and our own computer-based calculations point to an average incubation period of at least 10 years. For cases in which transmission was through healthy mucosa (e.g., most of the heterosexual cases) this period may be significantly longer with a considerable interval without measurable antibody titers and delayed infectivity.

Epidemiology

Today, cumulatively, the United States has had more than 61 000 reported AIDS cases (updated May 1988), about 55% of whom are dead. Underreporting is obvious. The number of infected persons in the USA is estimated at between 1 and 1.5 million.

South America and Europe have thousands of AIDS cases too. Worldwide, every country seems to have been struck (136 countries have reported AIDS cases to the WHO), but with marked differences in the dates of first onset. The situation in several tropical countries, in Central Africa, and in the Caribbean, where many millions are infected, can be regarded as disastrous and the spread of the epidemic extremely difficult to contain. When did the real size of the problem become apparent?

Faced with the first cases of this new, severe disease, the main reasons for serious concern were the lack of therapy and vaccine, the high mortality (80% after

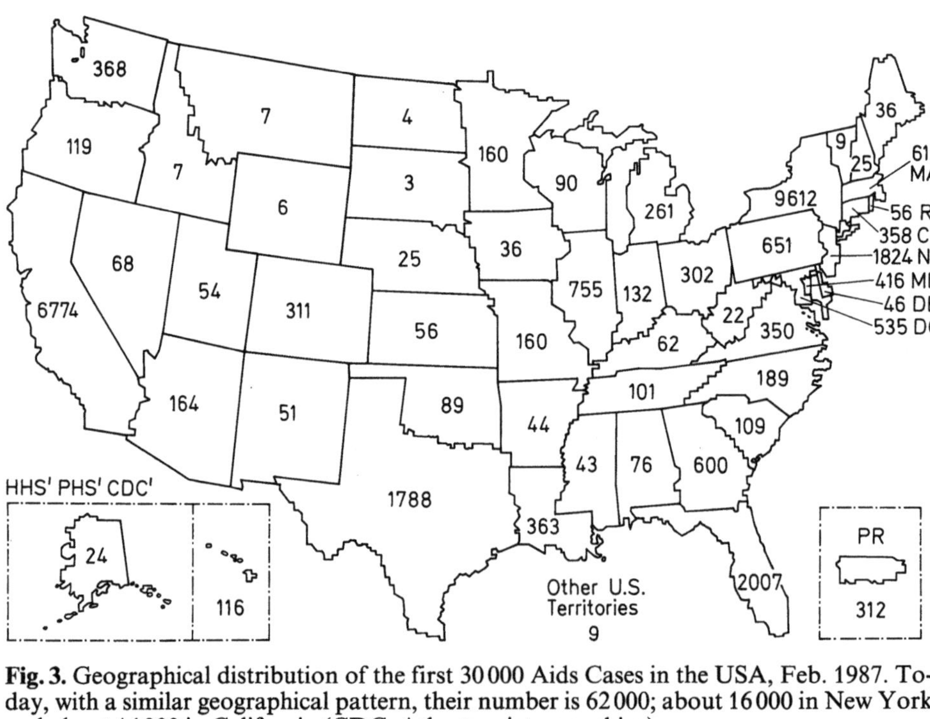

Fig. 3. Geographical distribution of the first 30 000 Aids Cases in the USA, Feb. 1987. Today, with a similar geographical pattern, their number is 62 000; about 16 000 in New York and about 14 000 in California (CDC, Atlanta, picture archive)

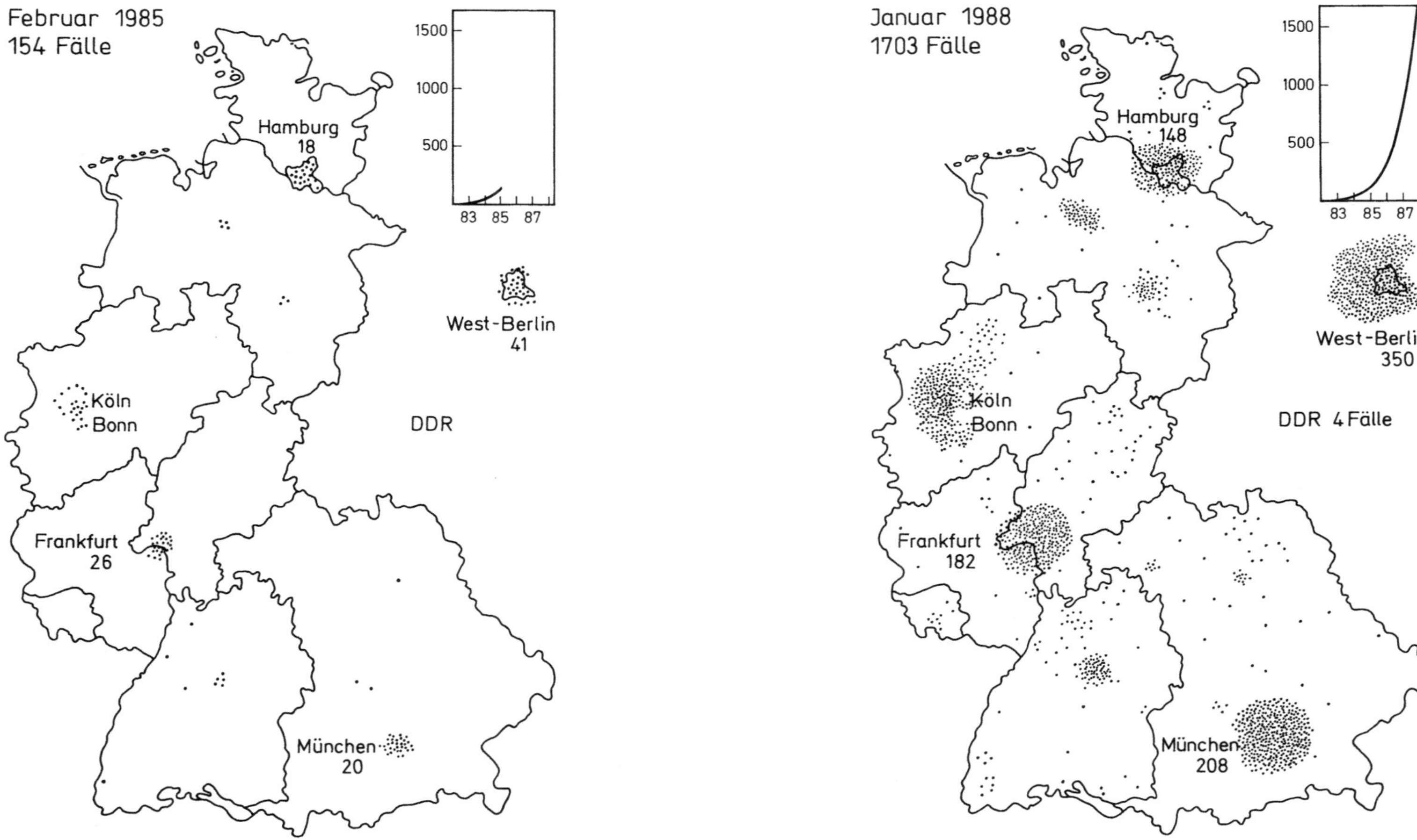

Fig. 4. Geographical distribution of Aids cases in the Federal Republic of Germany. There is a considerable underreporting (at least 50%). Single cases are moved in their position to inhibit case identification (Copyright 1988: Spektrum der Wissenschaft, Heidelberg) (Michael G. Koch: Aids – Vom Molekül zur Pandemie. Spektrum der Wissenschaft, Heidelberg 1987)

2 years' observation), and especially the rapid acceleration in the appearance of new AIDS cases. Making a preliminary prediction based on the first few hundred patients, the result was startling: for the year 1985 the expectation was about 10000 AIDS cases, cumulatively, for the United States alone. Nobody was willing to believe such a forecast, but the prediction proved deadly accurate. By the end of 1985 the real number of AIDS cases stood at about 15000. What are the prospects in Europe?

It seems as if the Western European countries follow the development of the AIDS epidemic in the United States with an approximate 2-year time lag, with the Eastern European countries being a further 3 years behind. Thus one thing is obvious: condoms may be virusproof, but borders are not.

It is crucial that we learn, from the experience of others, what will work and what will not. However, there are a lot of psychological hurdles to overcome, such as the "opportunistic inertia" that always tries to maintain today's tranquillity at the price of tomorrow's troubles. It is by just such "lenti-understanding" that countless calamities have been turned into catastrophies.

The situation in Haiti, the Bahamas, Bermuda, Barbados, Trinidad, and other Caribbean countries, some cities of Brazil and Mexico, and especially a major part of Central Africa seems to be far worse than officially admitted. This state of affairs may be due to the fact that these regions, and Africa in particular, were among the earliest to show signs of the spread of the disease. Indeed, the epidemic must be supposed to have started in the tropical "subsaharan-lymphoma belt," in a region in the vicinity of the East African great lakes. It was supposedly spread from monkey to man by injections of monkey blood into human genital tissues in order to boost sexual activity (reported in as early as 1973 by the African anthropologist Kashamura). The rapid spread of HIV today may even be due to other factors: sexual promiscuity, prostitution, low standards of health care, frequent scarification, and a high number of other uncontroled paramedical activities. Even the role of bloodsucking insect vectors has been discussed, but hitherto discounted. In Uganda, Zaire, Congo, Rwanda, Burundi, Tanzania, Zambia, as well as other countries in this region, HIV seems very widespread. Here the AIDS problem (with 2%–20% of the population infected) poses a major health problem, with a predictable negative impact on the socioeconomic and political structure of several countries, and, probably, on the population growth rate. Although some will not admit it, the epidemic is definitely out of control.

The risk of acquiring HIV infection from a blood donor in Kampala (Uganda) or Lusaka (Zambia) is today about 15%–20%. Despite that risk, mandatory blood-donor screening has not yet been established all over Africa. Up to now, many African countries have tried to dismiss the idea of a major epidemic and to create smokescreens around scientific data, possibly with the object of protecting tourism, trade, and foreign assistance. That policy has failed utterly in Haiti and is even doomed to fail in Africa.

We can state today that the AIDS epidemic in tropical countries is much more obviously linked to heterosexual activity than to the conventional "risk group" behavior we know from Europe and the United States. The different ways in which the virus spreads are still not completely elucidated. As the incubation period seems to be about 10 years, with a wide standard deviation of about 5–6 years, there result in the epidemiological curves unusual "smearing" effects called transients. These transients may confuse our perception of the true nature of certain epidemiological characteristics, which unfold in a delayed manner. These phenomena are explained and their consequences discussed elsewhere (González and Koch 1986; Koch et al. 1987; Koch and González 1987). An initial period of low infectivity will give rise to another special effect, called "crescent delay" (González et al., in press).

The incubation period we observe is necessarily lengthening all the time and has, from the very beginning, always been equal to the maximum duration allowed by our observation time. It may turn out to be even longer than now believed and is likely to vary with the mode of transmission and the amount of the primary infectious inoculum. For the first time in history, we are following the birth and growth of a new epidemic with a high level of scientific awareness; we should therefore remain open-minded about its future development and the scientific findings that are yet to come.

Some of the statements we are able to make today about predominant risk groups, the known modes of transmission, and the possibilities for protection against this severe infectious disease will be reviewed here. The character of the risk, more than its mere size, should – for the sake of our patients, for the protection of our staff and their families, and for the esteem of our profession – instill in us unconditional vigilance.

This virus has chosen for its survival the most essential cells in our immune system: the T-helper cells and the macrophages, the breakdown of which renders us helpless. To facilitate its spread the virus is linked to the two liquids that sustain life: blood and sperm. It affects the regulator of our behavior and judgement: the brain. And its transmission is associated with behavior extremely difficult to change or to refrain from: sexual contacts and drug abuse. This is an ominous combination.

Intimate contact is very difficult to influence and impossible to control. The fact that, especially in certain high-risk populations, there is a negative attitude towards collaboration with the health-care system, simply compounds these problems. The circle of persons at risk for infection with HIV has gradually widened to include:

1. Homo- and bisexual men
2. Intravenous drug addicts
3. Haitians
4. Hemophiliacs
5. Transfusion recipients
6. Africans from endemic regions
7. Artificially inseminated women
8. Transplant recipients
9. Prostitutes
10. Clients of prostitutes
11. Bodybuilders who inject drugs
12. People exposed to tatooing or other paramedical procedures
13. Health-care workers
14. Laboratory workers (virology)

15. Lesbians
16. Heterosexual partners of the above
17. Children of the above

Results from different parts of the Western world show that there have been remarkable changes of behavior in some of the high-risk groups, resulting in a decreasing rate of new infections, but that drug addicts, prostitutes, and their clients seem to respond poorly to educational efforts. AIDS case figures, as they represent some sort of "HIV archeology," are only marginally influenced by such recent changes. Reliable figures which could give an updated picture of the ongoing spread of HIV would require the complete and repeated testing of some randomly chosen samples of persons at varying degrees of risk and exhibiting different behavior; such data are as yet widely inaccessible or at worst lacking.

Today we can state that the main routes of virus transmission are (and will remain so, even if other minor routes subsequently appear):

1. Intimate contact with exchange of body fluid, mainly sexual activities
2. Needle sharing among drug addicts and comparable exposure to contaminated medical or paramedical equipment
3. Receiving contaminated blood or blood products, other cells, tissues or organs
4. Pregnancy (transmission from mother to child)

AIDS is less infectious than the well-known hepatitis B, but the modes of transmission are quite similar. There are considerably less virus particles in the blood of HIV carriers, but, unlike hepatitis B, the duration of the viremic stage extends over many years. HIV infection must be considered persistent and contagious for a person's entire lifespan. A theoretically possible steady state for this infection within the whole population is at present a long way off.

Concern is often focused on less common routes of infection, routes which usually do not become obvious until an epidemic is well advanced: 41 health-care workers with AIDS are supposed to have been infected in the course of their duties (74 more are under investigation, 20 are dead or lost to follow-up; CDC 1988), with some 23 more shown to be infected by caring for HIV carriers. Most of them were exposed to the infection through needle injuries, a few only through splashes of blood in the face or on their fingers. A worker in a virology laboratory became infected with HIV from an isolate in cell culture, possibly by contamination of his gloves and contact with mucosa in the eye or nose.

Among known infected persons are physicians and dentists who might have been exposed to needle pricks or other forms of occupational injuries; a mother infected by her baby; a Good Samaritan infected by a sick neighbor for whom she cared, supposedly through lesions (eczema) of her hands; a few children infected by their mothers' breast milk; an 8-year-old boy infected by his younger brother; two persons supposedly infected by a bite; four Australian women infected by careful artificial insemination; some lesbians presumably infected through oral-mucosal contacts; laboratory workers – and more than a thousand others, both HIV carriers and AIDS patients, for whom the mode of transmission remains unknown. Bearing this in mind and remembering the macrophages (e.g., Langerhans cells near the surface of the healthy mucosa) are the primary target cells most susceptible to HIV infection, the thesis that HIV must have access to

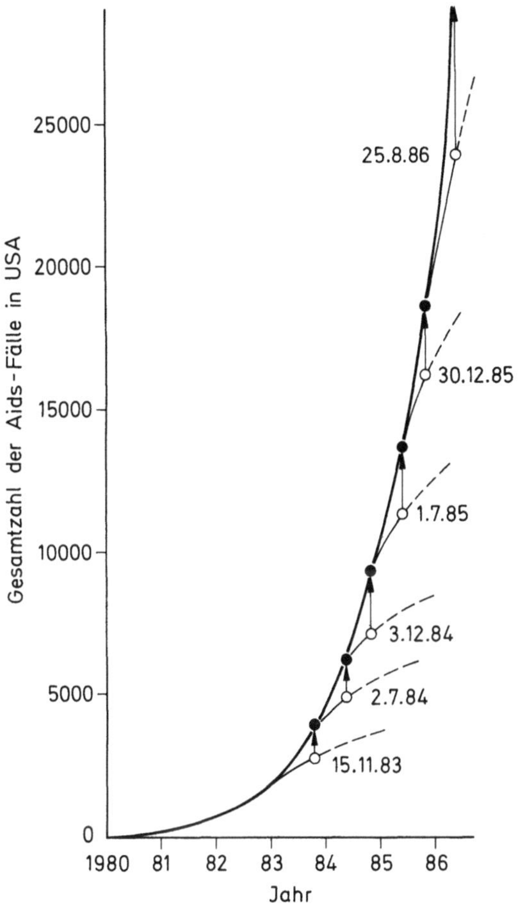

Fig. 5. Aids cases in the United States, based on the date of diagnosis, noted cumulatively, for different points in time (data from CDC, Atlanta). This is repeated for several years in the same diagram, thus giving a diachronical view. As the figures change with the course of time, corrections must be made for cases reported with delay, indicated by *stippled vertical arrows*. The *stippled prolongations of the preliminary curves* recall the spontaneous projections for different points in time. These expectations have never proved correct and supposedly, will not do so for some time to come (Copyright: Spektrum der Wissenschaft, Heidelberg 1987) (Michael G. Koch: Aids – Vom Molekül zur Pandemie. Spektrum der Wissenschaft, Heidelberg 1987)

the open bloodstream for transmission can no longer be maintained. Sexual mucosal contacts are likely to be sufficient for transmitting the virus.

Since HIV has been found in spinal fluid, blood and blood cells, sperm, various transplanted organs, vaginal secretions, saliva, breast milk, urine, amnion fluid, sweat, and tears, we have to be constantly alert to this infection and its possible routes of transmission maintaining our awareness as we learn. This means that the CDC's latest recommendations concerning precautions for health-care workers (CDC 1987) should be followed rigorously. Mucosal areas, and even healthy skin, should be protected in treating all patients (not just seropositives) when contact with any body fluid may occur. For surgeons, endoscopists, anesthetists, and dentists this doubtless means the wearing of gowns, goggles, mask, and gloves.

Patients with advanced-stage AIDS may be less contagious than the much more frequent subclinical or presymptomatic cases. Therefore it would be imprudent to restrict these precautions to the known-risk patient. Most HIV carriers, maybe 50 or more for every known AIDS case, will present to the health-care system without obvious indications of infection. These are the circumstances to which clinical routines have to be adapted.

Figure 5 shows how spurious, optimistic assumptions may emanate from uncritical interpretation of incomplete AIDS data. From the curve of AIDS cases known in the USA, at any point in time, based on the date of diagnosis, it is easy to derive the idea that the epidemic may be markedly slowing down, an impression that has repeatedly duped people all over the world – and still does so. Figure 5 shows, for several points in time in the past few years, how the curve has appeared to level off. Retrospectively, however, the necessary corrections of the AIDS case figures, due to delay in reporting, regularly reerect the steep (though not simply exponential) growth curve, thus more and more resembling the shape of the curve for AIDS cases based on the date of reporting. The preliminary data, based on the date of diagnosis, must still be adjusted even after 4–5 years and these corrections may be 30% more than the initial number.

To predict the effects of preventional measures and the outcome of behavioral changes in risk groups and in the general population, more sophisticated simulation models will be required. Such a program, AIDS Spread Simulations and Projections (ASSP) has just been completed and is being used, for example, in Switzerland and some other countries.

The growth curve for manifest AIDS cases is indeed continuously but moderately slowed down by positive transients, by saturation kinetics, by negative transients, and, ultimately, even by lowered rates of new infections (due to preventional measures and risk-reducing behavioral changes). The effects of the latter, however, will not be reflected by the number of new AIDS cases before 1991–1992. It is crucial not to lose sight of the unusual effects of the long incubation period, which is characteristic for lentiviruses.

Increasing numbers of patients will give rise to psychological and social problems of staggering dimensions, to questions concerning sexual habits and the possibilities of our influencing them by giving information and advice, to approaches for obtaining prognostic figures, necessarily based on what is known about man's intimate behavior. All this means that sexology will inevitably be involved in this rapidly growing field of professional concern.

Conclusion

To give a short summary of the points made here, we would like to emphasize the following features specific to the AIDS epidemic:

The Virus

We are confronted with a new and serious disease, the first lentivirus infection that, to the best of our knowledge, has ever struck mankind. The AIDS virus, HIV, is equipped to invade just those cell types which are of crucial importance for the efficiency (macrophages) and coordination (T-helper cells) of our immune system. Moreover it damages several other important cells (e.g., immature T cells, B cells, NK cells, hematopoietic cells, and certain brain cells).

The virus has many unusual features, including:

1. Antigenic shift
2. Antigen shedding
3. Molecular homologies to cellular structures
4. A predominantly intracellular existence, passing from one cell to another in (syncytial) intercellular cytoplasma bridges
5. A sophisticated regulation of replication (including self-inhibitory action)
6. The ability to survive in macrophages
7. The advantage of being assisted by antibody/complement-mediated opsonization when infecting macrophages.

The first property prevents fully developed immunity by rapidly changing the characteristics of the viral envelope; the second withdraws the virus from neutralizing antibodies and possibly directs such antibodies toward immunologically active host cells; the third enables the virus to bypass common immunological alarm systems and gives rise to multiple autoimmune reactions; the fourth allows the virus to spread without being accessible to circulating antibodies; the fifth gives the host organism a long period of survival, thus prolonging the time for viral spread within the host organism and to new individuals by 5–15 years; the sixth turns the ability of the host to find and to incorporate the pathogen into an advantage for HIV in finding its target cells; and the seventh uses immunological response for enhanced invasion of macrophages.

The lentivirus-specific survival in macrophages, cells that are designed to destroy pathogens by incorporation and lytic activity, has two more severe consequences. It undermindes the concept of a minimal infectious dose and may be responsible for total failure of vaccination efforts. Antibodies, by stimulating recycling of the virus and amplification within the phagocytic system, may no longer be useful, rather jeopardizing an immunological silence, which would give a chance of prolonged survival.

The isolation of about 4000 strains of this virus, which all seem to differ from each other, and the isolation of several virus variants from one single patient which even seem to develop increasing virulence in the course of a few years, gives an idea of the variability of HIV. The significantly different type HIV-2, which has recently been spreading from West Africa, has by now at least reached Europe and the Americas. (HIV's closest relative, SIV in apes, has, after just 1 year in cell culture, suddenly developed a new genetic variant with a new tropism, causing an intestinal disease, which is fatal within some weeks.) It is quite obvious that we are not dealing with a single virus. HIV behaves more like a moving target, a comet, the tail of which is rapidly broadening, fan-like, into a multitude of genetically different variants.

By integrating into the chromosome of the infected cell, the virus can save a copy of its genetic information, which "vanishes" into the host cell's genome. There, it cannot be selectively destroyed by conventional drugs. Infection is thus persistent and the contagiousness lifelong, as is the necessity for any conventional therapy. Frequent vertical infection gives the virus direct access to the next generation, which then must be treated as well.

The combination of "lenti" features with other properties of retroviruses give HIV the qualitites of a "smart" and insidious, well-adapted, intracellular parasite, the conbatting of which will need more skills and intelligence than our immune system has developed over millions of years. The long incubation time compensates for the inevitably lethal outcome, which otherwise would be a selectional handicap in the struggle for the virus' survival, by optimizing its spread. Therefore, this epidemic is not self-limiting by its high mortality, as is the case for many others (e.g., Marburg virus disease, Ebola fever, Lassa fever). Neither is there any reason to expect the epidemic to evolve in such a way as to become more benign in character.

Due to the circumstances mentioned we will, for a considerable time, lack both effective therapy and a protective vaccine. We have to plan for decades, not only for years. Risk-reducing advice will be our main prophylaxis during this period. That means we have to "vaccinate" those who are susceptible to infection with information.

The Disease

The mortality of AIDS is about 80% after 2 years, about 98% after 5 years. The average survival time after diagnosis is about 1 year, mainly spent in hospital. None of the more than 70 000 patients in the United States and Europe has ever recovered from the AIDS condition. That is, even by historical standards, exeptional.

The infected persons are persistent HIV carriers and seem to develop AIDS in a continuously increasing proportion, the final size of which cannot yet be determined. There are strong indications that most or all of them will develop the disease in the course of a long observation period, and several ongoing clinical follow-up studies show increasing evidence for such a serious final outcome.

AIDS is only a defined and late stage of a disease that has no name yet and shows a tremendous variety of prodromal stages (LAS, ARC) and other clinical pictures (AIDS dementia complex (ADC), autoimmune thrombocytopenia (ITP), lymphatic interstitial pneumonia (LIP), acute interstitial pneumonia (AIP), slim disease), some of which, though lethal, do not fulfill the CDC definition. The HIV infection even facilitates the development and aggravates the course of more common diseases such as tuberculosis, salmonellosis, or septicemia of various origins. The basic immune deficiency seems to trigger an ever widening variety of infections, malignancies, autoimmune diseases, and other unusual conditions in free combination with each other.

The affinity of HIV to the brain and other parts of the central nervous system, another typical feature of lentiviruses, becomes more and more obvious (ADC). It may lead to brain disease and death before the immune system is markedly damaged.

There are many complicated functions in the human organism we do not really understand until their breakdown unveils their crucial importance. The AIDS condition shows us in what an abundance of microbes we are incessantly forced to survive. The HIV-infected patient, whose immune system is continuously deteriorating, has to manage this under a gradually diminishing and finally vanishing protection.

The Epidemic

The epidemic has recently started and is spreading at an alarming rate. Many millions of people all over the world are already infected – people in more than 136 countries have been struck, even Canadian Inuit Eskimoes, Navajo Indians, Australian aborigines, people from Greenland, and inhabitants of the South American jungle and remote Pacific islands. There is not yet any proven method of containing the further spread of HIV efficiently.

The situation in some Central African countries and in certain parts of the Caribbean is fundamentally disastrous. A similar development seems to be going on in several urban regions (e.g., in Latin America) with extended slum areas. Ways in which one could stop the spread of the virus in slum populations are hard to imagine.

Political considerations often create smoke screens around the true epidemiological situation. Man's mind may balk at the implications of this development and therefore hesitate to project it into the future – nature, however, does not.

The obvious concentration of AIDS cases in certain risk groups in no way means a definite restriction of its spread. The term "risk group" may be useful for discussion and epidemiological surveillance, but should not induce unfounded complacency outside these groups. In reality, it already crossed their boundaries many years ago. There are no really distinct risk groups, but there is risky behavior that may cluster within certain sections of the population. The virus takes the chances it gets.

The real number of infected persons is difficult to evaluate due to the existence of antibody-negative virus carriers. These create essential problems for all necessary screening. Most virus carriers (maybe 90%) are today completely unaware of their condition. They contribute unintentionally and incessantly to the further spread of HIV.

The Spread of the Virus

The virus' existence is linked to the two fluids that sustain life: blood and sperm. Its spread is associated with behavior that is difficult to change. Transmission occurs through sexual contact, through contaminated instruments for drug abuse or paramedical activities, through blood and blood products, through transplanted organs, tissues, or donated sperm. Donor screening is crucial.

Macrophages in general (e.g., Langerhan's cells in the skin and macrophages in the lung and brain tissue) seem to be a widespread reservoir for the virus and indicate an unexpectedly high virus load in infected persons. This feature is also known from other lentivirus infections.

Recent studies have shown the existence of T4-positive cells (macrophages in various forms) in the healthy mucosa of the oral, vaginal, cervical, and rectal regions, and these cells have been found to be very susceptible to HIV and are infected early. Thus, the requirement for open wounds for virus transmission has become extremely questionable. Infection through normal mucosa (e.g., sexual contacts) may occur frequently.

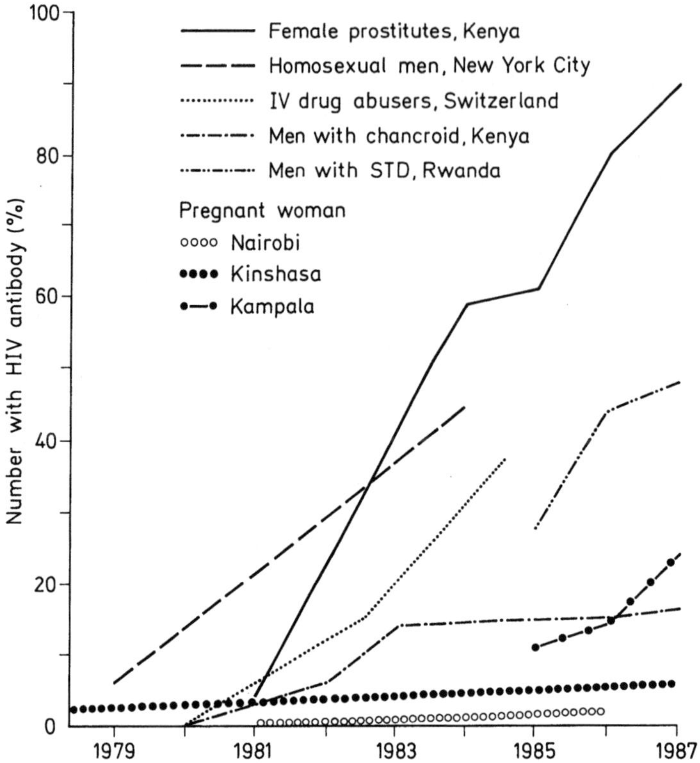

Fig. 6. Cohort and periodic cross-sectional studies of HIV seroprevalence in different population groups in Africa, Europe, and the United States

The latter mode of infection could give rise to very long incubation periods and lead to considerable delay in seroconversion (the development of measurable amounts of HIV-specific antibodies). This would explain the frequent detection of seronegative virus carriers, particularly among heterosexual partners, and indicate an additional invisible part of the epidemic.

The detection of HIV in cockroaches, mosquitos, tsetse flies, ticks, and other insects from two central African high-risk areas, and the proven survival of the virus in the common bedbug raise questions about the possibility of mechanical spread of the virus by insect vectors. (There is no indication that any insect would act as a biological vector for lentiviruses.)

It is not yet possible to specify the infectiousness of HIV. Transmission to health-care workers, though infrequent (23 published cases), has occurred, recently even as a result of blood splashes without injuries. About 40 other health-care workers have developed AIDS without any known mode of HIV transmission. Due to the possibility of longer seroconversion latency in cases with a low initial infection dose our actual conclusions are necessarily preliminary.

AIDS is spread as a sexually transmitted disease with some properties similar to hepatitis B. In the initial phase of every epidemic, however, we only see the main routes of transmission. Small alternative pathways will neither occur nor become consequential until the epidemic has reached certain dimensions. If at all, they will become visible after a considerable delay. This delay will be enhanced both by the unusually long incubation period of AIDS and by the very high frequency of sexual contacts, which for a long time might conceal some uncommon modes of transmission.

We have to consider, in general, that the mode and the initial dose of infection may be crucial for the duration of the incubation period. As we have initially seen mainly fast-developing cases, we might be biased towards a recurrent underestimation of the true length of the incubation period. Those repeatedly, and those massively infected would today be misleadingly predominant among the presently known AIDS cases.

AIDS has, readily and within less than 10 years, surpassed 28 of 30 notifiable infectious diseases in the United States which have had opportunities to spread for centuries. Thus it seems unreasonable to talk about very low infectiousness.

In comparison to the natural history of this infection (maybe 5–25 years), our rather short observation time (7 years) should make us cautious. Today, however, the lack of detailed knowledge is often converted into positive certainty, leading to premature and dogmatic statements.

Problems of Time Lag

The incubation period is unusually long and not yet definitively known. This gives rise to a surprising and treacherous gap between what is visible and what is the underlying reality, leading to a lack of motivation in making public health policies. In fact, a lot of published excitement has turned out to be only the storm before the lull.

The long incubation period is extremely variable, which results in uncommon "smearing effects" and a biasing acceleration in the number of initially appearing AIDS cases, called transients. These transients are insidious in that their passing by mimics a slow-down of the epidemic and thus may give rise to unfounded optimism. When this positive transient fades away after some 5–10 years, negative transients, based on saturation effects (an increasing lack of remaining, susceptible, not-yet infected persons) within certain subpopulations, begin to distort the curve. They continuously prolong the deceleration of the number of new AIDS cases, thus yielding an even stronger spurious reduction of the spread of the epidemic.

Finding sporadic AIDS cases retrospectively in the years 1960–1977 evoked the question of why the epidemic did not start then, but as late as 1981. The answer is, that it did start in the 1960s. To understand a lentivirus infection is to realize that the long, unnoticed slope of a slow exponential spread necessarily extends several decades back into the past.

The situation of the spread of the disease today reflects the spread of infection some 10 years ago. The situation of the spread of infection today will not become visible until 1998 or later. This means that the epidemic is always at a later stage than is apparent.

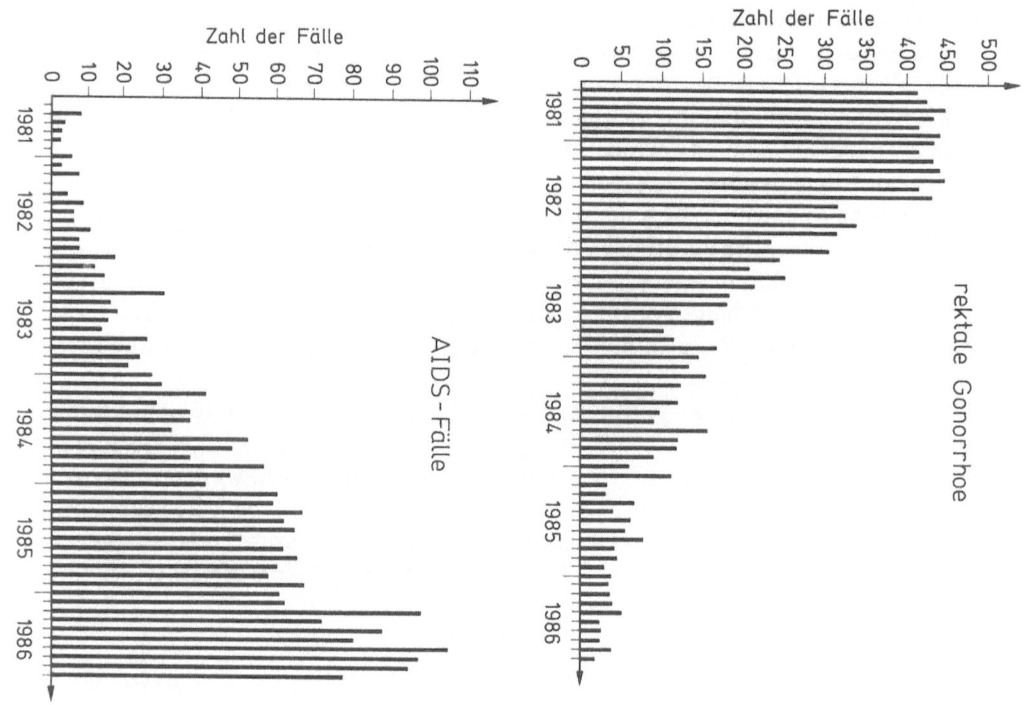

Fig. 7. San Francisco City Cohort Study: monthly reported, not cumulated cases of rectal gonorrhoea (above), changing dramaticly as an indication for markedly reduced risk taking behavior, and the development of new Aids cases (below), obviously independent of the behavioral changes above, due to a time lag of about 10 years (figures from W. Darrow, CDC, and D. Echenburg, San Francisco)

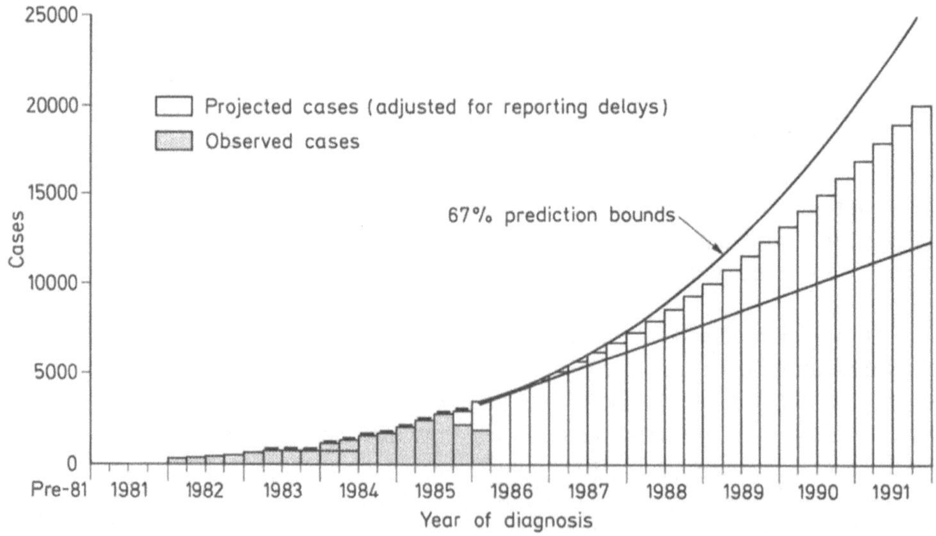

Fig. 8. Prognosis of Aids cases in the USA diagnosed quarterly until 1991 (CDC, Atlanta, picture archives)

Problems of Intervention

Intimate contact has always proved to be refractory to legislation and elusive to any form of control. Neither does drug abuse seem to be accessible for advice or legal surveillance.

Moreover, especially in certain risk groups such as intravenous drug addicts, not every virus carrier shares the normally unquestioned loyalty to the as yet uninfected population. There are, in fact, people who deliberately carry on the spread to virus. This lack of responsibility and solidarity will aggravate the problems we have to face.

The public has forgotten what an epidemic means and how it is fought. The old experiences have to be repeated and will lead back to well-known principles: find the sources, understand the modes of spreading – and interfere with both as fast as possible. It is difficult to save time by anticipating what is to come.

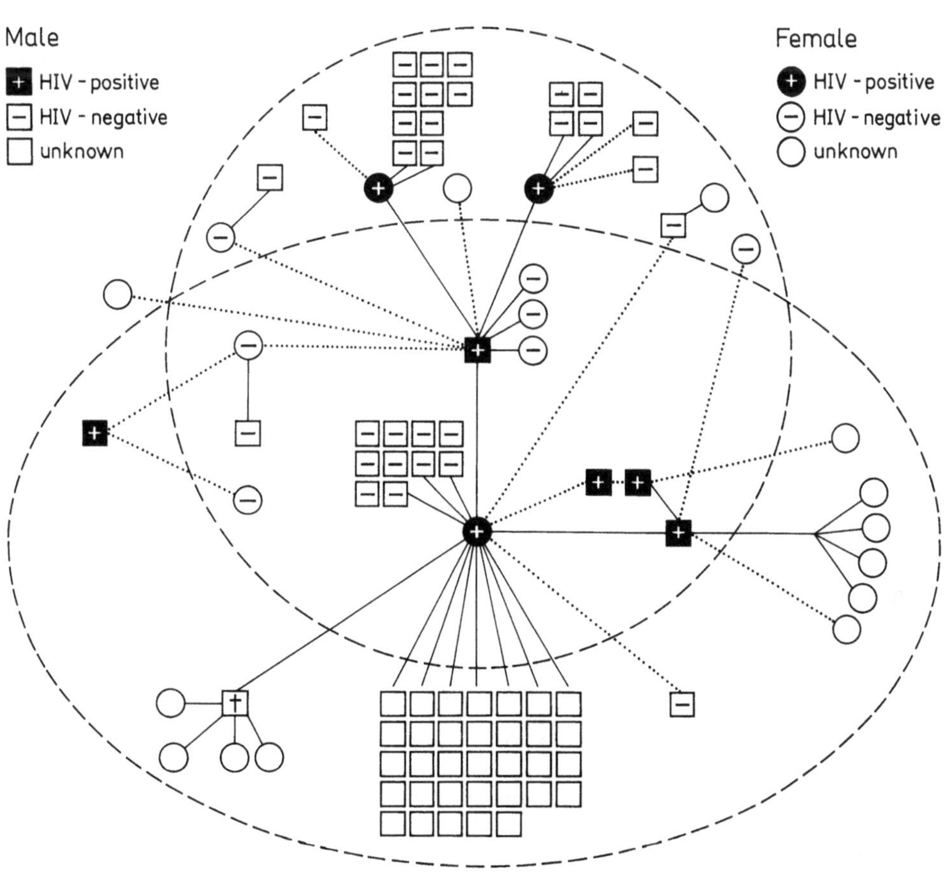

Fig. 9. HIV spread within the young population of a little town (17000 inhabitants) in Northern Sweden. Known contacts (about 50% needle sharing, 50% sexual contact, about 10% both) are marked by connecting lines; stippled lines: contacts after learning about the positive test result. Circle: the town Hudiksvall and vicinity. Ellipse: risk group of drug using (amphetamine) young population

There is much foreign experience from which great benefit can be derived, the utilization of which seems to be inhibited by opportunistic inertia, squabbles over competence, territorial thinking, reluctance to reconsider premature convictions, and other strong and widespread psychological biases. As Stanislaw Lec said, "Omitted actions sometimes give rise to a catastrophic lack of consequences."

The Scope of the Problem

The complex structure of this dynamic problem shows all the properties which – in the history of mankind – regularly result in a persistent lack of a thought-out solution. The medical situation does not look much better. We have not succeeded in fighting cancer, virus infections, chromosomal damage, autoimmune diseases, immune deficiencies, infectious brain atrophy, and aging of the cells. AIDS is a combination of these seven problems. Thus, of course, the solution is far away.

The infection is spreading throughout the world, inevitably, widely unnoticed, like an invisible and silent explosion in slow motion. After many years' delay follows a rumble of AIDS cases, the blazing final stages of long-term smouldering HIV infections. We have, today, no real idea how long this will go on.

References

CDC (1986) Reports on AIDS, published in the MMWR Jun 1981–May 1986. CDC, Atlanta, pp 178

CDC (1987) Recommendations for prevention of HIV transmission in health-care settings. MMWR 36 [Suppl 2S]

CDC (1988) AIDS and HIV among health-care workers. MMWR 37:229–239

CDC (1988) Update: acquired immune deficiency syndrome (AIDS) – Worldwide. MMWR 37:286–295

Ellrodt A, Le Bras P (1987) The hidden dangers of AIDS vaccination. Nature 325:765

Erfle V (1986) Möglichkeiten der Immunprophylaxe gegen die HTLV-III/LAV-Infektion. AIFO 1:117–133

Frösner GG (1988) Veränderungen der Inzidenz der AIDS-Erkrankung und geschätzte Prävalenz der HIV-Infektion in der Bundesrepublik Deutschland. AIFO 3:269–276

Gendelman HE, Orenstein JM, Martin MA, Ferrua C, Mitra R, Phipps T, Wahl LA, Lane HC, Fauci AS, Burke DS, Skillman D, Meltzer MS (1988) Efficient isolation and propagation of HIV on rCSF-1-treated monocytes. J Exp Med 167:1428–1441

González JJ, Koch MG (1986) On the role of transients for the prognostic analysis of AIDS and the anciennity distribution of AIDS patients. AIFO 1:621–630

Gonzáles JJ, Koch MG (1987) On the role of transients (biasing transitional effects) for the prognostic analysis of the AIDS epidemic. Am J Epidemiol 126:985–1005

Haase AT (1986) Pathogenesis of lentivirus infection. Nature 322:130–136

Healy MJR, Tillett HE (1988) Short-term extrapolation of the AIDS epidemic. J R Stat Soc 151 (in press)

Jaensson TGT (1985) Kan insekter sprida hepatit B-virus and AIDS-associeratretrovirus (LAV/HTLV-III)? Läkart 82:4133–4136

Karpas A (1987) Origin of the AIDS viruses. New Sci 67

Kashamura A (1973) Famille, sexualité et culture: essai sur les moeurs et les cultures des peuples des Grands Lacs Africains. Payot, Paris p 173

Koch MG (1987a) AIDS – die verdrängte Lentivirus-Pandemie. Spektrum Wiss 10:12–14
Koch MG (1987b) The anatomy of the virus. New Sci 46–51
Koch MG (1987c) HIV – die unvollendete Geschichte einer Virusentdeckung. Spektrum Wiss 7:14–15
Koch MG (1987d) AIDS – vom Molekül zur Pandemie. Spektrum Wiss 290
Koch MG, González JJ (1987) Transiente Phänomene – ein Exkurs über Aufmerksamkeitsfallen. AIFO 2:553–558
Koch MG, L'age-Stehr J (1987) Möglichkeiten der Prognose im Rahmen der AIDS-Epidemiologie. AIFO 2:94–99
Koch MG, L'age-Stehr J, González JJ, Dörner D (1987) Die Epidemiologie von AIDS. Spektrum Wiss 38–51
L'age-Stehr J, Schwarz A, Offermann G, Langmaack H, Bennhold I, Niedrig M, Koch MA (1985) HTLV-III infection in kidney transplant recipients. Lancet II:1361–1362
Noireau F (1987) HIV transmission from monkey to man. Lancet I:1498–1499
Pauza CD (1988) HIV-persistence in monocytes leads to pathogenesis and AIDS. Cell Immunol 112:414–424
Porterfield JS (1985) Antibody enhanced viral growth in macrophages. Immunol Lett 11:213–217
Robinson WE, Montefiori DC, Mitchell WM (1988a) Antibody-dependent enhancement of human immunodeficiency virus type 1 infection. Lancet I:790–794
Robinson WE, Montefiori DC, Mitchell WM (1988b) Will antibody-dependent enhancement of HIV-1 infection be a problem with AIDS vaccines? Lancet I:830–831
Schmidt CA, Fiek T, Neubauer A, Huhn D (1988) HIV-Infektion durch Nadelstichverletzung. Dtsch Med Wochenschr 113:76
Wolf H, Soutschek-Bauer E, Motz M, Modrow S (1987) Möglichkeiten der Entwicklung von Impfstoffen gegen die HIV-Infektion. AIFO 2:512–519
WHO (1987) AIDS Surveillance in Europe, Rep. No 16. WHO Collab Centre on AIDS, Paris

Psychosocial Aspects of AIDS

M. Fröschl, G. Hutner, J. Ring, and O. Braun-Falco

Dermatologische Klinik und Poliklinik der LMU, Frauenlobstr. 9–11
8000 München 2, FRG

In May 1981 the first cases of Kaposi's sarcoma and pneumocystis carinii pneumonia in young, formerly healthy homosexual men were reported. Apart from medical problems concerning the acquired immunodeficiency syndrome psychosocial issues play an important role in patient management. Many aspects of AIDS and its treatments are very stressful for the patient. Two important sources of stress are the youth of the population it affects and the high mortality rate. Especially the time when a patient learns about his or her positive HIV-antibody test is often a critical point for psychosocial intervention.

Almost suddenly a young man or woman is confronted with a potentially fatal illness. There are no sure answers for many of their questions especially concerning prognosis and treatment and, therefore, causing a feeling of uncertainty. They switch from renouncement and powerlessness on one hand to optimism and hope on the other. Moreover, there is the need for immediate changes in life-style. Leading a life conducive to health is often difficult for the patients. Modifying habits of eating, renunciation of smoking, caffein, or alcohol, and avoiding sunbathing greatly affects the life-style of HIV-infected persons. Changing sexual behavior should reduce the risk of transmitting the disease to others and reduce the risk of the infected individual of acquiring further infections that may exacerbate the disease.

The positive HIV-antibody test and its implications create immense feelings of fear and depression that could lead to suicide. During this time speaking about fear, despair, and sorrow can be helpful in avoiding an acute crisis situation. Sources of stress can be mainly of physical, social, or emotional origin. The appearance of symptoms such as weight loss, fever, diarrhea, fatigue, night sweats, or lymphadenopathy can be signs of the progression of this disease. These patients are confronted with all of the feelings experienced by any patient who approaches death including denial, fear, anger, ambivalence, hope, and the search for the meaning of existence.

Many of our patients are deeply afraid of symptoms of the CNS. HIV infection of the brain not infrequently causes a slow progressive dementia and leads to the need for extensive help.

Treatment of opportunistic infections or Kaposi's sarcoma has many side effects, for example, rash, drug fever, and leukopenia caused by high dosages of antibiotics or extensive fever in the case of interferon. Furthermore, patients cannot hope that treating these symptoms can cure the underlying immunodeficiency. Disfiguring skin diseases often lead to specific stress. Physical appearance plays an important role in our community, especially in the gay community.

Sexology
Eds.: W. Eicher, G. Kockott

Problems occur when lesions of the skin spread to the head, neck, and arms. Seborrheic dermatitis can be very stigmatizing. This harmless skin disease often causes many problems in social contacts. Kaposi's sarcoma is one of the definition criteria for AIDS. This disease can be easily identified by many people in the surrounding area of the patient. Covering lesions are often difficult, in particular when they occur on the face.

Social sources of stress can be found mainly in rejection of society, loss of work, and loss of friends and lovers. If AIDS patients try to be open and honest, they often risk rejection when they most need support.

The daily search for sensation by newspapers or other media concerning AIDS raises many emotional problems for HIV-infected persons.

Compared with other serious diseases, such as cancer, one can find significant differences regarding the acquired immune deficiency syndrome. The contagious nature, the sex-related aspects, and the fear of infection by the general public cause social rejection instead of social support, discrimination instead of sympathy, isolation instead of support by family and friends, and loss of one's job instead of employment. Therefore, HIV patients do not receive the same care and understanding that cancer patients get.

The fear of the symptoms and ongoing disease are accompanied by the fear of death. Most AIDS patients are between 25 and 40 years old and did not expect to be infected with a potentially fatal illness. They are young active persons who risk transition to symptom-wracked dying patients. Changes in sexual behavior can be extremely difficult when sex has been a major form of contact and communication. Guilt about past sexual behavior is another psychological problem described by HIV patients.

Besides these problems, HIV infection in women raises many specific difficulties in patient care. Many female patients are bringing up their child alone. So social rejection also becomes a problem for the child. The future of children of HIV-infected mothers is very uncertain. This situation is usually complicated by great financial problems.

The social network as created by homosexual men in the beginning of the epidemic is absent for women. Support groups are not available for female patients.

The risk of infection of the child during pregnancy seems to be quite high, and the course of the illness can be determined through pregnancy. That is why, as is now known, women should be told to use contraception regularly. Thus being HIV-positive at the present time means abandonment of the children. Because of the social role of women and the importance of appearance in our society, the fear of disfigurement is extremely high in female patients. Moreover, 84.6% of our women compared with 11.6% of our men are intravenous drug users. Stopping i.v. drug use is more difficult when infected and relapses are more frequent.

HIV infection not only raises problems for the infected individual but also for his or her family and friends. Many family members are confronted for the first time with their son's, brother's, or spouse's homosexuality, when they hear of their disease or they learn of their intravenous drug use. At the same time, they must cope with the possible death of their loved ones. The negative reaction of

Table 1. Problems after diagnosis

Fear of death
AIDS
Sexuality
Loss of friends
No future

society can also spill over to family or friends. Often the fear of contagion remains in spite of knowledge about the safety of social contacts.

For little while now we have begun to ask our patients with PGL or AIDS using a questionnaire about the psychosocial issues of their HIV infection. So far we have had the results from 25 patients. Seventeen of the patients reported that stress was extremely high after the diagnosis of HIV-positive, but in time the stress rate was decreased. Main problems after diagnosis are listed in Table 1. The fear of death and full-blown AIDS was mentioned by almost all of the patients. Changes in sexual behavior were difficult at first after diagnosis. Especially patients without a stable relationship have major problems with their sexuality. The loss of close friends is a period when psychosocial support is requested by all of the patients. They are often so afraid of becoming very ill or even dying that they do not believe they have a future left.

The answers to the question "what was helpful when you heard about your diagnosis" showed very clearly that speaking about diagnosis and problems with a physician, psychologist, friends, family members, or support groups was of great importance for patients. The maintenance of hope in all stages of their disease seems to be of great value for our patients.

Since February 1987 have attempted to establish a medical-psychosocial care system in our department, so called Münchner medizinisch-psychosoziale Beratung. Medical and psychosocial patient-management is being undertaken in the same unit. The possibility of close cooperation between physician, psychologist, and social worker as an integrated concept shows great benefits for the patients. The establishment of a structured support program and rapid solution to practical problems seems to be possible in this way.

The main problems of medical staff were the management of HIV-infected persons and safety precautions. The general public wanted to be informed in most cases about possible sources of infection.

In summary, HIV infection is not only a medical problem. Its psychological and social issues create many problems of patients themselves, their families and friends, medical staff, and last but not least society.

In September 1985 we established an AIDS-telephone, a medical phone counseling service. Up till 31st March 1988 we received more than 7500 phone calls.

Psychological Problems in Subjects with AIDS and Related Syndromes

M. Costa [1], F. Aiuti [2], I. Mezzaroma [2], S. Salvati [3], C. Simonelli [3], L. Solano [3], and M. Bertini [3]

[1] Istituto Italiano di Medicina Sociale, Via Pasquale Stanisl. Moncini 28, 00196 Roma, Italy
[2] Cattedra di Allergologia e Immunologia Clinica, Universitá „La Sapienza", Roma, Italy
[3] Dipartimento di Psicologia, Universitá „La Sapienza", Roma, Italy

Introduction

Acquired immunodeficiency syndrome may be differentiated from other contemporary public health problems due to a whole series of difficulties that subjects with AIDS have to deal with, and the terror it generates. AIDS, in fact, though having some elements in common with other untreatable and mortal pathologies, such as cancer, shows very peculiar features, being a new and infectious disease, therefore being perceived as threatening and prone to diffusion, linked with sex, and involving social groups (homosexuals and drug addicts) already burdened with social prejudice. It may also have devastating effects on many aspects of life in affected individuals and cause difficult problems in people who are in a personal, intimate, familiar relationship with the patient.

In spite of widespread interest on the part of science and mass media in AIDS, often focusing on the psychosocial impact of the disease, the psychological situation of patients and the opportunity to provide psychological support have generally been disregarded. The rare data which may be found on the subject, mainly in the North American literature, are about only the extreme aspects of the problem: interviews reported are in fact with patients who required psychological or psychiatric consultation, and who therefore were already in a state of particular mental distress (Dilley et al. 1985; Morin and Batchelor 1984; Perry and Tross 1984). To our knowledge, no systematic study has been performed aimed at a general analysis of needs and feelings in these patients. As to psychological support, only in the most affected areas, San Francisco and New York, are consultation centers for patients and their partners, relatives, and friends in existence. In Italy in particular we know neither of centers of this sort, nor of investigations on the subject. Our study was therefore aimed at performing an analysis of psychological problems faced by patients in the different phases of HIV infection, and possibly at developing strategies for intervention.

Methodology

Subjects

So far we have examined 16 subjects among those attending the outpatient clinic of the Center of Allergology and Clinical Immunology of the University of Rome,

Sexology
Eds.: W. Eicher, G. Kockott

Table 1. Diagnoses in 16 patients with AIDS

Diagnosis	Homo-sexual	Drug addicts	Hemo-philiacs	Hetero-sexual	Total
AIDS	2	1			3
ARC	3	2	1	1	7
LAS		1		2	3
Test positive	1	1	1		3
Total	6	5	2	3	16

in different phases of disease due to infection with HIV virus (see Table 1): at the time of the interview seven subjects had received a diagnosis of ARC, three of LAS, three of AIDS, and three were test positive but asymptomatic; they were all in fairly good general health. All risk categories are represented (see Table 1): 6 homosexuals, 5 drug addicts, 2 hemophiliacs, and 3 heterosexuals; 13 are males and 3 are females (2 drug addicts and 1 heterosexual). Cases of bisexuality are grouped with homosexuals, and ex-drug addicts are grouped with drug addicts. We believe that the set of problems met by test-positive individuals is very similar in all stages of disease (except of course during acute episodes): identical precautions and limitations affect their sexual activity, identical attitudes of fear and rejection are found in the "healthy" population, and their anxiety for their future is identical, threatened by the possibility of evolution into a worse phase or situation.

All subjects agreed to be interviewed by a psychologist, being given appointments on different dates, after a brief explanation of the purpose of the investigation on the part of the physician, who usually took care of them at the center (see "Instrument"). They were asked for their cooperation on a random basis after one of their follow-up visits. Until now 22 subjects have been invited to participate: 1 refused, 16 agreed and were present for the interview, and 5 agreed but were not present on the day of the appointment. Of these five (three drug addicts and two homosexuals), two gave no explanation for their absence while three later communicated to the center they had been ill. Results therefore are not biased by strong self-selection of subjects willing to cooperate.

Instrument

In order to avoid generating unrealistic expectations toward the interview or the psychologists, the referring physician made clear to subjects that the investigation was aimed at measuring adequacy and organization of health and social structures in respect to syndromes due to HIV infection, and at isolating areas of greater psychological distress in patients in order to develop appropriate support measures. The investigation was performed mainly through accurate interviews, lasting approximately 90 min, in the outpatient clinic where patients were habitually followed up. Before the interview, patients were administered a 16-item questionnaire focused on the following areas:

1. Modalities of communication of diagnosis and its impact on the subject
2. Consequences of the disease on life-style
   A semistructured interview followed, during which patients were encouraged to talk freely of their situation, on one hand, while trying on the other to obtain information from all subjects on some particular areas of experience, capable of highlighting feelings, opinions, and attitudes about the disease on the part of patients and others. These areas were:
3. Changes in sexual life-style
4. Changes in work
5. Attitudes of others in general
6. Attitudes and reactions of partners and relatives

Results

Impact of Diagnosis

Five patients received diagnosis in the institution where they are presently being followed up. Together with diagnosis they immediately received a series of information sheets and a treatment plan. All these patients reported a feeling of being "held" and reassured. The same was true for one patient who received diagnosis abroad, in a center specifically organized to deal with the problem of HIV infection, where he received, together with information and recommendations, immediate counseling with a psychologist.

Completely different was the situation for the other 11 patients, who received diagnosis, both as out- and inpatients, from institutions which had no facilities for dealing with the problem under all aspects, but only for performing the serological test. Only in one case was diagnosis followed by some explanation, although the problem of finding and contacting an institution capable of dealing with the problem remained with the patient. Even the three cases who learned of their situation as inpatients (of nonspecialized wards) found themselves alone with their diagnosis, at best with an indication of a specialized center they could consult. In the remaining eight cases diagnosis was received on an outpatient basis: on paper, by telephone, in one case attached to an "instruction booklet for AIDS patients" (?!). On the whole we are also left with the impression of a certain unwillingness to communicate positive test results to patients. In one case in which the patient failed to show up for 1 year after the test was made, no effort was made to contact him before he spontaneously came and asked for the result (in the false hope that if it were positive someone would have looked for him); in another case the patient read the diagnosis casually on his hospital record; in another still the patient, who periodically visited an institution for hemophilic problems, learned of his positive test result months after the test had been performed. This difficulty seems to be caused by uncertainty about what to do next, on the part of institutions not specializing in the problem.

The psychological reaction in nine of these patients is described in terms of "bewilderment," "where do I go now," "what can I do," "absolutely traumatic," and "despair." In two cases total denial of the result took place, waiting to perform the test again in a specialized structure. Since we considered only patients under treatment at a center, we obviously missed possible cases in which denial of the result was followed by no other test, so avoiding awareness of the possibility of infecting others.

Changes in Life-Style, Work, Attitudes, and Reactions of Others

Problems linked with social relationships, with work, and with the fear of exclusion emerge very clearly. Of 16 subjects only 1, test positive asymptomatic, spoke of his problem at work, with a collegue whom he greatly trusted, and who had always helped him with work problems linked with his being affected by hemophilia. He later regretted this confidence, since now he feels to be at this person's mercy. Twelve subjects told of their health situation to few friends they particularly trusted, obtaining a positive reaction of closeness and helpfulness. In one case, however, contact with a friend was completely lost after he learned of the patient's situation. In four cases simple acquaintances were informed directly from subjects, or learned the situation in some other way: flight or rejection was the reaction in three cases.

One subject stated having lost interest in friendship and three of being disinterested or finding difficulty in social relationships. Two explicitly reported having tried to sound to reactions of collegues and acquaintances, without revealing their own situation, and having experienced phobic reactions.

The area of family and couple relationships is more reassuring. All ten subjects who do have a partner reported finding very strong support in him/her, together with extreme acceptance. Fourteen subjects still hold relationships with their family of origin: of these only two failed to inform them. Of the 12 who told, 9 report having received great support, 1 finding some distrust in his father, 1 being disappointed with insufficient support on the part of his father, who together with his mother seemed worried mainly about the grandchildren being at risk, 1 finding his parents only materially helpful, being uncapable of deep, emotional communication. Four subjects informed no one else but their partner or family of origin.

At the time of interview nine subjects had a job, four were studying, and only three were unemployed. This datum strongly opposes against the view of the AIDS patient as a dropout. Problems due to AIDS and related syndromes, however, appear to have a strong impact on work activity. Of the unemployed, one had to leave his job following diagnosis of LAS due to risk of infections implied in traveling in Third World countries; another had to quit because in his conditions work had become too heavy. Of the nine working subjects five (three with ARC and two with AIDS) reported marked difficulties due to physical debilitation and a decreased work capacity. Two test-positive asymptomatic subjects reported no change, while two subjects, one test positive and one with LAS, reported greater activity, which they explained as a way of avoiding anxiety due to diagnosis. Disinterest in work was reported by two subjects (one with AIDS and one with ARC); of these one reported even experiencing hostile feelings toward his activity.

All subjects, except those working on their own, were anxious about the possibility of not being able to dissimulate their condition in the future in the case of aggravation of their disease, which would cause difficulty in justifying long absence from work, or in the case of the appearance of evident pathological signs such as Kaposi's sarcoma.

Sexual Life

This area showed remarkable alterations following diagnosis. We can generally say that, although there are no medical contraindications, one due precautions are adopted, almost all subjects report a drastic reduction of sexual activity especially in the period immediately following diagnosis. A heterosexual subject, for example, refrained from sexual intercourse with his wife for 3 months; another, heterosexual but without a stable partner, preferred complete abstinence from occasional sexual relationships in the fear that the partner might flee once informed of his health problem, or that rupture of the condom might endanger her.

We are confronted with a loss of libido that is something more than lack of interest for sexuality; the feeling of the interviewer was that a barrier of fear and despair had risen between subjects and their sexual striving. In all cases the idea of sexuality is fraught with fear of "infecting" and destroying the object of desire: Eros is turned into Thanatos. In this connection, a young homosexual whose sexual life before discovery of the disease was quite lively and joyful, reported a sense of confusion also at a cognitive level at the discovery that the same element, in this case sperm, until a short time before considered under an extremely positive light, had drastically become a persecutory element. Only one homosexual, a 46-year-old subject, reported having reduced sexual activity, more to protect himself from further infection than to protect others.

Homosexuals as a group have in most cases already experienced the impact with other sometimes serious sexually transmitted diseases during their sexual life: in three cases syphilis is mentioned directly. This might be one of the reasons for their coping rather adequately with their situation and for their being very well informed about diagnosis and prognosis of the different diseases, including AIDS. What happened in our country, as already in San Francisco (Haeberle 1986), is that the first to mobilize against the disease were the homosexuals, showing a solidarity considered fundamental for the definition of their identity and a more responsible and active attitude in taking care of diffusing correct information about prophylactic measures to be adopted (Ferracini 1985). Drug addicts, on the other hand, show less cohesion and find less support than homosexuals in their group.

Diagnosis of the disease, in homosexuals as in drug addicts, is often linked, in phantasy or in reality, with revelation of the activities characterizing these groups, and this increases anxiety due to being "caught" in a socially disapproved practice (homosexuality or drug abuse). These problems are in fact reported by subjects who, following diagnosis had or wanted to communicate to their family members an aspect of their lives which until then they had successfully and purposely kept unknown. We may infer that the disease might be at least partly elaborated as punishment for having broken a rule. In this connection we may quote the episode of a young woman whose sexual activity before diagnosis was quite promiscuous while afterwards she reported appreciating "moderation," since she discovered that sexuality "is an important and serious matter."

Both homosexuals and heterosexuals (a subject reported his difficulty in telling his wife about the extramarital relationship through which he was infected) connect the disease to a risky sexual choice, while transgression in drug addicts seems to have to do more with a search for pure pleasure, independent of an object. Being "different" and transgressive together with other people, directly in the case of hetero- and homosexuals, indirectly through the exchange of a syringe/phallus in addicts, is no more a way of finding pleasure, but can only be a source of mortal disease.

A similar situation is found in hemophilics, who equally experience a loss of libido, in fear of infecting others, although the disease in their case has no apparent link with transgressive behavior. Depressive attitudes are present, as if guilt feelings were present in any case.

Conclusions

The data reported are partial, since we mean to continue the investigation by interviewing a greater number of subjects, especially in categories less represented in the present work, such as test-positive asymptomatic subjects and heterosexuals. Some ideas and recommendations may, however, be derived. Learning of test results on HIV infection seems to cause more negative reactions when it takes place outside a structure capable of supplying immediate help. The obvious recommendation is that the test be performed only in such structures. The daily life of patients, in both sexual and other aspects, seems to be affected, by guilt feelings, phantasies of being dangerous to other people, and phantasies of having somehow deserved the disease as punishment. All these feelings add an unnecessary burden to patients who are already faced with severe physical illness and motivated anxiety for their survival. For these reasons psychological support, individually or in groups, seems highly indicated, at the moment of diagnosis and in later stages. Partners of patients in our sample also seem so heavily involved that they could also very probably benefit from psychological support.

Our subjects expect, probably with reason, fear and rejection attitudes at work. Accurate information could be of great help in putting the phenomenon in the correct light.

References

Dilley JW, Ochitill HN, Perl M, Volberding PA (1985) Findings in psychiatric consultations with patient with AIDS. AM J Psychiatr 142:82–85

Ferracini R (1985) AIDS. Edizioni Gruppo Abele, Torino

Haeberle EJ (1986) Prevenzione AIDS: il punto di vista sessuologico. Quaderni di sessuologia e scienze psicobiologiche 1:9

Morin SF, Batchelor WF (1984) Responding to the psychological crisis in AIDS. Public Health Rep 99:4–9

Perry W, Tross S (1984) Psychiatric problems of AIDS inpatients at the New York Hospital: preliminary report. Public Health Rep 99:200–205

Psychotherapy in AIDS Patients

I. Rechenberger[1] and H.-G. Rechenberger[2]

[1] University Dermatology Division, Moorenstr. 5, 4000 Düsseldorf, FRG
[2] Psychotherapy Clinic, Nettelbeckstr. 3, 4000 Düsseldorf, FRG

In our works as physicians on the wards and in the outpatient department of a University Dermatology Division and in the same work at a hospital for psychotherapy, we came into contact with patients manifestly suffering from AIDS as well as with members of risk groups, e.g., homosexuals. In some cases, these persons live in fear of becoming infected with AIDS or already being infected. In some cases, they suffered from the consequences of such an infection. We included psychotherapeutic strategies in our considerations as to how nevertheless to help these patients within limits, despite our being powerless against this disease up to now. Even if the number of our patients who in this way received more supportive than curative treatment is not yet very great, we should like to present here an initial communication on our observations as well as results in the hope that we can thus make a contribution (even if modest) to dealing medically with this disease.

In the treatment of HIV-positive patients with therapy oriented to depth psychology, it became necessary for us to modify psychoanalysis. Depending on the stage of the disease, we found that it is better to deal with these patients not only in terms of their capacity to undergo psychotherapy, but also with regard to the prognostic objective. We were able to help patients of group 0 in accordance with the Walter Reed classification, i.e., homosexual patients who are still negative for HIV, but who are exposed to a high risk of infection, to adopt a lower-risk behavior. Thus, for example, a homosexual patient in an exposed position who already realized that his social existence was threatened was enabled by psychoanalysis to find a woman who accepted, in mutual agreement, the importance of a young man's presence in his experience. A stable marriage was thus arrived at in which both partners found satisfactory means of sexual and social self-realization. The risk of a HIV infection was thus eliminated.

We have refrained from a classification according to Walter Reed, because it has been shown that the clinical picture can deteriorate under treatment. We prefer a classification into the following three groups:

1. Patients with behaviors which indicate the presence of risk factors and who expose themselves to the danger of an infection, but who are not yet infected with the HIV virus
2. HIV-positive patients without discernible symptoms
3. HIV-positive patients with symptoms

In group 1, in our opinion the task is to attain reduction of the risks of infection as soon as possible in that the patient is helped to establish stable partnerships.

Sexology
Eds.: W. Eicher, G. Kockott

In group 2, we hope to delay the manifestation and pronounced development of the clinical picture by improvement of libido economy and to channelize promiscuous behavior in such a way that the danger of infection for unsuspecting partners is reduced. In one patient of this group, a severe contact problem could be improved to such an extent by psychoanalytically oriented therapy that he no longer frequented and thus endangered random partners, e.g., in public toilets.

In addition, a limited restructuring of the personality should be at least aimed for. Whereas we were formerly inclined as psychologists to classify patients with homosexual, promiscuous, or perverse behavior as in general relatively unaccessible to psychoanalysis, this view has been modified. Today, we are convinced that we can attain an alteration of the personality structure by psychoanalysis in suitable risk patients. The therapist must know that little is to be achieved by use of fear in therapy, since the sexual urge increases the more intensely the more fear is released. For this reason, special attention should be paid to the manifestation and handling of aggressive impulses. As a result, it can often be achieved that an aggressive impulse is released verbally and corresponding acting-out manifested in endangering unsuspecting partners is dispensed with.

Patients who are fatally infected without playing an active role themselves, e.g., from blood or plasma derivatives, must carry out work of grief and can thus also profit from therapy oriented to depth psychology.

Special problems result for patients of group 3: Anxieties can be intensified by the usual somatic diagnosis and therapy. Many patients are afraid of becoming medical guinea pigs and therefore do not undergo the necessary routine investigations. Withdrawal of these patients (also from social groups) is not only to be regarded as resignation, but also as self-protection from stimulation of the behavioral patterns from which they have developed the disease. On the one hand, these patients teach us that surrogate satisfaction with persons of the same intention brings about superficial release of tension, but that, on the other hand, the so far subliminal stimulation thus becomes even more lasting and more pressing. In these persons who are becoming increasingly more ill, pregenital needs are most prominent. Owing to this regression, sexual reference persons lose their high importance and pregenital needs occur and must be accepted.

It is of course to be observed that a high percentage of patients of group 1 do not take advantage of the offer of psychotherapy. It was also observed that patients visit therapists without being prepared to attempt treatment seriously. Those patients who nevertheless commenced a psychoanalytically oriented therapy had the chance of learning retrospectively to cope partially with aggressive, selfish-destructive, and perverse impulses and thus to deal with them better than was previously the case. In these patients, the therapist with his own (often well-founded) fears finds himself in trouble too. For example, one patient stated that he carried out manipulations on his anus when going to the toilet before the therapy session, in order to infect the therapist when shaking hands. Sometimes the desire to infect the therapist orally with contaminated food also became manifest. The poorer the prognosis, the more the apathy of the patient's own destructiveness toward noninfected persons can increase in these patients. In therapy, the anger of the patient with regard to his fate should be worked on. Special attention must also be paid to the countertransference, which often fluctuates between anxiety and pity. It is striking how frequent persons in the environment, including the physician inadvertently endanger themselves in that they grasp infected needles and injure themselves. Special attention is to be paid to countertransference, since it is simply not true that it is motivated by anxiety and pity alone, but it rather stimulates substantial aggressive and destructive tendencies in the treating physician himself.

With this form of psychoanalytically oriented therapy, we not only hope to be able at least temporarily and partially to help patients with AIDS, but also to reduce or gradually eliminate the (in some cases justified) fears of the social environment.

AIDS and The Response of American Religious Institutions

R. T. Francoeur [1] and N. A. Scherzer [2]

[1] Fairleigh Dickinson University, Madison, New Jersey, USA 07940
[2] Essex County College, Newark New Jersey, USA 07102

Introduction

Religious institutions have been no different from other institutions within our society in their slow response to the AIDS epidemic, mainly because initial victims were not acceptable to the churches or society, namely, IV drug users and homosexuals. Despite this, considerable grassroots energy and personnel are committed to working with patients with AIDS (PWAs).

Bishop Quinn: "The Church has a long courageous tradition of making present the compassionate healing freeing love of Christ to the sick and dying. It has been especially present in times of plagues, tragedies and terrible illness. The Church has never hesitated to appoint special ministers... Much more remains to be done. We need a change of heart."

Bishop Quinn is particularly concerned that persons with AIDS (PWAs) have dealt with their own homosexuality for years, but, suddenly, now that they are dying of AIDS, their families are confronted with a loved one's homosexuality. This is a major challenge for the ministry to PWAs, to help families become reconciled with a gay family member and to deal with the ultimate tragedy of the death of a loved one in the family.

Three Sources of Conflicts: Why Have Religious Institutions Been Slow To Respond to the AIDS Epidemic?

Doctrinal

Biblical interpretations on: (1) homosexuality: Most PWAs are gay. To deal with gay PWAs, one must confront and deal with their social structure and their gay life-styles. (2) Heterosexual promiscuity, i.e., premarital especially teenage sex and extramarital sex become an issue when advocating safer sex practices.

Intrainstitutional

Within almost every denomination and church group, there is a radical division between conservative, fundamentalists, evangelical, and orthodox and the more liberal, less literal interpreters of the bible. To conservatives, what is more important is that condoms are a license to primiscuity and homosexual relations which

Sexology
Eds.: W. Eicher, G. Kockott

are in conflict with church doctrine. To the liberal, what is important is balancing doctrine, interpersonal concern, and above all the gospel of care and compassion, comforting and consoling the sick (Rev. Michael Galvan, consultant for the National Council for Catholic Bishops).

Some religious liberals, like the Unitarian minister who handed out condoms, might say the preservation of life is paramount. If it takes a condom to save a life, use a condom. However, in Januar 1987, an Episcopal Diocese of Newark New Jersey Task Force recommended creation of new rituals and ceremonies to celebrate gay unions.

Institutional Images as Reflected by Media

Recently there has been much concern about the public image of the church, especially the possibility of gay clergy and AIDS among the clergy. The religious institutions, however, are now very much open to scrutiny by the press because of the AIDS crisis and their work in AIDS ministry. Reporters want to know (1) about gay clergy and the risk of AIDS in that population, (2) AIDS education, and (3) how AIDS ministry accommodates the emotional and social needs of gay PWAs. Religious institutions see these inquiries as a threat to their institution and are reluctant to engage in activities that would result in disapproval by higher officials or parishioners. Negative effects on financial support and church attendance are also feared.

Examples of This Conflict

Doctrinal Conflict on Gay Life-Styles and Consequent Lack of Dialogue with the Gay Community

A major clash exists between Catholic Church doctrine, as expressed in the Vatican's October 1986 pastoral guidelines on homosexuality, and Dignity, a noncelibate Catholic gay group endorsing gay life and safe sex. Dignity chapters have been expelled from church facilities in some dioceses, but not all as yet. The crucial question is whether any bishops will continue to allow Dignity chapters to use church facilities. In April 1987, Dignity was expelled by Archbishop Roach of St. Paul, Minneapolis, despite the bishop's support of AIDS ministry and his liberal reputation. The critical dioceses to watch are Chicago, San Francisco, and Milwaukee. Jesuit and other priests in New York City are now required to seek chancery permission before saying mass for any gay group on or off church property.

Three two developments have further alienated the gay communities from the Catholic Church and added to the distrust.

1. Gay communities nonreception of Priest's Senate of San Francisco: 1983 statement of Ministry and Homosexuality in the Archdiocese of San Francisco, because all consultation and dialogue with gays had been refused.
2. Proposition 50 in New York City prohibiting employment discrimination against gays successfully opposed by Archdiocese. On one the hand the Church does not want to employ gays, but offers to heal them.

3. A public relations and media war between officials arranging for Pope John Paul II's visit to the United States this fall and gay communities has documented the uneasiness of church leaders to deal with homosexuals as persons. Efforts are clearly being made to keep the Pope's route and schedule secret to avoid any gay demonstration. Considerable difficulty has emerged as local church officials try to arrange for the Pope to meet an AIDS victim without running the risk of a gay demonstration. Gay leaders view these efforts as a safe out, having the Pope meet a nearly dead gay person but not healthy, normal everyday gay men and women.

AIDS Prevention, Education, and Condoms

In February 1987 the California Catholic Conference asked the bishops to decide if the conference should support a bill that would mandate AIDS education program in all public schools, grades 7–12. A film produced by Walt Disney Productions discusses risks of AIDS from vaginal, oral, and anal sex, and IV drug use. The film also discusses availability of condoms to prevent AIDS virus transmission. Bishops claim presentation of condoms as a means to prevent AIDS implicitly sanctions promiscuity. The church prohibits condom use because they are a contraceptive, and recommending their use implies endorsement of premarital promiscuity.

"The only safe sex is in a monogamous relationship within marriage." Sr. Catherine McNamee, director of National Catholic Educational Association.

Only Oakland CA plans to discuss condoms in their parochial schools. "I don't see how you can avoid it. It's a medical fact. It's how we interpret the facts that is important. At this time in history, if we're going to work with the faith lives of youth, we have to do it in the society in which people live, and it is a society very much concerned about AIDS. If we're afraid to talk about condoms, and all the other issues AIDS raises, then we're really missing it. And in the meantime, people are dying." Sr. Rosemary Hennessey, Catholic school superintendent.

Final Outcome. Bishops approved the film for public schools and agreed to its use in parochial schools.

Media Conflicts and Church Politics

Some obvious negatives – A lot of what happens comes down to: *Can it be done quietly, without openly bucking Rome?* Then, go ahead. If it gets in the papers, forget it!!!

Archbishop Roger Mahony, Roman Catholic Archdiocese of Los Angeles, announced it would not allow an AIDS education group to hold seminars in its churches because the organization condones the use of condoms. "In the issue of AIDS, such use implies either heterosexual promiscuity or homosexual activity. The church approves of neither." Everything appeared to be going smoothly with the conference until the Los Angeles Herald Examiner carried a headline "To fight AIDS, Church Sanctions Condoms." This is believed to have triggered cancelation.

As a result, the diocese refused to allow the meeting in church facilities, nor did it allow distribution of AIDS information in the 160 Spanish-speaking parishes in the diocese.

The message: do whatever you want, just don't put it in the newspaper or on the evening news!!! If what you are doing is contrary to church doctrine, i.e., allowing gays to cohabit in a hospice, and this becomes public, the Bishop will have to put a stop to it.

But There Are also Some Media Positives

In Januar 1987, 38-year-old David Hefner (Protestant) and his Catholic wife Maria were refused permission to renew their civil marriage vows by the rector of St. Patrick's Cathedral in a small wedding with only four guests. Father John Clermont, associate pastor, told them it would "be a privilege for him to celebrate the wedding" and had already set a date for February 14 when a higher authority in the diocese canceled permission. After considerable TV and newspaper coverage, Cardinal O'Connor reversed the decision and the couple had their wedding.

Media Reports About Gay Clergy and AIDS in the Clergy

There have been several stories in *The National Catholic Reporter* and other religious publications on gay priests.

Newsweek Cover Story. Richard Sipe (Maryland psychologist, former priest) held 1500 interviews between 1960 and 1985 and concluded that about 20% of 57000 American Catholic priests are gay and half of these are sexually active. Since 1978, Sipe believes the number of gay priests has increased significantly to about 40%. Estimates for Episcopal clergy run as high as 50% in such urban dioceses as San Francisco and New York (*Newsweek*, 2/23/87, p. 58).

Such stories make clergy reluctant to work with gay PWAs for fear of being labeled gay themselves.

But the Denial Response Continues in Some Areas. Church officials continue to enrage the gay community as their responses to such stories highlight a deep homophobia among the clergy and hierarchy, e.g., John Cardinal O'Connor, New York: "If I believed some of the newspapers and some of the articles I read, I'd fear for my safety right now because of sitting with seven other bishops who have nothing in mind but to assault me sexually..." Cardinal O'Connor also denies knowing of any NY priests who have died of AIDS, despite widespread knowledge of specific priests who have died of AIDS. Is the Cardinal so isolated he does not know the facts, or is this a coverup? Bishops of Fresno and Los Angeles deny reports of gay priests and ask people to "trust their priests."

"I suspect the homophobic reaction many priests express in dealing with PWAs springs from a fear of their own covert and unfaced homosexual orientation." (Joe DeBenedictis, NJ Dignity AIDS Pastoral Team).

Conflicts Revealed in Pastorals Issued by Catholic Bishops

All adhere to the Vatican line, but with important and clearly different nuances. All talk about being nonjudgmental and reaching out. Some oppose condoms and AIDS prevention that accepts life-styles, other say nothing about this. A parent or lover talking with O'Connor (NY), Bernadine (Chicago), and Quinn (SF) would certainly get different messages. Refer O'Connor's statement 20 May comparing AIDS and fire. When asked whether AIDS was God's punishment. "That would take a prophet and I'm not a prophet. If I put my hand in the fire, it's going to get burned. Is that a punishment from God? I suppose we could say 'yes' if we say God gave us common sense and God makes it possible to know what fire is and God gives us the ability to put our hand in it or not" (*Star Ledger* 10 March 1987). This is not being nonjudgmental, and it certainly does not facilitate communications between the church and the gay communities.

In Chicago, Cardinal Bernadin's pastoral was praised by several Catholic groups headed by sisters and brothers, but also criticized as "too little, and a bit late."

Mother Teresa of Calcutta

Hospices for PWAs run by Mother Teresa of Calcutta's Sisters in New York and Washington have been severely and widely criticized by gay groups as lacking in understanding of PWA needs. Her hospices apply a third world ascetic mentality to Americans, with very tight regulations and screening on all visitors, even priests, and reading material. Gays, lovers, homosexual reading materials, and Dignity chaplains are not welcome. There is superb medical care, but across the board application of religious poverty, i.e., no TV, no rugs, etc. But, her hospices do provide for last-stage AIDS care. They are great in providing terminal care and in dealing with death.

But AIDS hospices run by an order of Brothers founded by mother Teresa, in Philadelphia and Los Angeles, are very sensitive to the social and emotional needs of PWAs. (Contact Mark Prantner, 212-228-2239.)

Summary

Few AIDS victims return to their religions, yet many seek transcedence (Bill Kenkelen, NCR).

"Only a small group go back to the religion they were raised in when they become ill with the life-threatening disease." "They've see the church as rejecting and abandoning them, a church of moralists and theologians. I try to expose them to a church of love and compassion" (Sr. Patrice Murphy, director AIDS supportive care at St. Vincent Hospital, NYC).

Gallup polls indicate the majority of men 20–40 years old do not attend religious services regularly, but alienation among gay men is even higher. "Most gay men have found that in order to accept their sexuality, they've had to put God in the closet" (Steve Martz, Chicago AIDS counselor). A significant percentage of gay men with AIDS come from Catholic backgrounds, in San Francisco,

40% + of 2000 AIDS patients. Bill Nelson (SF General Hospital: "Many AIDS patients cling to life until they achieve some sort of peace and reconciliation. Some people end up dying angrily and unhappily because they don't achieve this. Some achieve it through traditional religion. But most find what they need in more shamanistic, ambiguous philosophies. Their bodies are wasted and dying, and so they struggle to find a place of existence above this life."

Many AIDS patients who cannot find their way back to the religions they were raised in, or other traditional religions, turn to New Age guru Louise Hays. Books, tapes, and videos emphasize visualization of love and healing energy soaking every cell of their bodies; urged to look on death as a positive change. This is acceptable to many AIDS counselors in traditional religions.

However, conflicts, dissent, and disputes are still a productive process, because they raise consciousness of the issues. Also, given the American Democratic mentality, authoritarian condemnations of gay life-styles and safe sex practices are counterproductive in some segments. Political conservative advocacy is turning off many religious people.

However, if AIDS becomes a holocaust, the conservative agenda could succeed in a violent swing of the pendulum toward the conservative agenda, i.e., no safe sex, no condoms, no dealing with gay life-styles or teenage sexuality except by "say no."

What is Being Done (Not Comprehensive, but Typical Examples)

In religious groups with doctrinal conflicts, much grass roots pastoral ministry for PWAs is going ahead without higher institutional inspiration or support.

Public Education and Information

1. *AIDS: the church responds* by William Johnson and William Stackhouse. Report of United Church of Christ educational and ministry efforts for PWAs. Emphasis (Planned Parenthood Federation. Summer 1986, pp 13–14).
2. May and November 1986 National Days of Prayer and Healing, sponsored by the National Council of Churches. Led by the Episcopal Church. Information packets for AIDS victims, their families and lovers.
3. *America magazine* a full issue of this Jesuit weekly on AIDS in February 1987.
4. AIDS Fact Sheet Pastoral Care Guide prepared by Presbyterians for Lesbian/Gay Concerns.
5. *Shanti Project*. Religious support services for people with AIDS and their loved ones. Not church-affiliated, founded 1981 as a development of Kubler-Ross' workshops on death and dying. San Francisco. Publishes a directory of over 1500 national, state, regional, county, city, and international AIDS service groups. (890 Hayes Street. SF, CA 94117)
6. *Christianity and Crisis*. 19 May 1986. James B. Nelson (Presbyterian theologian, St Paul Minneapolis) Cover article: "Responding to, Learning from AIDS." There have been many workshops, conferences, and resource packets.

7. *"AIDS: Responding to the Crisis."* A special May 1986 issue of *Health Progress*, Journal of the Catholic Health Association. Very positive, with no homophobia.
8. *A Civil Counterpoint:* The state of New Jersey Directory of AIDS Resources has been published without Chap. 1, which many presume would have contained discussion of *safe sex* and condoms, but political sensitivities and hopes made such a chapter inadvisable. There are blue and orange covered versions, one with safer sex and condoms, the other leaving these topics out.

Political: Two Sided

Positives: The Lyndon LaRouche Referendum: Strong public opposition to the Lyndon LaRouche referendum to quarantine AIDS persons from Jewish and Catholic Bishops, and Protestant leaders helped defeat this move. The San Diego Catholic Bishop called it "morally intolerable" in a pastoral read in all churches.

Also: *Opposition to Mandatory AIDS Testing.*

Negative: Opposition to AIDS education with condom information in most cases; e.g., Bishop of Vermont opposed condoms in state prisons. The bishop lost.

Hospices and Residential Programs

Convents and residential facilities converted to serve PWAs: Los Angeles, San Francisco, Detroit, Greenwich Village, and Washington. Two counterpoints to hospices run by sisters of Mother Teresa of Calcutta's stand out in reports from gay groups

1. St. Mary's Hospital in San Francisco, Fr. Michael Lopes. Early and very sensitive hospice program for gay PWAs. But he works under Episcopal sponsorship and his AIDS work is volunteered time in addition to his work as a full-time parish pastor.
2. Sr. Patrice Murphy, director AIDS supportive care at St. Vincent Hospital, NYC. One million dollars in free care given to PWAs; $ 50000 donated by the Archdiocese.
   Both welcome lovers of PWAs and are nonjudgmental.
3. St. Michael's Hospital, Newark, NJ; excellent care for pediatric PWAs.
4. The New York Governor announced canceling a state-funded facility for prisoners with AIDS at the Metropolitan Hospital and a switch to St Clare's Hospital. $ 550 a day at St. Clare's vs. $ 1260 cost at the Metropolitan, and costly delays in building at the Metropolitan. St Clares Hospital was dying but now a 22-bed facility is to be expanded to 60 beds. Seventy prisoners currently have AIDS in NY state.

Nuns in Kentucky forced a change in state laws to allow AIDS patients in nursing homes. Damian House in Washington DC is run by a noncanonical religious order of gay priests and brothers, some with AIDS or ARC, but also indirectly supported with money by the Archdiocese of Washington. New Ways Ministry, Mount Rainier, Maryland. Two full issues of their newspaper were devoted to AIDS issues and the Catholic church.

Interfaith Councils for AIDS Ministry

A major national development. Los Angeles, San Francisco (Houston et al.).

Houston Clergy Consultation for AIDS has developed an extensive interfaith operation of education and of care for AIDS victims. Co-coordinators Ronald H. Sunderland and Rev. Earl E. Shelp (Southern Baptist) sparked its development in late 1985. Ninety-five religious congregations are directly involved, a dozen of them intensively. This includes 15 home "respite teams" of 200 members. Other congregations do home visiting and provide food. Homecare respite teams provide meals, practical nursing, cleanup tasks, transportation, friendship, and encouragement as well as changing bedclothes. One hundred and fifty Houston congregations, Protestant, Roman Catholic, Eastern Orthodox, and Jewish, sponsored AIDS Awareness and Intercessory Prayer Sabbath in February 1987.

By February 1987, Houston had had about 1000 AIDS cases; 600 have died, and 450 current cases are under review. (21 February 1987, Associated Press.)

Interfaith Councils offer an important referral resource when doctrinal conflicts arise or when publicity leads higher authorities to step on grass roots effects.

Special AIDS Ministry Programs Within Denominations

The National Episcopal effort led the way for mainstream churches by mandating that AIDS education programs be in place by March 1986.

Seattle Catholics: 24 priests and laypersons involved in AIDS counseling and care.

Chicago: an AIDS Pastoral Care Network with a Jesuit director, 30 counselors, and over 50 PWAs.

AIDS ministry directors have been appointed in many Catholic dioceses and Protestant churches.

One innovative approach in the Catholic tradition is *noncanonical* orders. Sisters for Christian Community (over 700, founded in 1971); brothers (about 25, founded in 1976). Minimal control by church authorities leaves them free to work with PWAs, e.g., Joe De Benedictis, NJ Dignity Pastoral Team member.

Union of American Hebrew Congregations

The Union of American Hebrew Congregations, a reformed Jewish group with 1.25 million members, endorsed AIDS education including safe sex education in their schools, summer camps, and youth publications. A group of rabbis and laypersons are being trained as AIDS counselors in 13 regions.

Hardline Fundamentalists

Even the hardline fundamentalists are taking a few positive actions.

- Liberty Federation (Moral Majority) lobbied for increased federal funding for AIDS research.

- Jerry Falwell invited Surgeon General Koop to speak at his Liberty College even though he mentioned condoms and safe sex.

Two Examples of an Interfaith Trend

Union Theological Conference in New York City 20 March 1987

Cosponsored by Social Justice and Roman Catholic Theology, Union Theological Consultation on Homosexuality, Lesbian/Gay Caucus, and Union Theological Seminary: Bishop Paul Moore (Episcopal) was given an award for prophetic leadership in the gay/lesbian community. John McNeill (gay Jesuit), Rev Ellen Barrett (Lesbian Episcopal priest), and John Boswell were speakers.

Interfaith Conference on AIDS and ARC for Clergy and Caregivers San Francisco 21–22 March 1987

Sponsored Rabinical Conference, Catholic and Episcopal Bishops. Cosponsors: Catholic Social Services AIDS/ARC Program, Lutherans, Episcopal Diocese of CA, Shani Project. Speakers from 20 local and national religious groups: Baptist, Evangelical Lutheran, United Methodists, Christian Churches of CA, NAACP, Board of Rabbis, Lutheran Church in America (middle of the road), Lutheran Church Missouri Synod (conservative), Presbyterians, Imam Faheen Shuaibe (Moslem), Metropolitan Community Churches, World Council of Churches. Episcopalians, Civils Rights and Human Services Commission, National Baptist Convention, Hartford Zen Center, Church and Society Division-World Council of Churches (Geneva), AIDS Interfaith Network, Rama Krishna Order Vedanta Society, Foundation of Tao, Buddhist, and Metaphysical Alliance.

Of 34 very interesting topics, including families, children, women, Hispanics, native American, Asians, Latino, blacks, and intravenous drug users. Read the list of workshops!!!! (handout) There were *simultaneous workshops at a Lutheran church and Catholic cathedral*, which hosted the conference.

Great, but not one workshop on *gays* or *safe sex*! Only one lonely use of the word "gay" in the 16-page program and that in the identification of a speaker as a member of the "Gay American Indians." No workshops on safer sex, nor any mention of condoms.

This was a political compromise in response to expected objections from the Black Episcopal Church, Missouri Synod Lutherans, and conservative Catholics.

In the closing sermon at this first of its kind interreligious conference on AIDS, David Gosling of the World Council of Churches, Church and Society Division, quietly but angrily said the Roman Catholic Church is the "greatest obstacle" in the worldwide battle against AIDS. "... they [the Vatican] say nothing, and that certainly is an immorality." Criticism of the Catholic church and concern for Catholic "troubles" and "troubled" Catholics was a constant, underlying tension throughout the conference. San Francisco's Archbishop Quinn agreed to be a sponsor and host the conference at his Cathedral, "but then the people around him kept trying to put the brakes on, because they were afraid of a backlash." "Prominent Episcopal, Baptist and Jewish leaders spoke with anger and passion about the curches' failure to fully help people who are drug abusers or gay." (*National Catholic Reporter*, 3 April 1987, Bill Kenkelen, special report, p 28).

Summary

1. The Churches have a significant function in dealing with AIDS, primarily in the hospital and hospice setting. However, in AIDS education and prevention, a common but not universal factor is a conflict between doctrine and reality. Protection of sexually active persons against AIDS, safe sex practices, is essential, even if they do not fit into the categories morally acceptable to the churches. Churches will increasingly have to deal with PWAs and their life-styles, with gays, swingers, extramarital sex, premarital sex, etc., without instilling guilt and being judgmental, either overtly or covertly.

2. When AIDS become more common in the heterosexual community than among gays, the churches will be much more comfortable dealing with it and be able to relegate the gays to their usual minority role. However, for the next 5 years, the number of gay PWAs will increase exponentially, forcing the churches even more to deal with their families, and the gay social and political environment. Ministry to PWAs will increasingly have to be channeled through Dignity, Damian House, and other religious-oriented gay groups.

AIDS has given the moral preaching of monogamy, celibacy, and premarital virginity a new life and force.

But, also, AIDS will force the churches to provide a more comprehensive sex education for the clergy and in the parochial schools.

The unknown factor is how the churches, especially Catholic, will react when AIDS hits their clergy and bishops in undeniable numbers. "Unfortunately, churches only seem to be getting involved once AIDS really hits home." Marcia Ludwig, a Presbyterian from San Jose, reported that a Presbyterian church in San Jose which opposed a 1984 effort to study Presbyterian homosexual needs is not getting involved after burying their fourth AIDS victim in the parish (*NCR* 3/3/87).

Suggestions

1. Need for full-time clergy to be supported by churches in AIDS ministry.
2. Networking with other agencies to improve medical and emotional care for PWAs.
3. Support of AIDS and safe sex education in the schools.
4. Deal with homophobia in clergy, hierarchy, and laity.
5. Churches must involve their congregations in creating respie teams, as they have done in Houston.
6. Interfaith cooperation is needed to handle conflicts and provide options for those seeking care in a pastoral setting.

Congressional Testimony for the Republican Leadership Task Force on Health Care: AIDS

T. L. Crenshaw

3750 Riviera Drive, Suite 1, San Diego, California 92109

The United States leads industrialized societies in AIDS cases but not in prevention of AIDS. Our nation is used by foreign countries as an example of what not to do. Many smaller countries, from Swaziland to England, have surpassed our limited preventative efforts although their population of infected individuals is minuscule compared with ours.

AIDS is a preventable disease that we are allowing to spread throughout our country at a speed that jeopardizes our very survival and threatens our economic stability. We could lose one fourth of the world's population before we gain control of this epidemic, even if we act swiftly now. If not, it may be more.

I am not an alarmist but I am alarmed. I am not a political activist but I have become politically active. I am not funded or subsidized but am so concerned that I am working full-time for AIDS prevention in the nation and the world.

We are in a war against AIDS and so far the AIDS virus is winning. Today there are ten times more cases of AIDS in heterosexuals than we had in the homosexual community just 5 years ago. In our major cities, 50%–70% of homosexuals are already infected with the AIDS virus. Heterosexuals seem to be repeating their history. There are 14000 teenagers infected in New York City alone and 37000 nationwide (verbal report from CDC). Our children are bearing the burden of society's mismanagement of prevention. Sexually active teenagers are the most significant risk group of all. Adults have been battling among themselves instead of protecting the next generation.

We must change our approach to the management of this pandemic dramatically. We have not done a good job to date. We are not now doing what needs to be done. The number of infected people contradicts anyone who suggests otherwise. We have been illogical and ineffective. When 90% of those infected and contagious to others do not know it and continue to spread it, how can we hope to stop the progression of this disease? There is no cure and no vaccine.

Each individual must find the courage to be tested, then exercise the discipline to remain negative or, if positive, to avoid spreading the disease to others. Being tested is not enough. Responsible sexual behavior is essential. We must use all rational resources available to us.

Our society is in grave danger, not from AIDS but from the experts who have consistently misread this epidemic, disregarded the evidence of Africa, been unwilling to apply traditional epidemiological methods (such as routine testing and contact tracing) – from gay leaders who have resisted measures that might limit or inhibit sexual freedoms; from the conservative right who have fought AIDS education in schools and on television; and from ourselves who have been unwill-

Sexology
Eds.: W. Eicher, G. Kockott

ing to face reality and change our sexual practices radically enough or rapidly enough.

The AIDS virus is formidable and lethal but no longer the major danger. Political decisions, public health decisions, and medical decisions will determine the outcome of this epidemic. Up until now many laws have been passed that favor the survival of the virus. Ideally, the management of this epidemic should be free from politics and in the hands of physicians. However, politics has played the major role in the course of this disease and it now rests in the hands of politicians to undo the damage that has been done and to steer a healthier course with courage and good judgment in order to win the war against AIDS. This is an unwelcome challenge and a grave responsibility for nonmedical people. However, common sense is an invaluable resource in any crisis and I will help to point out how well it can be applied – even in the face of medical complexities – to get control of this epidemic, why it has been lacking, and how to correct that void.

No Freedom of Speech

It is difficult to get a clear picture of the facts about prevalence and research because there is no freedom of speech about AIDS. Every scientist dealing with the controversial AIDS issue is subject to attack from one side or the other.

There is hardly a leader in the field who has not received death threats or been subjected to character assassination by those who disagree with their point of view. Many require increased security or bodyguards when they lecture or appear in public, regardless of which view they represent. Researchers holding unpopular views cannot obtain grant support. Teachers risk losing tenure; public health officials who disagree openly with prevailing policies risk losing their jobs. Is it any wonder that many are not speaking up? I have never before had the experience in medicine where I most commonly receive one statement on the record and another point of view off the record that is quite contradictory.

But this form of pressure does not just apply to professionals. Anyone expressing the "nonprevailing" view is also subject to character assassination or ridicule. They are called hysterical, alarmist, or irresponsible.

People are judged and criticized, instead of the opinions they hold. In the process the issues are clouded. Many toes are testing the water before wading in and speaking their minds. For example, in Atlanta, the meetings over the qustion of mandatory testing had to be ended early because of the unprofessional and rowdy behavior of extremist groups. Many who initially intended to support mandatory testing were intimidated into changing their views. Scientists who raise the question of insect transmission, saliva transmission, or casual transmission are generally ostracized. Anyone who questions the wisdom of infected children attending school is labeled an hysterical parent, and anyone who suggests the appropriateness of mandatory testing under any circumstance is considered either foolish or dangerous. Name calling and character assassination have replaced rational deliberation. These are known occupational hazards of politics but scientists are ill equipped to cope with them.

When the scientific and public health issues of AIDS are subject to such cynicism, criticism, and risk, you cannot expect many people to speak their opinion honestly and openly if the consequences are loss of job, loss of income, loss of substantial votes, or loss of credibility. Scientists holding views opposed by gay activists, AIDS patients, civil libertarians, conservatives/religious advocates, and others are actually experiencing discrimination so severe that it affects their ability to make a living and provide for their families.

Until there is more freedom of speech about AIDS, reflected in professional discussions between differing points of view with objective and open-minded analysis of data, little progress will be made and the information that reaches Congress, the press, and the public will be so garbled or contradictory as to be uninterpretable.

Politics of AIDS

AIDS, virtually neglected by politicians 4 years ago, has become the leading issue determining the election of public figures in our country from the President to the local Board of Supervisors. But the politics began long ago. Doctor Gallo and the Pasteur Institute have a history of discord over naming of the virus and ownership of testing rights. When we first began to recognize AIDS as a contagious disease, Dr. James Curran and Dr. Donald Francis at the Centers for Disease Control differed in their approach. Doctor Curran preferred research and epidemiological tracking and Doctor Francis fought for aggressive prevention through education. Doctor Curran prevailed. Research and knowledge have thrived, but the lack of emphasis on effective prevention efforts has cost millions of lives. At the CDC there has been sabotage of experiments and accusations of suppression of information.

The most interesting and unfortunate politics at the CDC have been the politics of labeling – the artificial and misleading distinctions between AIDS, ARC, and confirmed asymptomatic infection. Reporting and recording only AIDS cases has enabled the Public Health Department to minimize the scope of the problem and create a false sense of security by talking in terms of thousands of cases instead of millions. As long as ARC and HIV-positive status are nor reportable conditions, the epidemic seems under control – the numbers manageable. This is a false picture.

The CDC has also been subjected to outside political pressures, resulting in manipulation of statistics. Haitians were included, excluded, and then included again as a high-risk group, as one example. Another political misrepresentation is that no one outside of high-risk groups has become infected. This statement has remained true only because every time a new group was discovered, such as prostitutes, it was quickly labeled as a new high-risk group until heterosexuals with multiple partners finally became a high-risk group too. That includes most of the "baby-boomer" generation and means that the concept of high-risk groups is obsolete, because now the majority of Americans fall into one of the high-risk groups. If we are going to be talking in terms of risk groups, we should be concentrating on low-risk groups.

Politics of Big Business

The economic politics have been no less troublesome. The big business of blood banking caused delayed screening of blood for almost a year beyond the proven value of testing and continues to claim greater safety of transfusions than is warranted. Until recently, the option of autologous transfusions (giving your own blood for elective procedures) has been difficult although clearly in the best interests of the motivated patient. The blood blanking industry has also successfully obscured the fact that most hospitals have the facility to suction and filter a person's own blood during surgery if unexpected blood loss occurs. It is then given back to the patient while on the operating table. It is curious that there has been so little discussion of this readily available technique at the medical or public level. It is expensive and requires prior setup; however, research funds could certainly have been directed long ago toward making this procedure more economical and more readily available. The same is true regarding blood substitutes, many of which are available but the public is not being informed. It would be to the disadvantage of the blood bank industry.

Politics of Special Interest Groups

Many special interest groups continue to argue among themselves and with others in an effort to avoid association with AIDS, obscuring an accurate picture of this disease. Africa has consistently refused to reveal figures, refused to cooperate with World Health Organization research teams, and boycotted conferences that intended to report these statistics. Haiti has pressured the United States to protect them from the stigma of being a high-risk group. Gay activists and civil libertarians have been most aggressive in resisting traditional public health measures for management of the AIDS epidemic by frigthening people into believing that these measures inevitably lead to secret lists, quarantine, and concentration camp atmospheres.

Africa would hate to have it known that AIDS was spread by mosquitoes. It would ruin their tourist trade. Gays would not want it known that AIDS was spread by casual contact for fear that they would be ostracized. The extreme right does not want sex education in schools or condoms advertised on television for moral reasons. Blood banks want the blood supply to appear safe and condom companies want condoms to appear safe to promote the sale of condoms. There are just a few of the special interest groups that have a strong bias to protect regardless of the facts. With pressures of this magnitude, it is not difficult to understand how data can be suppressed or distorted.

Consequences of Politics

Laws have been passed initiated by Art Agnos in California that have swept the country and ensure the spread of AIDS. These laws forbid contact tracing, forbid a physician to tell another physician caring for the same patient that that partient is infected, forbid telling a spouse that their husband or wife is infected, and forbid doing a screening test for AIDS without the written consent of the individual. This is the only blood test in the history of medicine that cannot be performed by law.

Because there are both criminal and civil charges that can be brought in addition to financial damages against physicians who do not follow these guidelines (laws), the majority of physicians avoid the blood test altogether. One physician told me, "I could get thrown in jail and sued for everything I am worth if may nurse misfiles a report. I can't take the chance so I send them somewhere else." In New York, where there is the highest prevalence of AIDS, the test is the hardest to acquire.

The politics of AIDS has prevented other forms of infection with the AIDS virus (asymptomatic HIV infection and ARC) from being reportable to the Public Health Department, has prevented physicians from doing the blood test when they feel it is indicated, has prevented health professionals from communicating with each other, and has forbidden physicians to protect the lives of sexual partners of those infected with the virus. Under these circumstances, it is not possible to stop the spread of this disease.

Economics of AIDS

- The World Health Organization estimates conservatively that there are 10 million individuals infected with the AIDS virus worldwide today and predicts 100 million by 1991. If the disease continues to spread at the same rate, 1 billion will be infected by 1996 and 10 billion by 2001. The world population is only 5 billion. Those who have been sexually exclusive for over a decade would probably survive. Economically the loss of a tremendous segment of our population will be enormous, not to mention the tragedy in loss of lives.
- The annual AIDS health care cost to the United States is estimated to be $ 66.4 billion/year by 1991.
- The estimate of indirect costs attributable to productivity loss among AIDS patients will rise to $ 55.6 billion in 1991. Nonpersonnel costs for research, education, screening, and general support services are expected to rise to $ 2.3 billion in 1991.

All of these figures are low. They can be multiplied by a factor of between 10 and 100 because they reflect AIDS cases only and do not include ARC or those who are infected yet asymptomatic. Patients are hospitalized for ARC and die of ARC without ever being classified as having AIDS. Multiply these billions of dollars by 10 and already overwhelming figures become almost unmeasurable.

Even using the most conservative figures, if they are partly true the AIDS epidemic has the potential to destabilize our economy and consequently our political system. The Centers for Disease Control claim 1.5–2 million people infected with AIDS in America today. Their figures have been historically low and significant underestimates; however, using these figures, assuming that the majority will become ill, consider the fact that in America we have only 1.3 million hospital beds to treat all medical conditions.

We are not prepared, we have not planned. And such strenuous effort has been made to ensure that we cannot be sure how many people are infected, that it perpetuates a state of paralysis. Because of those who do not want generalized, massive testing, we cannot trust the figures that we have. A perfect "Catch 22": Those opposed to testing say the numbers do not justify testing, but as long as they obstruct widespread testing we cannot get accurate numbers. Consequently we can continue to debate how serious and how extensive this disease truly is until there is no choice but to react and cope. We have the capacity to be proactive but are still deliberating about whether it is more cost effective to screen our population or to treat AIDS patients once they are already ill.

A History of False Information, Overstatements, and Underestimations

The majority of the experts addressing you confidently today not so many years ago just as confidently were making statements to the effect that:

- This is only a homosexual disease transmitted through anal intercourse. There is no risk to heterosexuals (in spite of the strong suggestion of heterosexual spread in Africa).
- This disease is not easy to get. It requires multiple partners and an impaired immune system.
- Women can get AIDS from men but men cannot get AIDS from women.
- Health care workers are not at risk. You cannot get AIDS from needle stick.

All of these statements have been made by a variety of experts, all experts upon whom you still rely today. All of these statements have been proven untrue. AIDS is not a homosexual disease. It is a sexually transmitted disease – heterosexually, vaginally, anally, from male to female and from female to male. Multiple partners increase your risk but one exposure to an infected person can cause disease. Compromised immune systems make you more susceptible to AIDS as well as any other infection but are not a prerequisite for becoming infected. Infections have occurred among health care workers, not only from needle stick but more recently from blood splash. How many times have you heard these so-called experts say "All modes of transmission are known and understood. You don't need to worry. Don't be irrational"? And yet, there has always been a 3%–10% category of "other," reflecting cases that cannot be explained by known routes of transmission. These have been discounted by catchall phrases like, "Obviously these people lied and were simply refusing to acknowledge the true risk category they were in." It is so easy to bias the interpretation of data in this disease, especially since AIDS initially affected homosexuals, IV drug abusers, and prostitutes. These groups have high incentive not to admit to their illegal or socially less acceptable behaviors. When prostitute activity was first reported by the military, again, the initial conclusions were deception – actual homosexuals who refused to admit their practices for fear of expulsion from the Navy. These oversimplistic reactions delayed appreciation and recognition of the facts.

The main question is, "Which is the bigger lie?" – from those individuals who truly deceive the professionals about their risky behavior, or the professionals who deceive themselves and conclude that everyone who does not fit into their preconceived notions is lying.

The most incurable flaw of logic in the analysis of the AIDS epidemic has been the "no case yet" reasoning. The "no case yet" fallacy operates in the following way: "There has been no reported or confirmed case of (heterosexual transmission, insect transmission, casual transmission, saliva transmission, etc.), therefore it does not happen." Too often it happens. The next statement from those who previously insisted it was impossible is, "Well, yes, it happens, but it is so rare that you can disregard it." Eventually the progression of the disease and the reality of its course of transmission speaks for itself but by that time our unwillingness to accept reality and prepare for it has cost many lives to be unnecessarily lost.

Scientific Contradictions

1. Scientists suggest that AIDS was transmitted from the green monkey to man by monkey bites or humans eating monkeys. The same scientists state that bites cannot transmit the virus from human to human and that it is impossible to acquire AIDS by eating in restaurants, yet babies can get the disease from nursing.
2. One can become infected from one needle stick and even blood splash. The AIDS virus has been found in 50 insects in Africa including the mosquito but most scientists conclude that it cannot be spread by insect vectors.
3. The scientific consensus currently believes saliva transmission does not occur. The same scientists suggest in the recent blood splash case that blood splashed in the mouth was thought to be the source of transmission. Blood is often found in the mouth through brushing teeth, dental flossing, or gingivitis (inflammation of the gums). If saliva transmission occurs, it may actually be blood to blood.
4. School children cannot be routinely tested for the AIDS antibody but the law requires certain vaccinations that are contraindicated for someone infected with the AIDS virus. Therefore, the only way to find out if a school child is infected is to vaccinate them and watch helplessly as they die.
5. The AIDS test is reliable for testing the blood supply but unreliable for testing human beings.

Today's Myths

1. Myth: Mandatory testing will drive people underground and they won't get tested.
   Truth: 90% of those infected (numbering in the millions) do not even know it; they are already underground. We cannot do much worse. Eventually those who become ill will need hospital care, medical treatment, and will have to get tested. Mandatory testing in certain circumstances will not drive individuals underground, but have the opposite effect. It will simply enable us to predict more clearly our future medical needs.

2. Myth: AIDS is hard to get.
   Truth: If AIDS is so hard to get then why are so many people already infected? AIDS is much easier to get than originally believed.
3. Myth: Condoms are safe sex.
   Truth: Already Dr. Margaret Fischl has demonstrated a 30% failure rate for condoms in vaginal intercourse, and prostitute studies have suggested a 50% failure rate for anal intercourse. Condoms with an infected person are deadly.
4. Myth: The AIDS test is inaccurate.
   Truth: The AIDS test is one of the most accurate tests of its kind known to medicine. However, no test diagnoses a disease, and most tests have false positives and false negatives. Confirmatory tests are necessary and to be expected.
5. Myth: Only 30%–50% will go on to develop AIDS.
   Truth: There is no one who can say that the majority of infected individuals will not become sick and die. Most experts including Doctor Gallo, Doctor Krim, and myself agree that up to 100% of infected individuals could eventually die of AIDS or related conditions.
6. Myth: You cannot change or legislate sexual behavior.
   Truth: You can. The people making these statements are not experts in the complexities of human sexual behavior. It is true that you cannot monitor compliance with sexual laws – or for that matter any law. We have laws against murder yet people still commit murder. The law is an enforceable guide. It has power as an expected social protocol. We are not utilizing this powerful resource to help us against the deadliest threat to human beings in modern times.
7. Myth: Central nervous system involvement leads only to depression, fatigue, and sleepiness.
   Truth: Central nervous system infection with the AIDS virus can infect any part of the brain and can lead to any mental impairment depending upon the zones of the brain infected, including violent and aggressive behavior, schizophrenia, and impaired judgment, as well as depression, fatigue, and sleepiness.
8. Myth: It is not important if you are in a high-risk group, it is whether or not you are participating in high-risk behavior.
   Truth: The concept of high-risk behaviors is the most dangerous of all. Any sexual behavior whatsoever with an infected person is high risk. The only safe sex is sex with someone who is not infected. The high-risk group is simply a mathematical probability. Among Haitians and homosexuals you are still more likely to be exposed to someone who is infected than among white heterosexual males. However, the infection is currently so widespread that the usefulness of mathematical probabilities is becoming more and more limited, especially now that heterosexuals with multiple partners are considered a high-risk group.
9. Myth: Homosexuals are doing an excellent job of education and prevention, follow their example.

Truth: In our major cities the majority of homosexuals are infected with the AIDS virus. Many are still living like lemmings, more concerned about their sexual freedoms than their health. Gay leaders are telling them that condoms are safe sex. Bath houses, toilets, and X-rated film houses are still well attended. Most of the sexual activity is unprotected sex. In San Francisco, over 70% (conservatively speaking) of the homosexual community is already infected. In Los Angeles it is 45%–55%. In San Diego it is 35%–45%. With numbers like these, how can anyone say that they are doing a good job of prevention?

10. Myth: The modes of transmission of the AIDS virus are known.
    Truth: The recent blood splash cases demonstrate the inaccuracy of this statement. The percentages and numbers in the "other" category confirm it. *There is still much to be learned about this epidemic.* However, too many authorities in their effort to reassure a worried public overstate their case.

Major Issues that Have not yet Been Effectively Addressed

1. Perhaps the most important and the most difficult is the CNS impairment in AIDS patients that occurs, sometimes before any other symptoms develop. Our entire political approach to the AIDS epidemic depends upon the judgment of the infected person not to knowingly or unknowingly infect others. When the virus affects the brain they cannot be expected to use good judgment. This reality must be confronted by politicians, physicians, and the lay public.
2. Airplanes are the most significant threat to society's survival. The ease and speed of world travel made possible by our modern technology makes this disease more dangerous to human beings than any other in history. In the past, inconvenient modes of travel or the impossibility of travel to certain corners of the Earth ensured that even airborne plagues would only affect a small segment of the human race. Now, because of rapid travel, a disease that takes much longer to cause death, that is not as acutely virulent as plagues of the past, is a greater threat to the survival of the human race.

Common Sense Solutions

1. During the past 6 years our society has done a remarkable job in funding research and treatment and this must continue. However, it has done an abysmally inadequate job of preventing spread of disease as proven by the numbers we now face. Prevention efforts must take at least equal priority. *Sex education on a massive scale must be implemented, not just talked about.*
2. The artificial distinctions between asymptomatic infection, ARC, and AIDS should be eliminated. For public health purposes, anyone who is infected (a confirmed antibody positive) is considered contagious and should be handled accordingly. In order to stop the spread of this disease *it is essential that all forms of HIV infection be reportable to public health departments with confidentiality* but not anonymity.

3. *Wide-range antibody testing on a voluntary basis for all segments of society* – old, young, heterosexual, homosexual, child, adult – *should be encouraged*, and *mandatory or routine testing should be implemented under special situations.* Required testing is appropriate: On admission to drug rehabilitation and alcohol programs, on hospital admission, prior to marriage, with pregnancy, in prisons, for immigration, and for health care workers. As we learn more, it may become appropriate to include other groups. *Children should be tested on school admission prior to any required vaccinations.*
4. *Contact tracing to the fullest extent that manpower allows should be instituted.*
5. *Existing laws, both criminal and civil, should be enforced in cases of intentional transmission to discourage this behavior.*
6. *Physicians should be required to inform sexual partners of someone who is infected and existing laws that make this illegal or criminal should be eliminated.*
7. Safe sex practices currently being recommended should be discarded in favor of clear and more accurate recommendations such as:
   - There is no safe sex with an infected partner, only degrees of risk.
   - The only safe sex is sex with someone who is not yet infected.
   - Do everything humanly possible to ensure that your partner is uninfected before establishing a sexual relationship including blood testing as often as neccessary and the use of condoms and spermicides for at least a year and/or until you are secure about your partner's trustworthiness.
8. There should be counseling of all those who test negative about how to remain negative and counseling of positives to prevent spread of disease. Once infected, tough love measures should be employed. These include the following: *Anyone infected with the virus should be advised not to have sex with anyone*; the degree of risk involved with an uninfected person is unacceptable, and it is medically contraindicated for them to have repeated sexual relationships with someone else who is infected for fear that they will accelerate the progression of their own disease.
9. *Promote celibacy for teenagers, exclusivity, monogamy, and trustworthiness for the sake of health.* If some groups encourage this behavior for moral reasons do not object. The net effect is the same.
10. *Recommend condoms in conjunction with spermicides in addition to, not instead of, these measures* as a protection against the potential untrustworthiness of a partner, whether married or single. They should be used in addition to testing, celibacy, monogamy, etc.
11. *It is critical that we get the civil rights issue into perspective or we will all die a very democratic death.* Protecting the civil rights of some while infringing on the civil rights of others is resulting in greater numbers of infected people. *Our society cannot let the exercise of the rights of someone who is infected cause someone else to become infected.* The civil rights issue has been adopted by those who are infected while in truth civil rights belong to everybody – even the healthy. We must protect the civil rights of the healthy as well as the civil rights of the ill.

12. *Recognize that sexual behavior can change if the motivation is sufficient and if public leaders expect and recommend it. Death is a powerful motivator. Tell the public the whole truth.* The present message, "Calm down, don't panic, but do change your sexual behavior," will not work psychodynamically. To motivate sexual behavior change, one must alarm and concern people enough to motivate change, then calm them down with an action plan that demonstrates how they can stay healthy.
13. Promote the concept of quality monogamy. Many people confuse the terms, "monogamy" and "monotony," thinking they are synonyms. It is important during this difficult time to make the best of what we have. *Quantity sex is over but quality sex is not.*

Conclusions

Unless these issues are confronted and effectively implemented, there is little hope of stopping the spread of AIDS. The majority of people who are infected and contagious to others do not know it and continue to spread the disease to others at a geometric rate. While we argue about the magnitude of the numbers, they grow. Until this situation is corrected, all other measures are relatively meaningless.

Our nation needs courageous and definitive leadership. Politicians will be judged as harshly for what they did not do as for what they did do. It is your responsibility to change the course of this epidemic now. Without your support, medicine and public health systems alone are inadequate. Your action or inaction will determine the course of history.

Subject Index

W. Eicher, Mannheim (Ed.)

Plastic Surgery in the Sexually Handicapped

1988. Approx. 140 figures. Approx 150 pages.
Hard cover. ISBN 3-540-19131-3

This book considers in particular the diseases which result in sexual handicap and which can be treated by reconstructive surgery.
Breast surgery, including congenital anomalies and reconstruction after amputation, genital malformations, from congenital anomalies in the vaginal area and of the penis through to the deformities of intersexuality and aplasia of the vagina, changes due to genital prolapse in women, the lost penis syndrome and impotence with vasosurgical and prosthetic remedies, and genital transformation in the case of transsexualism (both male-to-female and vice versa) are the main topics of value to plastic, pediatric, and vascular surgeons as well as to urologists and gynecologists with regard to surgical technique.
The features are, however, of equal importance to all other physicians who are involved in sexual medicine and so have to be well informed on the subjects of diagnostics and possible therapies. They include general practitioners, specialists in internal medicine, andrologists, gynecologists, urologists, pediatricians, and – not least – psychiatrists and psychotherapists.

Springer-Verlag
Berlin Heidelberg New York
London Paris Tokyo

Springer

MIX
Papier aus verantwortungsvollen Quellen
Paper from responsible sources
FSC® C105338
FSC
www.fsc.org

If you have any concerns about our products,
you can contact us on
ProductSafety@springernature.com

In case Publisher is established outside the EU,
the EU authorized representative is:
Springer Nature Customer Service Center GmbH
Europaplatz 3, 69115 Heidelberg, Germany

Printed by Libri Plureos GmbH
in Hamburg, Germany